THE EPIDERMIS IN WOUND HEALING

DERMATOLOGY: CLINICAL & BASIC SCIENCE SERIES
Series Editor Howard I. Maibach, M.D.

Published Titles:

Protective Gloves for Occupational Use
Gunh Mellström, J.E. Walhberg, and Howard I. Maibach

Bioengineering of the Skin: Water and the Stratum Corneum
Peter Elsner, Enzo Berardesca, and Howard I. Maibach

Bioengineering of the Skin: Cutaneous Blood Flow and Erythema
Enzo Berardesca, Peter Elsner, and Howard I. Maibach

Bioengineering of the Skin: Methods and Instrumentation
Enzo Berardesca, Peter Elsner, Klaus P. Wilhelm, and Howard I. Maibach

Bioengineering of the Skin: Skin Surface, Imaging, and Analysis
Klaus P. Wilhelm, Peter Elsner, Enzo Berardesca, and Howard I. Maibach

Bioengineering of the Skin: Skin Biomechanics
Peter Elsner, Enzo Berardesca, Klaus-P. Wilhelm, and Howard I. Maibach

Skin Cancer: Mechanisms and Human Relevance
Hasan Mukhtar

Dermatologic Research Techniques
Howard I. Maibach

The Irritant Contact Dermatitis Syndrome
Pieter van der Valk, Pieter Coenrads, and Howard I. Maibach

Human Papillomavirus Infections in Dermatovenereology
Gerd Gross and Geo von Krogh

Contact Urticaria Syndrome
Smita Amin, Arto Lahti, and Howard I. Maibach

Skin Reactions to Drugs
Kirsti Kauppinen, Kristiina Alanko, Matti Hannuksela, and Howard I. Maibach

Dry Skin and Moisturizers: Chemistry and Function
Marie Loden and Howard I. Maibach

Dermatologic Botany
Javier Avalos and Howard I. Maibach

Hand Eczema, Second Edition
Torkil Menné and Howard I. Maibach

Pesticide Dermatoses
Homero Penagos, Michael O'Malley, and Howard I. Maibach

Nickel and the Skin: Absorption, Immunology, Epidemiology, and Metallurgy
Jurij J. Hostýneck and Howard I. Maibach

THE EPIDERMIS IN WOUND HEALING

Edited by

David T. Rovee
Howard I. Maibach

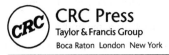

CRC Press
Taylor & Francis Group
Boca Raton London New York

CRC Press is an imprint of the
Taylor & Francis Group, an **informa** business

CRC Press
Taylor & Francis Group
6000 Broken Sound Parkway NW, Suite 300
Boca Raton, FL 33487-2742

First issued in paperback 2019

ISBN-13: 978-0-8493-1561-9 (hbk)
ISBN-13: 978-0-367-39463-9 (pbk)

A CIP record for this book is available from the British Library.

Library of Congress Cataloging-in-Publication Data available on application

**Visit the Taylor & Francis Web site at
http://www.taylorandfrancis.com**

**and the CRC Press Web site at
http://www.crcpress.com**

Series Preface

Our goal in creating the *Dermatology: Clinical & Basic Science Series* is to present the insights of experts on emerging applied and experimental techniques and theoretical concepts that are, or will be, at the vanguard of dermatology. These books cover new and exciting multidisciplinary areas of cutaneous research, and we want them to be the books every physician will use to become acquainted with new methodologies in skin research. These books can be also given to graduate students and postdoctoral fellows when they are looking for guidance to start a new line of research.

The series consists of books that are edited by experts, with chapters written by the leaders in each particular field. The books are richly illustrated and contain comprehensive bibliographies. Each chapter provides substantial background material relevant to its subject. These books contain detailed tricks of the trade and information regarding where the methods presented can be safely applied. In addition, information on where to buy equipment and helpful Web sites for solving both practical and theoretical problems are included.

We are working with these goals in mind. As the books become available, the efforts of the publisher, book editors, and individual authors will contribute to the further development of dermatology research and clinical practice. The extent to which we achieve this goal will be determined by the utility of these books.

Howard I. Maibach, M.D.

Preface

Just 30 years ago, the book *Epidermal Wound Healing* was published. That collection of papers from leaders in the field presented an interdisciplinary view of various aspects of wound healing. The primary focus, while on the epidermis, did not exclude interaction with other tissues. At the time of that work, little of the emerging data on wounds was being applied clinically. Today, many of the so-called advanced wound therapies can be traced back to the ideas presented by the group of contributors to *Epidermal Wound Healing*. These include the use of film, hydrocolloid, and gel dressings, which have brought about the acceptance of "moist wound healing" to prevent dehydration necrosis in the wound and enhance epithelial migration for early wound closure. The moist environment has also been employed to reduce inflammation and subsequent scar formation in the dermis. One aspect of these dressings, which was not predicted by the work in 1972, was their utility in enhancing autolytic debridement in chronic wounds, such as decubitus, venous, and diabetic ulcers. Also included in the original publication was the early work on growth factors and their potential applications to wound therapy. Today, clinicians are able to employ platelet-derived growth factors (PDGF) and tissue-engineered living skin products, which deliver an array of other growth factors.

The availability of new biological techniques and a renaissance of interest in both acute and chronic wound healing have led to a tremendously improved understanding of the cellular and chemical complexities of the healing process. We have begun to appreciate that much of what we have learned based upon acute wound healing does not always apply to the chronic wound. With this realization, much of today's clinical and research practice focuses on decubitus ulcers, venous ulcers, and diabetic foot ulcers.

Surprisingly, the original text from 1972 remains the only book focused on epidermal healing and is still frequently cited, even though there have been many further advances. The purpose of this second book on the topic is to update the information available on the epidermis, present a selection of the newest findings, and stimulate original research and development in wound therapy. Our intent is to focus on biological advances that improve our knowledge and lead to new opportunities for research and clinical applications in wound healing.

David T. Rovee, Ph.D.
Howard I. Maibach, M.D.

Editors

David T. Rovee, Ph.D., began working in the field of wound healing during his graduate education at Louisiana State University and Brown University, and has maintained this interest throughout a long career in the pharmaceutical, medical device, and biotechnology sectors. He has been instrumental in the development of new approaches in wound care, surgical devices, and dermatologicals while working in the laboratory and later in managing research and development programs in the medical industry. He has been the editor of the journal *Wounds: A Compendium of Clinical Research and Practice* since 1992. Dr. Rovee continues working with healthcare companies as an outside director and a consultant.

Howard Maibach, M.D., is a professor of dermatology at the University of California, San Francisco and has been a long-term contributor to experimental research in dermatopharmacology and to clinical research on contact dermatitis, contact urticaria, and other skin conditions.

Contributors

Magnus S. Ågren
Åagren Dermaconsulting ApS
Humblebaek, Denmark

Oscar M. Alvarez
University Wound Clinics, LLC
Bronx, New York

Leslie Baumann
Department of Dermatology and
  Cutaneous Surgery
University of Miami School of
  Medicine
Miami, Florida

Jill Holly Bigelman
Department of Dermatology and
  Cutaneous Surgery
University of Miami School of
  Medicine
Miami, Florida

Laura L. Bolton
ConvaTec
Skillman, New Jersey

Carlos A. Charles
Department of Dermatology and
  Cutaneous Surgery
University of Miami School of
  Medicine
Miami, Florida

Jeffrey M. Davidson
Department of Pathology
Vanderbilt University School of
  Medicine
Nashville, Tennessee

Robert H. Demling
Burn Center
Brigham & Women's Hospital
Boston, Massachusetts

Kevin Donohue
Department of Dermatology
Roger Williams Medical Center
Providence, Rhode Island

Anna Drosou
Department of Dermatology and
  Cutaneous Surgery
University of Miami School of
  Medicine
Miami, Florida

William H. Eaglstein
Department of Dermatology and
  Cutaneous Surgery
University of Miami School of
  Medicine
Miami, Florida

Elof Eriksson
Division of Plastic Surgery
Brigham & Women's Hospital
Boston, Massachusetts

Vincent Falanga
Department of Dermatology
Roger Williams Medical Center
Providence, Rhode Island

Giovanni Gaggio
Department of Energetics
University of Pisa School of Medicine
Pisa, Italy

Jonathan A. Garlick
Department of Oral Biology and
  Pathology
School of Dental Medicine
State University of New York at
  Stony Brook
Stony Brook, New York

Mitchel P. Goldman
Department of Dermatology
University of California
La Jolla, California

Monica Halem
Department of Dermatology and
  Cutaneous Surgery
University of Miami School of
  Medicine
Miami, Florida

Patricia A. Hebda
Children's Hospital of Pittsburgh
University of Pittsburgh
Pittsburgh, Pennsylvania

Thomas K. Hunt
Department of Surgery
University of California at
  San Francisco
San Francisco, California

Robert S. Kirsner
Department of Dermatology and
  Cutaneous Surgery
University of Miami School of
  Medicine
Miami, Florida

Howard I. Maibach
Department of Dermatology
University of California at
  San Francisco School of Medicine
San Francisco, California

Stephen Mandy
Department of Dermatology and
  Cutaneous Surgery
University of Miami School of
  Medicine
Miami, Florida

Lucy K. Martin
Department of Dermatology and
  Cutaneous Surgery
University of Miami School of
  Medicine
Miami, Florida

Diego Mastronicola
Department of Dermatology
University of Pisa School of Medicine
Pisa, Italy

Patricia M. Mertz
Department of Dermatology and
  Cutaneous Surgery
University of Miami School of
  Medicine
Miami, Florida

Holly Rausch
Roger Williams Medical Center
Providence, Rhode Island

Marco Romanelli
Department of Dermatology
University of Pisa School of Medicine
Pisa, Italy

David T. Rovee
The Rovee Group
Cambridge, Massachusetts

Vlad C. Sandulache
University of Pittsburgh School of
  Medicine
Pittsburgh, Pennsylvania

Greg Skover
Johnson & Johnson Consumer and
  Personal Products Worldwide, Inc.
Skillman, New Jersey

James M. Spencer
Department of Dermatology
The Mount Sinai School of Medicine of
  New York University
New York, New York

Tor Svensjo
Department of Surgery
Kristianstad Central Hospital
Kristianstad, Sweden

Stephen Thomas
Surgical Materials Testing Laboratory
Princess of Wales Hospital
Bridgend, South Wales, United Kingdom

Marjana Tomic-Canic
New York University School of
  Medicine
New York, New York

Jan Jeroen Vranckx
Division of Plastic and Reconstructive
  Surgery
Leuven University Medical School
Leuven, Belgium

Feng Yao
Division of Plastic Surgery
Brigham & Women's Hospital
Boston, Massachusetts

Hongbo Zhai
Department of Dermatology
University of California at San Francisco
San Francisco, California

Table of Contents

PART IV   *Physical and Chemical Factors Affecting Repair*

PART V   *New Approaches to Understanding and Treating Wounds*

Part I

Cellular and Biochemical Issues

1 Human Skin-Equivalent Models of Epidermal Wound Healing: Tissue Fabrication and Biological Implications

Jonathan A. Garlick

CONTENTS

1.1 INTRODUCTION

The development of human tissue models to advance our understanding of the integrated sequence of events during wound repair requires the ability to engineer tissues that faithfully mimic their *in vivo* counterparts. In general, *in vitro* studies of reepithelialization have often been limited by their inability to simulate wound repair as it occurs in humans. For example, wound models using skin explants[1–4] or monolayer, submerged keratinocyte cultures[5,6] demonstrate limited stratification, partial differentiation, and hyperproliferative growth. These culture systems have been helpful in studying keratinocyte migration in response to wounding[7] but have been of limited use in studying the complexities of keratinocyte response during wound repair, as these cultures do not provide the proper tissue architecture to study wound response as it occurs *in vivo*. Biologically meaningful signaling pathways, mediated by the linking of adhesion and growth, function optimally when cells are spatially organized in a three-dimensional (3-D) tissue but are uncoupled and lost in two-dimensional culture systems.[8] It is therefore essential that 3-D cultures, which display the architectural features seen in *in vivo* tissues, be adapted to model and further understand the biological behavior of wounded keratinocytes in their appropriate tissue context.

In the last decade, the development of tissue-engineered models that mimic human skin, known as skin equivalents (SE), has provided novel experimental systems to study the response of keratinocytes to wounding.[9–13] The SE is an *in vitro* tissue that consists of a stratified squamous epithelium grown at an air–liquid interface on a collagen matrix populated with dermal fibroblasts. This generates 3-D, organotypic tissues that demonstrate *in vivo*-like epithelial differentiation and morphology, as well as rates of cell division similar to those found in human skin.[14,15] Such engineered human tissues have been adapted to study the healing of human wounds *in vitro*[10] and have been found to simulate the chronology of events that occurs during reepithelialization in human skin.[16]

This chapter will describe the adaptation of SE cultures to study wound healing of human keratinocytes that have been developed to mimic this process from the initiation of keratinocyte activation until restoration of epithelial integrity. This will be accomplished by reviewing previous studies using wounded SEs that have defined key response parameters, such as growth, migration, differentiation, growth-factor response, and protease expression. These applications demonstrate the utility of these human-like tissues in studying phenotypic responses that are characteristic of the switch from a normal to a regenerative tissue during wound healing. It is hoped that by describing human tissue models which recapitulate the *in vivo* wound response, further study of the nature and fate of keratinocytes activated and mobilized during reepithelialization will be facilitated.

1.2 MORPHOLOGIC ASPECTS OF THE RESPONSE OF WOUNDED SKIN EQUIVALENTS

Immediately after keratinocyte injury, epithelium at the wound edge undergoes a sequence of coordinated temporal and spatial events that prepare these cells for new tissue formation. These initial phenotypic changes characterize a preparative phase that precedes migration into the wound site. This phase of wound response has been defined as the stage of "keratinocyte activation," during which the injured epithelium responds to wound injury by reprogramming patterns of gene expression to prepare for reepithelialization.[17] The "activated" keratinocyte thus undergoes a shift from a program of differentiation to one leading to directed and sustained migration and proliferation, which is then followed by stratification and differentiation.

The morphologic appearance of wounded SEs that occurs during these events has been studied in several investigations.[10,18,19] Figure 1.1 demonstrates a schematic of the construction of SEs that describes how these cultures have been adapted to study wound healing. Color Figure 1.2* shows the appearance of such a wounded culture 6 d after wounding. The generation of this model has demonstrated wound response that recapitulated many of the morphologic events known to occur during cutaneous reepithelialization *in vivo* and thus provides an opportunity to study the appearance of wound keratinocytes during the various stages of reepithelialization and epithelial reconstitution (Color Figure 1.3). At 8 h, a wedge-shaped epithelial tongue two to three cells in thickness was seen at the edge of the wound margin (Color Figure 1.3A) in a tissue in which wound margins could be seen at the transition from a double layer of collagen matrix to a single layer (Color Figure 1.3, arrows). By 24 h, the wound floor was completely covered with a monolayer or bilayer of keratinocytes in the center and a more stratified epithelium toward the wound margins (Color Figure 1.3C). This showed that the stage of reepithelialization was complete and that stratification could now occur adjacent to the wound margins. Tissue stratification continued at 48 h, and by 4 d post-wounding a multilayer epithelium was generated. At 6 d after wounding, the reepithelialized surface demonstrated a fully stratified epithelium (Color Figure 1.3F) that was similar to nonwounded epithelium. This chronology of events during reepithelialization was very similar to those reported in earlier *in vivo* studies.[16,20–22] Other studies have shown similar spatiotemporal patterns of repair upon wounding of SEs.[9,11] Geer and co-authors have shown that cells in wounded SEs initiated migration as an epithelial tongue by 48 h after wounding and were completely reepithelialized within 72 h.[11] Falanga et al. showed that wounded SEs initiated migration after 12 h, that reepithelialization was complete by 48 h, and that a well-stratified epithelium had reformed by 96 h after wounding.[9] The consistency of epithelial response in these three studies demonstrates the ability to adapt a variety of SE-based models to study wound response in a manner that mimics that seen *in vivo*.

1.3   PROLIFERATIVE RESPONSE TO SKIN-EQUIVALENT WOUNDING

Following the response of wounded SEs in organotypic culture provides an opportunity to directly measure the proliferation of keratinocytes during various stages of wound response. Cell growth in wounded SEs can be determined by incubation of cultures with bromodeoxyuridine (BrdU) several hours before cultures are processed to determine the labeling index (LI), which is measured as the fraction of BrdU-positive basal cells. Previous studies have shown that the proliferative activity of SEs during reepithelialization had two distinct temporal and spatial phases. The first of these occurs during early reepithelialization, as the wound floor is being covered with the epithelial tongue. During this stage, proliferation is limited in the migrating epithelial tongue but is elevated at the wound margins. The second phase of proliferative activity occurs after coverage of the wound is complete, as epithelium in the center of the wound undergoes stratification. No BrdU labeling was seen in the tip

---

* Color figures follow page 110.

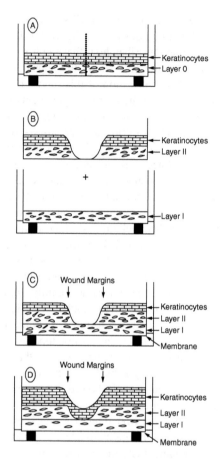

FIGURE 1.1 Construction of composite organotypic coculture wounding model. A) Schematic of stratified keratinocyte sheet growing on contracted collagen matrix containing fibroblasts (Layer II). This organotypic culture rests on a semipermeable membrane and is nourished with medium from below, thus resting at an air–liquid interface. An incisional wound is formed by cutting through the epithelium and collagen matrix (dotted line). B) The wounded culture is then transferred onto a second collagen matrix that has undergone contraction (Layer I). C) The resultant composite co-culture consists of two layers of contracted matrix and one layer of epithelium. Wound margins are seen at the transition zone from layer I to layer II and are noted with arrows. D) Reepithelialization occurs as wounded keratinocytes migrate onto the collagen in layer II and is then followed by stratification of the tissue to reconstitute a fully stratified epithelium that covers the wound bed.

of the wound edge at the earliest time point (8 h after wounding) (Color Figure 1.4), suggesting that these cells were nonproliferative and had assumed a migratory phenotype. This finding is in agreement with skin explant studies, which show that migration can be initiated as an active process independent of proliferation.[6] Proliferative activity in the epithelium of the wound margin peaked at 24 h after wounding, as LIs were as high as 50% in the epithelium of the wound margin and reached 80%

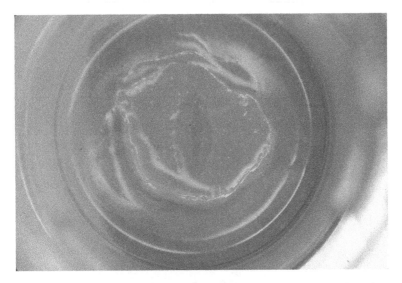

FIGURE 1.2 Appearance of wounded skin equivalents grown in organotypic culture at an air–liquid interface. An organotypic culture transferred to a second collagen gel after an incisional wound is seen 6 d after wounding. The shape of the original wound is elliptical, and the wound is nearly closed in the center.

in the center of the wound epithelium. This burst of mitotic activity in the wound margin was transient, since the marginal epithelium returned to lower levels of growth activity at 48 h after wounding. These findings matched previous *in vivo* studies demonstrating a similarly delayed and transient increase in proliferative activity at the wound margin beginning after initiation of migration.[16,21] The finding that proliferation at the wound margin was higher than in the epithelium more distal to the margin suggested that cells were displaced from the wound margin onto the wound floor upon their proliferation. The observation that suprabasal cell migration was followed by a proliferative response in adjacent cells supports the suggestion of Winter that mitotic activity is, in part, a response to cell migration.[16] The movement of suprabasal cells at the edge of the wounded epithelium would leave that tissue somewhat denuded and would be analogous to the elimination of suprabasal cells by tape stripping. During the later phase of proliferation that occurred after wound coverage, mitotic activity continued to remain high in the wound epithelium at 4-h and 4-d time points (Color Figure 1.4). This elevated mitotic activity led to stratification of the wound epithelium even after the proliferative rates in all other areas of the epithelium returned to baseline levels.

Proliferative response of SEs to wounding has also been evaluated using Ki67 as marker of cell growth. Geer et al. found a similar pattern of growth to that described above, as was seen by a delayed and transient elevation of Ki67 expression at the wound edge.[11] In this study, Ki67 expression decreased significantly after wound closure as maturation and differentiation of the epithelium occurred. A similar pattern of Ki67 expression was seen in a study performed by Falanga et al.[9] Using

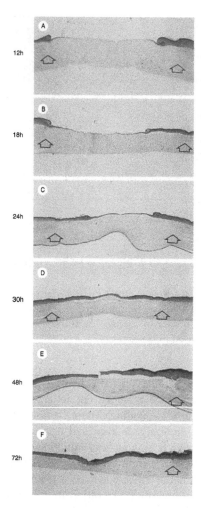

FIGURE 1.3 Morphology of skin eqiuivalents at various points after wounding. Wounded skin equivalents were stained with hematoxylin and eosin at (A) 12 h, (B) 18 h, (C) 24 h, (D) 30 h, (E) 48 h, and (F) 72 h after wounding. Two phases of epithelial response can be seen. The first phase extends from the earliest migration of epithelium (A,B) until the wound is completely covered by a thin epithelium (C). The second phase of stratification begins at 30 h (D) and is complete when the tissue is of similar thickness to that of the unwounded epithelium at the wound margins (F). Open arrows demarcate the wound margins. (Original magnification × 10.) (See color figures following page 110.)

an innovative approach to characterize proliferative activity following SE wounding, these authors confirmed their findings on the spatial distribution of Ki67-positive cells in wounded SEs by assaying for the presence of S-phase nuclei using flow cytometry. To accomplish this, epithelial cells were separated from the underlying connective tissue in the SE by thermolysin treatment and were then disaggregated. It was found that SEs demonstrated a roughly twofold decrease in their fraction of S-phase cells after wounding. These findings are in agreement with other SE studies

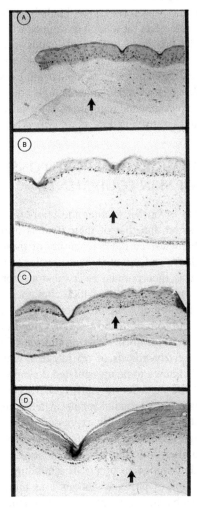

FIGURE 1.4 Proliferative activity of reepithelialized wounds at various points after wounding. Wounded skin equivalents were labeled with an 8-h pulse of BrdU, stained with a monoclonal antibody to BrdU, and counterstained with hematoxylin at (A) 8 h, (B) 24 h, (C) 48 h, and (D) 4 d after wounding. While few BrdU-nuclei are seen shortly after wounding (A), a sharp increase in proliferative activity is seen in both the wound and in the adjacent wound margins 24 h after wounding (B). This proliferative activity is maintained in the wound by 48 h as the tissue stratifies (C). Proliferation is considerably less at 4 d post-wounding when the reepithelialization process is complete (D). The arrows demarcate the wound margins. Labeling Index (LI) was calculated as the percentage of basal nuclei labeled with BrdU. Wound margins are demarcated by arrows. (Original magnification × 50 for A, B, and C and × 66 for D.) (See color figures following page 110.)

described above and with *in vivo* findings that have characterized the shift of wounded keratinocytes from a proliferative to a migratory phase shortly after wounding.

The proliferative indices and rates of reepithelialization observed in these SE models are somewhat greater than those seen in wounds with scab formation *in vivo,* as the organotypic model presented here is analogous to a wet rather than a dry healing environment. A wet environment is more conducive to an accelerated healing response[16,20,23,24] and likely explains the more rapid healing response seen in wounded SEs compared to *in vivo* wound repair. Interestingly, the proliferation of wound epithelium is subject to environmental regulation, as the growth response was shown to be sensitive to growth factor regulation, as described below.

1.4   KERATINOCYTE MIGRATION IN RESPONSE TO WOUNDING OF SKIN EQUIVALENTS

In vivo, wound response is known to alter the temporal and spatial patterns of integrin receptor expression and that of their ligands during reepithelialization. Several studies have characterized the distribution of these proteins during reepithelialization of wounded SEs. Geer et al. have developed an SE model for wound repair in which fibrin was incorporated as a substrate for reepithelialization by generating fibrin gels in the wound bed, which contained physiologic concentrations of fibrinogen and thrombin.[11] The presence of fibrin was found to accelerate keratinocyte activation and to reduce the time of wound closure when compared to controls that did not contain fibrin. This promotion of reepithelialization was associated with the *de novo* synthesis of $\alpha 5$ integrin, which is not expressed in mature epithelium and is known to be upregulated during wound response *in vivo*. Both with and without the presence of fibrin gels, $\alpha 5$ was expressed at higher levels in migrating cells in the epithelial tongue when compared to cells distal to the wound, while $\alpha 2$ integrin was equally expressed in these two regions. Expression of $\alpha 5$ decreased significantly in nonwounded tissue but remained elevated in the center of the wound after 96 h. Integrin upregulation in response to wounding of SEs has also been determined in other SE wounding models.[12,13] It has also been shown that expression of proteins that serve as integrin ligands needed for cell migration, as well as basement membrane components, is also altered during reepithelialization of wounded SEs. Expression of laminin 1 has been found to be delayed somewhat during early reepithelialization, as migrating cells at the tip of the epithelial tongue did not express this protein, and expression was seen closer to the wound margin. However, all basal cells expressed laminin 1 after wound closure, suggesting that keratinocytes can synthesize their own basement membrane proteins upon completion of the migratory phase of reepithelialization. Interestingly, the earliest stage of keratinocyte migration was associated with the expression of laminin 5 in the epithelial tongue, as this protein was seen in basal and suprabasal cells at the tip of the forming epithelial tongue.[25] These studies using wounded SEs have shown that following wounding, keratinocytes were activated to express an altered distribution of integrin receptors and their associated ligands, both to facilitate migration shortly after wounding and to stabilize the epithelium through assembly of new basement membrane after wound coverage was complete.

1.5 GROWTH FACTOR RESPONSIVENESS AND SYNTHESIS IN WOUNDED SKIN EQUIVALENTS

SE models of wound repair facilitate the determination of the synthesis and response of surface keratinocytes to soluble growth factors, as it is possible to directly assay their effect on reepithelialization by adding these soluble factors to culture media. *In vivo* studies have previously shown that growth factors, such as transforming growth factor (TGF)-β1,[18,19] can modulate reepithelialization and wound repair through autocrine or paracrine pathways.[26,27] Systemic administration of TGF-β1 is known to accelerate cutaneous wound healing,[28] while topical administration inhibits epithelial regeneration at elevated doses[29] and can stimulate epithelial regeneration at low doses.[14,30–32]

The temporal response of wounded SEs to TGF-β1 was determined in the presence of active doses of this growth factor that are known to be present in the *in vivo* environment shortly after wounding.[26] It was found that addition of 2.5 ng/ml TGF-β1 to cultures at the time of wounding delayed reepithelialization and reduced hyperproliferation. Twenty-four hours after wounding, nontreated cultures had undergone reepithelialization, while TGF-β1–treated cultures showed only a thin tongue of elongated cells moving onto the wound surface. Proliferation in this tongue, as detected by BrdU incorporation, was considerably lower than that seen in the wound epithelium not treated with TGF-β1. This delay in reepithelialization was shown to be transient, as TGF-β1–treated cultures had completely reepithelialized by 48 h after wounding. This TGF-β1-induced shift towards a migratory response and delayed reepithelialization was found to be dose-dependent, as a progressively greater delay in reepithelialization was observed 24 h after wounding at increased doses of TGF-β1. For example, complete reepithelialization and stratification had occurred within 48 h, even in the presence of 7 ng/ml TGF-β1, where epithelial proliferation was completely suppressed. This suggested that reepithelialization at this concentration was primarily due to the stimulation of keratinocyte migration. These studies confirmed *in vivo* studies on the effects of TGF-β1 on the wound environment that have shown its ability to induce enhanced migration and a dose-dependent effect on epidermal regeneration.[33]

These studies used either foreskin[19] or gingival[18] keratinocytes to demonstrate that the TGF-β1–induced delay in reepithelialization was due to a reduced hyperproliferative response at the wound margins. Although the LIs were lowered two- to fourfold by the presence of 2.5 ng/ml TGF-β1, the level of proliferation was still considerably higher than that of nonwounded control cultures treated with TGF-β1, demonstrating that wounded keratinocytes were refractory to the known TGF-β1–induced inhibition of proliferation.[27] This supports the view that keratinocytes activated after wounding are not subject to the same inhibitory effects that TGF-β1 has been shown to exert on nonwounded cultures. Similarly, the addition of TGF-β1 enhanced the migratory phenotype of wounded SE cultures. This confirms previous findings from studies performed using simple, monolayer culture systems, as it has been shown that migrating keratinocytes upregulated their repertoire of migration-associated integrin receptors and their extracellular matrix ligands in response to TGF-β1 in order to facilitate their movement.[33] Thus, the use of SE wounding models has demonstrated that TGF-β1 alters reepithelialization by modifying both proliferation and migration. Keratinocyte activation following wounding is therefore thought to be a prerequisite to facilitate the switch from a normal to an activated, regenerative epithelial cell phenotype.[17] TGF-β1 may then modulate this altered cell phenotype by enabling a dose-dependent control of proliferation and migration in order to modulate the phenotype of the activated keratinocyte during different stages of reepithelialization.

Falanga et al. studied the production of growth factors and proinflammatory cytokines by reverse transcription polymerase chain reaction (RT-PCR) after wounding of SEs and found a sequential program of expression of these proteins.[9] Expression of cytokines interleukin (IL)-1α, IL-1β, IL-6, IL-8, IL-11, and tumor necrosis factor (TNF)-α was turned on shortly after wounding and peaked shortly thereafter. In contrast, levels of growth factors, such as insulin growth factor-2, TGF-β1, and platelet-derived growth factor-B (PDGF-B), increased subsequent to this point at 48 to 72 h after wounding. These levels of expression were closely correlated with protein levels of these soluble factors as determined by enzyme-linked immunosorbent assay (ELISA) analysis of supernatants from wounded SEs. Taken together, these studies demonstrated the utility of SEs in determining the presence of and response to soluble factors in patterns that simulated the events known to occur *in vivo.*

1.6 PROTEASE ACTIVATION IN WOUNDED SKIN EQUIVALENTS

The matrix metalloproteinase (MMP) family of proteinases acts to degrade all components of the extracellular matrix (ECM).[34] During reepithelialization, such degradation directs tissue remodeling and facilitates removal of damaged tissue, thus paving the way for migration of keratinocytes over dermal connective tissue in the wound bed. *In vivo,* cutaneous wounds demonstrate the spatially and temporally coordinated expression of MMP-1 (Type I collagenase)[35,36] and MMP-10 that are expressed at the migrating edge of keratinocytes, while MMP-3 (stromelysin 1) was found to be expressed just distal to these cells.[37] In migrating gingival keratinocytes, expression of MMP-9 (92 kDa Type IV collagenase) was found to be elevated.[38] The distinct compartmentalization of these degradatory enzymes in response to wounding suggests that they play specific functions during reepithelialization.

To determine if this *in vivo* pattern of MMP expression was also present upon wounding of SEs, expression of MMP-1 ribonucleic acid (RNA) expression was assayed by *in situ* hybridization. Wounding of SEs showed that MMP-1 RNA was expressed only in keratinocytes that were actively repopulating the wound. At 8 h after wounding, only keratinocytes that had initiated reepithelialization and were in contact with the Type I collagen on the wound surface were positive for MMP-1. Similarly, at 24 h after wounding, expression of MMP-1 RNA was only detected in the center of the wound and not in nonwounded keratinocytes at the wound margin (Color Figure 1.5). At later time points, MMP-1 expression was no longer seen in either keratinocytes in the center of the wound or at wound margins.

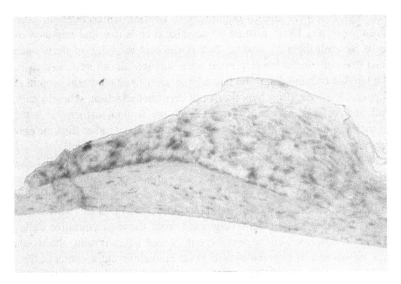

FIGURE 1.5 MMP-1 RNA expression is restricted to migrating keratinocytes covering the wound. Basal keratinocytes at the leading edge of the epithelial tongue express MMP-1 RNA, as detected by *in situ* hybridization 4 d after wounding. Keratinocytes distal from the wound edge demonstrate no MMP-1 RNA expression. Thus, only keratinocytes in contact with Type I collagen on the wound surface express this protease. (See color figures following page 110.)

These findings suggested that only keratinocytes that were in direct contact with the Type I collagen in the wound bed could activate MMP-1 expression, as this connective tissue interface did not contain the basement membrane components that were present under keratinocytes found at the wound margins. As these basement membrane components were not present on the substrate on which reepithelialization occurs, it appeared that activated keratinocytes turned on expression of MMP-1 to promote remodeling of extracellular matrix proteins as cells moved over the wound bed. Expression of MMP-1 was terminated upon synthesis of new basement membrane components in the center of the wound, as initial assembly of basement membrane structure occurred at this site. In this light, the initiation of reepithelialization onto a Type I collagen substrate served as an activation signal to direct wound repair and activated protease expression and activity. Thus, the remodeling of the dermal–epidermal interface was an essential step in the restoration of epithelial attachment and renewed stabilization at the basement membrane zone.

1.7 PATTERNS OF KERATINOCYTE DIFFERENTIATION IN WOUNDED SKIN EQUIVALENTS

The ability of wounded keratinocytes to alter their expression of markers of keratinocyte differentiation have been studied in wounded SEs.[10] Expression of both keratins 1 and 10 (K1, K10) was seen at the edge of the epithelial tongue at 8 h after wounding, in both suprabasal and basal cells at the wound edge. In addition, cells in this position also expressed involucrin, supporting the view that cells initiating migration were already committed to terminal differentiation. This initial epithelial tongue was likely formed by suprabasal cells that had migrated over the basal cells beneath them to assume their position at the edge of the tongue. This suggested that cells initiating migration were suprabasal, differentiated cells at the wound edge that became displaced laterally in order to attach to the wound surface. This supports the "leap-frog hypothesis" of reepithelialization, wherein suprabasal cells roll over cells adjacent to them to reach the wound surface.[16,20] It therefore appears that migration is initiated as a multilayer cell sheet rather than the epidermal monolayer proposed by the "sliding model" of reepithelialization.[16]

At 24 h post wounding, the wound bed was covered by an epithelial sheet and cells expressing K1, K10 were no longer seen in a basal position. This suggested that migration was initiated by differentiated cells but was maintained by proliferating cells and their progeny as the epithelial tongue covered the wound floor. It is likely that these replicating cells originated from these proliferative cells at the wound margin described above and were displaced laterally onto the wound bed. No K1, K10 was seen in suprabasal cells in the epithelium at the center of the wound after 24 h, suggesting that its expression was delayed during stratification due to the hyperproliferative nature of the regenerating epithelium in this region. However, involucrin was correctly expressed immediately upon stratification in cells directly above the basal layer in the wound epithelium, even when only two cell layers were present. This demonstrates that cells became committed to terminal differentiation in the reepithelializing tissue shortly after covering the wound and as soon as stratification occurred.

1.8 SUMMARY

This chapter has demonstrated the utility of SEs as biologically relevant models of epithelial wound response by demonstrating the following:

1. The proliferative, migratory, and synthetic response of wounded, "activated" keratinocytes can be monitored in a "controlled" culture environment.
2. The phenotype of keratinocytes during the wound response in SEs closely mimics that seen upon cutaneous wounding.
3. The absence of *in vivo* factors such as a variety of mesenchymal cells in SEs allows the response of keratinocytes to wounding to be directly determined.
4. The wound milieu can be easily modified in SEs in order to study the effects of agents, including potential therapeutic agents, that may alter the course of wound response.

Different adaptations of SE technology for wounding models in several independent studies have shown similar responses, thus suggesting the broad adaptability of these tissue models for the study of wounding. In summary, these engineered tissue models using SEs have thus demonstrated that the first cells to initiate migration are nonproliferating, terminally differentiated keratinocytes that form an epithelial tongue by moving laterally onto the wound floor. This loss of cells from a suprabasal position may be partially responsible for the proliferative response that occurs at the wound margins. At this stage, progeny cells from this proliferative edge displace proliferative cells centrally into the elongating epithelial tongue that partially covers the wound floor. At the same time, nondividing cells continually migrate and, together with the progeny of proliferating cells, advance to completely cover the wound floor. These early changes mark a phenotypic switch from a proliferating, nonwounded epithelium to one in which cell migration is predominant. Once reepithelialization is complete, the proliferative phenotype becomes dominant again as cell division induces stratification. As cells re-form a multilayer tissue, keratinocyte differentiation of cells at the center of the wound floor lags behind that of the areas closer to the wound margins as cells first undergo terminal differentiation near the wound margins. Finally, proliferative activity continues to be high in the wound epithelium even after the wound margins return to baseline levels of mitotic activity. This allows the wound epithelium to stratify to a thickness similar to that of the nonwounded epithelium. Keratinocyte activation following wounding is thought to be a prerequisite to sustain cell proliferation and to enhance cell migration *in vivo*.[17] These effects are coincident with the switch from a normal to an activated, regenerative epithelial cell phenotype that occurs following wounding and has been simulated and studied using SE technology.

1.9 FABRICATION OF SKIN-EQUIVALENT WOUND HEALING MODEL

1. Growth media for submerged cultures used to prepare cells for skin-equivalent cultures
   a. *Medium for keratinocytes grown in submerged culture* — Primary keratinocytes can be grown in commercially available, serum-free media or using irradiated 3T3 feeder layers and serum-containing medium according to the following formulation.
      i. Dulbecco's modified eagle medium (DMEM)/Ham's F12 medium (Gibco, BRL) (3:1).
      ii. Fetal bovine serum (FBS) 5% (Hyclone Laboratories).
      iii. Penicillin–streptomycin (Sigma, St. Louis, MO) — Dissolve 2.42 g penicillin and 4.0 g streptomycin in 400 ml $2 \times$ dH$_2$O to make a 100× stock, filter sterilize, aliquot, and store at –20°C.
      iv. HEPES (Sigma) — Dissolve 47.24 g in 250 ml 2× dH$_2$O to make a 100× stock. Filter sterilize, aliquot, and store at –20°C.
      v. Adenine (ICN, Aurora, OH) — Dissolve 0.972 g in 2.4 ml of 4 *N* NaOH; bring volume to 400 ml with 2× dH$_2$O to make a 100× stock (18 m*M*), filter sterilize, aliquot, and store at –20°C.
      vi. Cholera toxin (ICN Inc.) — Dissolve 1 mg in 1 ml 2× dH$_2$O, add this to 90 ml DMEM with 10 ml FBS to make a 1000× stock (1.2 $\times 10^{-7}$ *M*), filter sterilize, aliquot, and store at –20°C.

vii.Epidermal growth factor (cat. no. GF-010-9, Austrial Biological, San Ramon, CA) — Dissolve 10 μg/ml in 0.1% BSA to make a 1000× stock, filter sterilize, aliquot, and store at –20°C.

viii.Hydrocortisone (Sigma) — Dissolve 0.0538 g in 200 ml 2× dH$_2$O to make a 500× stock (7.4 × 10^{-4} M), filter sterilize, aliquot, and store at –20°C.

ix. Insulin (Sigma) — Dissolve 50 mg in 10 ml of 0.005 N HCl to make a 1000× stock (5 mg/ml), filter sterilize, aliquot, and store at –20°C.

b. *Medium for 3T3 fibroblasts as feeder cells for submerged keratinocyte cultures* — The clonal growth of keratinocytes requires cocultivation with metabolically active, nonproliferating feeder layers of 3T3-J2 fibroblasts. When cells are 90% confluent they are trypsinized, pelleted with centrifugation at 2000 r/min for 5 min and irradiated by a gamma source of 2000 Ci (Cs-137, 100% = 1215 r/min) for 6.5 min. Irradiated cells are then plated at a density of 2 × 10^6/p100 in keratrocyte complete media (KCM) before keratinocytes are added.

   i.   DMEM (Gibco, BRL)

   ii.   Bovine calf serum 10% (Hyclone Laboratories)

   iii. Penicillin–streptomycin (Sigma)

   iv. HEPES (Sigma)

2. Preparation of skin-equivalent cultures

a. *Fibroblasts for skin-equivalent cultures* — Fibroblasts are first isolated from human foreskins by using the connective tissue remnant after dispase separation of keratinocytes used for submerged culture. The connective tissue is then rinsed twice in phosphate-buffered saline (PBS) and placed in a 15-ml conical tube with 1 ml of collagenase in collagenase buffer. This mixture is incubated at 37°C for 30 min and is agitated every 5 min. Trypsin/ethylenediamine tetra acetic acid (EDTA) mixed in a 1:1 ratio is added for 10 min at 37°C, at which time 1 ml of fibroblast culture medium is added to inactivate the trypsin and cells are counted. These fibroblasts are grown so that they are densely confluent one day before the collagen matrix is to be cast. At this time, passage the cells at high density so they will regrow to full confluence the next day when they will be added to the collagen matrix. This extra passage ensures that a high fraction of fibroblasts are proliferating at the time of initiation of matrix construction.

   i. Reagents for isolation of fibroblasts from human foreskins

      A. Collagenase buffer (130 mM NaCl, 10 mM Ca acetate, 20 mM HEPES. Adjust to pH 7.2 and filter sterilize.).

      B. Dispase — Make 10× stock by dissolving 5 g in 200 ml double-distilled H$_2$O, filter sterilize, store at –20°C.

      C. Collagenase (Worthington Biochemical) (3 mg/ml in collagenase buffer).

      D. Trypsin — prepare as a 1% stock by mixing 10× PBS (200 ml), 2 g glucose, 2 g trypsin, 0.2 g penicillin, and 0.2 g streptomycin.

Dissolve these components in the PBS and then bring to 2 l with
2× dH$_2$O, filter sterilize, aliquot, and store at −20°C.
E. EDTA — prepare as a 0.2% stock by dissolving 2 g in 1 l PBS
and adjusting the pH to 7.45 with 4 N NaOH; autoclave and store
at room temperature.
F. PBS — prepared as a 10× stock by dissolving 1.6 kg NaCl, 165
g Na$_2$HPO$_4$, 40 g KH$_2$PO$_4$, and 40 g KCl in 20 l 2× dH$_2$O.
ii. Fibroblast culture medium for growth of fibroblasts to be incorporated into collagen gels
A. DMEM (Gibco, BRL)
B. FBS 10% (Hyclone Laboratories)
C. Penicillin–streptomycin (Sigma)
D. HEPES (Sigma)
b. *Fabrication of collagen gel for skin-equivalent cultures* — To construct
the collagen matrix, mix the following components on ice to generate
acellular and cellular collagen layers for the SE. The goal is to create
a thin layer of acellular collagen that will act as a substrate for the
thicker layer of cellular collagen. This will prevent the cellular collagen
from contracting completely and pulling off the insert.
i. Keeping all components on ice, mix the acellular matrix components
in the order listed in Table 1.1. The color of the solution should be
from straw-yellow to light pink; any extreme variations in color
may indicate a pH at which the collagen may not gel. If the final
solution is bright yellow, slowly titrate sodium bicarbonate drop by
drop until the appropriate color is noted. Add 1 ml to each insert,
making sure the mixture coats the entire bottom of the insert. Once
the gel has been poured, it should stand at room temperature, without
being disturbed, until it polymerizes (10 to 15 min). As the gel
polymerizes, the color of the matrix will change to a deeper pink
color.

TABLE 1.1
**Components for the Collagen Matrix with Incorporated Dermal
Fibroblasts**

	Acellular Matrix for 6 ml (1 ml/insert)	Cellular Matrix for 18 ml (3 ml/insert)
10X DMEM	0.60 ml	1.65 ml
L-Glutamine	0.05 ml	0.15 ml
Fetal bovine serum	0.70 ml	1.85 ml
Sodium bicarbonate	0.17 ml	0.52 ml
Collagen	4.60 ml	14.00 ml
Fibroblasts	—	4.5×10^5 cells in 1.5 ml fibroblast media

ii. While the acellular matrix layer is polymerizing, trypsinize and resuspend fibroblasts in fibroblast culture medium to a final concentration of 3.0×10^5 cells/ml. Resuspend these cells fully, since it will be harder to resuspend them properly once mixed with collagen.

iii. For the cellular matrix, again keep all components on ice, and mix in the order indicated above. Again, if the color needs to be adjusted, carefully titrate in a small amount of sodium bicarbonate. The fibroblasts should be added last to ensure that the mix has been neutralized by the addition of collagen so that the cells are not damaged by an alkaline pH. Mix well and add 3 ml to the insert; allow it to gel at room temperature without disturbing for 30 to 45 min. When the gels are pink and firm, they are covered with 12 ml of fibroblast culture medium and incubated for 4 to 7 d until the gel no longer contracts. A raised, mesa-like area is seen in the center of the matrix; the keratinocytes will be seeded there.

iv. Reagents for fabrication of collagen gels with foreskin fibroblasts.

A. Confluent cultures of human foreskin fibroblasts

B. Six-well deep tissue culture tray containing tissue culture inserts with a 3 μm porous polycarbonate membrane

C. Sterile bovine tendon or rat tail acid-extracted collagen

D. 10× minimum essential medium with Earle's salts (cat. no. 12-684F, BioWhittaker)

E. Newborn calf serum (Hyclone Laboratories)

F. L-Glutamine (200 mM) (cat. no. 17-605E, BioWhittaker)

G. Sodium bicarbonate (71.2 mg/ml)

H. Fibroblast culture medium

c. *Skin-equivalent culture medium* — Use keratinocytes from feeder layer cultures when they are no more than 50% confluent in order to minimize the number of differentiated cells seeded onto the collagen gel. Thoroughly remove the 3T3 feeder cells from the culture by incubation in PBS/EDTA (1:1 ratio) for 2 min followed by gentle rinsing. Take care not to leave the culture too long in PBS/EDTA, as small keratinocyte colonies may detach. Rinse with PBS until the 3T3s have been removed.

i. Trypsinize the keratinocyte colonies with trypsin/EDTA (1:1 ratio) for 5 to 10 min and add cells to a 15-ml tube so that 5×10^5 keratinocytes will be plated in each insert. Centrifuge the cells at 1500 r/min for 5 min.

ii. Remove all fibroblast medium from the inserts containing the contracted collagen matrices.

iii. Resuspend the keratinocytes so that they can be plated in a small volume with each insert receiving 50 ul of suspension containing 5 $\times 10^5$ keratinocytes. This can be done by eliminating all residual supernatant above the pellet. Use a sterile plastic 1 ml pipette with the appropriate volume of Epidermalization I medium to lift the

TABLE 1.2
Media Formulations for 1l Total Volume (All Volumes are in ml):

	Epidermalization I	Epidermalization II	Cornification (at airlift)
DME	725	725	474
F12	240	240	474
L-glutamine	20	20	20
Hydrocortisone	2	2	2
ITES	2	2	2
O-phos	2	2	2
CaCl$_2$	2	2	2
Progesterone	2	2	—
Serum	1(cFCS)	1(FCS)	20(FCS)

pellet and transfer it to a sterile Eppendorf tube. Then use a 200 or 1000 ul pipetteman to gently resuspend the cell pellet in the Eppendorf tube. The cell suspension can then be placed in the central, raised, mesa-like portion of the contracted collagen gel with a 200 ul pipetteman.

iv. Do not touch the plate for 1.5 to 2 h while the keratinocytes adhere. At this point, add 12 ml of Epidermalization I medium (~10 ml in the well and 2 ml on top of the keratinocytes), and incubate cultures at 37°C, 7% CO$_2$.

v. Cultures are fed for 7 d in the following way (media formulations are shown in Table 1.2).

A. Epidermalization I medium — submerged in 12 ml, first 2 d

B. Epidermalization II medium — submerged in 12 ml, next 2 d

C. Epidermalization II medium — grown at the air–liquid interface by feeding with 7 ml for 3 d

vi. Reagents for skin-equivalent culture medium

A. DMEM Base Modified (catalog no. 56430-10L, JRH Biosciences, Lenexa, KS).

B. Ham's F12 (Gibco, BRL).

C. L-Glutamine (BioWhittaker); 200 mM is a 50× stock.

D. Hydrocortisone (Sigma).

E. Insulin–transferrin–triodothyronine (ITT) (Sigma) 500× stock:

1. Bovine insulin — Dissolve in 0.0001 N HCl to a final concentration of 5 μg/ml.

2. Human transferrin — Dissolve in double-distilled H$_2$O (2× H$_2$O) to a final concentration of 5 μg/ml.

3. Triiodothyronine — dissolve in acidified ethanol, dilute with double-distilled dH$_2$O to a final concentration of 20 pM.

F. Ethanolamine–O–phosphorylenanolamine (EOP) stock (500×).

1. Ethanolamine (Sigma) — reconstitute with 2× dH$_2$O to 10^{-4} M.

       2. O-phosphorylethanolamine (Sigma) — dilute with 2× dH_2O
         to 10^{-4} *M*.

     G. Adenine (Sigma) — Dissolve 0.18 m*M* (500× stock) in acidified
       water warmed in a 37°C water bath.

     H. Selenious acid (Aldrich) — Dissolve 5.3×10^{-8} M (500× stock)
       with 2× dH_2O.

     I. Calcium chloride — Dissolve 132.5 μg/ml (500× stock) in 2×
       dH_2O.

     J. Progesterone — 2 n*M* solution is a 500× stock.

     K. FBS (Hyclone):

       1. Chelated newborn calf serum — Stir 100 ml serum with 10
         g Chelex 100 for 2 h and filter sterilize.

       2. Newborn calf serum (NBCS).

  3. Wounding of skin equivalents

    a. *Generation of wounds in skin equivalents* — SEs are wounded 7 d
      after keratinocytes are seeded onto the collagen matrix. One week
      before cultures are to be wounded, an additional collagen matrix is
      fabricated as described above. This will be used as the substrate onto
      which the wounded SE will be transferred.

     i. Aspirate all medium from the SE, remove the insert from the six-
       well plate and place it upside down onto a sterile p100.

     ii. Use the scalpel to cut out the entire polycarbonate membrane around
       the periphery of the insert. Place the cut-out SE onto a p100 so that
       it rests on its polycarbonate membrane.

     iii. Trim the culture with the scalpel several millimeters from its raised,
       mesa-like region. This removes parts of the SE without keratinocytes
       (since keratinocytes are initially only seeded on the center mesa of
       the matrix) and facilitates removal of the culture from the insert
       membrane for transfer.

     iv. Place the scalpel's edge directly in the center of the culture and rock
       the blade back and forth in order to create an incision 1.2 cm in
       length. This incision completely penetrates the epidermis, collagen
       matrix, and membrane. The culture should not be completely cut in
       half and the two sides are to be kept attached.

     v. Use the forceps to gently lift the edge of the culture so that it
       separates from the polycarbonate membrane. At this time bring a
       dental mirror, which will serve as a spatula, close to the culture and
       drag the culture onto the mirror with a long forceps, leaving the
       membrane behind. The transfer will be facilitated if the mirror is
       slightly moistened with medium.

     vi. Unfold any wrinkles in the culture by moving it back and forth on
       the mirror using the forceps. Once the culture is smooth, pull one
       side of the culture slightly over the edge of the mirror; this is the
       site where the culture will be transferred onto the new matrix.

     vii.Bring the mirror directly over the second collagen matrix and lower
       it inside the insert so that the edge of the mirror and the culture are

in contact with the matrix. Slide the culture onto the collagen using the forceps as the mirror is pulled away slowly, leaving the culture on the collagen matrix.

viii. Using the forceps, tease apart the incision in order to create an elliptical space between the two halves. This elliptical space will be 2 to 3 mm at its greatest width. The transferred culture must be kept completely free of any folds or wrinkles.

ix. Maintain the culture at air/liquid interface by adding 7 ml of Epidermalization II medium to the outer well. Incubate at 37°C with 7% CO_2, and change the medium every 2 d until the end of the experiment.

b. *Processing of skin equivalents* — Skin equivalents are fragile if handled improperly and require special care during tissue freezing and processing. The following steps should ensure that samples can be efficiently cryosectioned without artifactual damage.

i. Cultures are rinsed twice in PBS, and SEs are separated from the plastic culture insert with a scalpel blade. The incision should include the polycarbonate membrane, as specimens will be easier to handle if still on the membrane. At this point, the wound can be sectioned longitudinally to provide equal halves for formalin and frozen processing.

ii. Immerse the SE for frozen section analysis in 2 *M* sucrose at room temperature for 1 h. This will remove some of the water from the collagen matrix and prevent fracture artifact upon freezing. After removal from sucrose, the SE should be noticeably firmer (should not flop over when standing on edge). As an alternative, SEs may be kept overnight at 4°C, but incubation for any longer than this may result in the culture becoming somewhat brittle and difficult to cut.

iii. A slow freezing technique in which the sample is frozen in liquid nitrogen vapor is preferred, rather than snap freezing in liquid nitrogen. This can be accomplished by using a 3/4 in. bottle cap as a template to make a mold of that cap with aluminum foil. Fill the mold with embedding compound to a thickness of 1/2 in., place it on a test tube rack, and place the rack in a styrofoam box filled with liquid nitrogen to just below the upper surface of the rack.

iv. In order to embed the tissue specimen on edge, the embedding compound must be cooled to increase its viscosity. Place the aluminum mold on the rack so that it starts to chill in the liquid nitrogen vapor. Within 30 sec, the embedding material turns white near its edges and should be sufficiently viscous in the center to allow the culture to be stood on edge. If necessary, hold the SE upright with a forceps. The SE will freeze within several minutes, and specimens can be placed in a pill box for storage at –70°C.

REFERENCES

1. Freeman, A.E. et al., Growth and characterization of human skin epithelial cell cultures, *In Vitro,* 12, 352, 1976.
2. Hintner, H. et al., Expression of basement membrane zone antigens at the dermo-epibolic junction in organ cultures of human skin, *J. Invest. Dermatol.,* 74, 200, 1980.
3. Marks, S. and Nishikawa, T., Active epidermal movement in human skin *in vitro, Br. J. Dermatol.,* 88, 245, 1973.
4. Stenn, K.S., The role of serum in the epithelial outgrowth of mouse skin explants, *Br. J. Dermatol.,* 98, 411, 1978.
5. Stenn, K.S. et al., Multiple mechanisms of dissociated epidermal cell spreading, *J. Cell Biol.,* 96, 63, 1983.
6. Stenn, K.S. and Milstone, L.M., Epidermal cell confluence and implications for a two-step mechanism of wound closure, *J. Invest. Dermatol.,* 83, 445, 1984.
7. Woodley, D.T., O'Keefe, E.J., and Prunieras, M. Cutaneous wound healing: a model for cell-matrix interactions, *J. Am. Acad. Dermatol.,* 12, 420, 1985.
8. Bissell, M.J. and Radisky, D., Putting tumours in context, *Nat. Rev. Cancer,* 1, 46, 2001.
9. Falanga, V. et al., Wounding of bioengineered skin: cellular and molecular aspects after injury, *J. Invest. Dermatol.,* 119, 2002.
10. Garlick, J.A. and Taichman, L.B., Fate of human keratinocytes during reepithelialization in an organotypic culture model, *Lab. Invest.,* 70, 916, 1994.
11. Geer, D.J., Swartz, D.D., and Andreadis, S.T., Fibrin promotes migration in a three-dimensional *in vitro* model of wound regeneration, *Tissue Eng.,* 8, 787, 2002.
12. O'Leary, R., Arrowsmith, M., and Wood, E.J., The use of an *in vitro* wound healing model, the tri-layered skin equivalent, to study the effects of cytokines on the repopulation of the wound defect by fibroblasts and keratinocytes, *Biochem. Soc. Trans.,* 25, 369S, 1997.
13. O'Leary, R., Arrowsmith, M., and Wood, E.J., Characterization of the living skin equivalent as a model of cutaneous re-epithelialization, *Cell Biochem. Funct.,* 20, 129, 2002.
14. Bell, E. et al., Living tissue formed *in vitro* and accepted as skin-equivalent tissue of full thickness, *Science,* 211, 1052, 1981.
15. Parenteau, N.L., Skin equivalents, in *The Keratinocyte Handbook,* Leigh, I.M. and Watt, F.M., Eds., Cambridge University Press, Cambridge, 1994, pp. 45–56.
16. Winter, G.D., Epidermal regeneration studied in the domestic pig, in *Epidermal Wound Healing,* Maibach, H.I. and Rovee, D.T., Eds., Year Book Medical Publishers, Chicago, 1972, pp. 71–112.
17. Coulombe, P.A., Towards a molecular definition of keratinocyte activation after acute injury to stratified epithelia, *Biochem. Biophys. Res. Commun.,* 236, 231, 1997.
18. Garlick, J.A. et al., Re-epithelialization of human oral keratinocytes *in vitro, J. Dent. Res.,* 75, 912, 1996.
19. Garlick, J.A. and Taichman, L.B., Effect of TGF-beta 1 on re-epithelialization of human keratinocytes *in vitro*: an organotypic model, *J. Invest. Dermatol.,* 103, 554, 1994.
20. Krawczyk, W.S., A pattern of epidermal cell migration during wound healing, *J. Cell Biol.,* 49, 247, 1971.
21. Matoltsy, A.G. and Viziam, C.B., Further observations on epithelialization of small wounds: an autoradiographic study of incorporation and distribution of 3H-thymidine in the epithelium covering skin wounds, *J. Invest. Dermatol.,* 55, 20, 1970.

22. Odland, G. and Ross, R., Human wound repair. I. Epidermal regeneration, *J. Cell Biol.*, 39, 135, 1968.
23. Hertle, M.D. et al., Aberrant integrin expression during epidermal wound healing and in psoriatic expression, *J. Clin. Invest.*, 89, 1892, 1992.
24. Martinez, I.R., Fine structural studies of migrating epidermal cells following incision wound, in *Epidermal Wound Healing*, Maibach, H.I. and Rovee, D.T., Eds., Year Book Publishing, Chicago, 1972, pp. 323–342.
25. Garlick, J., personal communication, 2003.
26. Cromack, D.T. et al., Transforming growth factor beta levels in rat wound chambers, *J. Surg. Res.*, 42, 622, 1987.
27. Nathan, C. and Sporn, M., Cytokines in context, *J. Cell Biol.*, 113, 981, 1991.
28. Cromack, D.T., Pierce, G.F., and Mustoe, T.A., TGF-beta and PDGF mediated tissue repair: identifying mechanisms of action using impaired and normal models of wound healing, *Prog. Clin. Biol. Res.*, 365, 359, 1991.
29. Mustoe, T.A. et al., Growth factor-induced acceleration of tissue repair through direct and inductive activities in a rabbit dermal ulcer model, *J. Clin. Invest.*, 87, 694, 1991.
30. Ksander, G.A. et al., Exogenous transforming growth factor-beta 2 enhances connective tissue formation and wound strength in guinea pig dermal wounds healing by secondary intent, *Ann. Surg.*, 211, 288, 1990.
31. Levine, J.H. et al., Spatial and temporal patterns of immunoreactive transforming growth factor beta 1, beta 2, and beta 3 during excisional wound repair, *Am. J. Pathol.*, 143, 368, 1993.
32. Parenteau, N.L. et al., Epidermis generated *in vitro*: practical considerations and applications, *J. Cell Biochem.*, 45, 245, 1991.
33. Zambruno, G. et al., Transforming growth factor-β1 modulates β1 and β5 integrin receptors and induces the *de novo* expression of the $\alpha v \beta 6$ heterodimer in normal human keratinocytes: implications for wound healing, *J. Cell Biol.*, 129, 853, 1995.
34. Brinckerhoff, C.E. and Matrisian, L.M., Matrix metalloproteinases: a tail of a frog that became a prince, *Nat. Rev. Mol. Cell Biol.*, 3, 207, 2002.
35. Saarialho-Kere, U.K. et al., Distinct localization of collagenase and tissue inhibitor of metalloproteinases expression in wound healing associated with ulcerative pyogenic granuloma, *J. Clin. Invest.*, 90, 1952, 1992.
36. Saarialho-Kere, U.K. et al., Cell-matrix interactions modulate interstitial collagenase expression by human keratinocytes actively involved in wound healing, *J. Clin. Invest.*, 92, 2858, 1993.
37. Saarialho-Kere, U.K. et al., Distinct populations of basal keratinocytes express stromelysin-1 and stromelysin-2 in chronic wounds, *J. Clin. Invest.*, 94, 79, 1994.
38. Makela, M. et al., Matrix metalloproteinases (MMP-2 and MMP-9) of the oral cavity: cellular origin and relationship to periodontal status, *J. Dent. Res.*, 73, 1397, 1994.

2 Epidermal Repair and the Chronic Wound

Marjana Tomic-Canic, Magnus S. Ågren, and Oscar M. Alvarez

CONTENTS

2.1 INTRODUCTION: IMPORTANT DIFFERENCES BETWEEN ACUTE AND CHRONIC WOUNDS

Any epithelium artificially given a free edge....As in wounding will spread if provided with the proper substratum.

J.P. Trinkaus[1]

The term "chronic wound" implies slow progress and long continuance. This term is often misinterpreted because there is no steadfast definition, and it is not known how much time a wound must remain open before it is classified as chronic. The classical theory is that chronic wounds are caused by an abnormality or disease condition that directly or indirectly affects the skin or its blood supply. Chronic wounds are often referred to as dermal ulcers. Most common are pressure ulcers, venous ulcers, diabetic (neuropathic) ulcers, and ischemic (arterial) ulcers. Less common are inflammatory ulcers (caused by inflammatory disorders, which by their nature can directly produce cutaneous erosion), ulcers secondary to malignancy, ulcers caused by an abnormality of red blood cells (hemaglobinopathy), and ulcers caused by impaired immunity. Although no formal definition exists for "chronic wound," it is generally agreed that a wound may be classified as chronic if it has remained open for longer than 2 months.

It is commonly assumed that chronic wounds are deviations of the normal wound repair process. However, this approach is simplistic and less than satisfactory. Chronic wounds are quite different from acute wounds and possess characteristics that are inherent in their presentation (Table 2.1). In contrast to acute wounds, chronic wounds do not follow the predictable ordered sequence of events (phases) of wound repair.

Normal wound repair has been arbitrarily divided into three phases:

1. Inflammation (early and late)
2. Tissue formation (reepithelialization and granulation)
3. Tissue remodeling (matrix formation and scarring)

TABLE 2.1
Important Differences between Acute and Chronic Wounds

Chronic Ulcer	Acute Wound
Slow, nonhealing, long duration	Usually from trauma
Underlying cause	Predictable phases
Prolonged/consistent inflammation	Short inflammatory phase
Bacterial contamination/bio-burden	Heals in <45 days
Unbalanced proteinases and inhibitors	Infection delays repair
Cellular senescence	No pathology

TABLE 2.2
Abnormalities of Chronic Dermal Ulcers

Category	Defect	Ref.
Provisional matrix	Rapidly degrading provisional matrix	4, 5
Extracellular matrix	Increased neutrophil elastase	4
Wound fluid	Increased gelatinolytic activity and superactive gelatinases	23, 24, 180
	Decreased α-1antitrypsin activity	5, 207
	Decreased levels of TIMPs	28, 86, 200
	Unbalanced MMPs (MMP-2, 8, and 9)	184–186, 189, 220
Bacterial colonization	Prolonged inflammation	31
Bio-burden	Increased levels of inflammatory cytokines (TNFα, IL-1, IL-6)	30
Cellular senescence	Decreased growth capacity of repairing cells	33, 179, 202
	Increased levels of beta-Gal	32
	Decreased response to growth factor stimuli	179, 202
	Upregulation of elastase/matrix degradation	211
Keratinocytes	Impaired keratinocyte activation cycle	170, 172
	Increased expression of collagenases	14, 188, 191, 192
	Expression of stromelysin 1 and 2	20, 194

The phases of normal repair are not mutually exclusive and overlap considerably in time with one another.[2] In chronic wounds, the sequence of events is disrupted, and the wound appears to be "stuck" in the inflammatory phase. Inflammation is a highly effective component of the innate response of the body to infection or injury. The inflammatory response is an important consequence of injury and one that normally leads to repair and restoration of function. As recently as 1970, inflammation was perceived as an entirely beneficial host response. It has become apparent, however, that inflammation can contribute to the pathogenesis of a large number of diseases. For example, neutrophil infiltration, if not controlled, contributes to tissue injury and necrosis.[3] In chronic wounds an abundance of neutrophil proteinases is present,[4] indicating a chronic inflammatory response. Proper balance between proteinases and inhibitor levels is crucial to the resolution of prolonged inflammation and subsequent wound reepithelialization.

Although the inflammatory phase of the wound healing process has received a great deal of attention (from a research prospective), most of the investigative efforts have dealt with the onset of inflammation. Little is known about the processes by which inflammation normally resolves. Understanding how inflammation resolves will provide therapies that assist the mechanisms favoring the closure of chronic (nonhealing) and slowly healing dermal ulcers.

In chronic wounds the provisional matrix (supporting the growth of repairing cells) is degraded rapidly. This degradation is due to increased levels of serine proteases (neutrophil elastase) combined with a decreased activity of α1-proteinase inhibitor (α1-antitrypsin), a potent regulator of fibronectin.[5] The inhibitor protects fibronectin from degradation by neutrophil elastase in chronic wounds. α1-Antitrypsin is intact and functional in acute wounds, but it is degraded and inactive in chronic wounds. Elastase, the physiologic target of α1-antitrypsin, is up to 40 times higher in chronic wound fluids. Thus, the nonfunctional α1-antitrypsin fragments are incapable of inhibiting the neutrophil elastase that is responsible for fibronectin degradation in chronic wounds.[4] Interestingly, degradation of α1- antitrypsin was observed in patients with chronic inflammatory disorders such as pulmonary emphysema and rheumatoid arthritis.[6,7] Of the mammalian enzymes, the following matrix metalloproteinases (MMPs) have been shown to have α1-antitrypsin–degrading activity: MMP-8, MMP-3, MMP-7, and MMP-9.[8-11] Increased levels of MMP-2 and MMP-9 have been shown in chronic wound fluids.[12]

Throughout the wound healing process, there is significant connective tissue turnover in order to prepare the matrix for epithelial coverage. The matrix reconstruction process is mediated by MMPs, which are a family of zinc-dependent endopeptidases that include collagenases, gelatinases, and stromelysins.[13,14] MMPs are secreted by cells as zymogens; upon activation, MMPs as a group are capable of degrading all major extracellular matrix (ECM) components, including fibrillar collagens.[13] MMPs are inhibited by specific cell-secreted proteins, tissue inhibitors of metalloproteinases (TIMPs) that bind the active sites of MMPs noncovalently but with high affinity, resulting in an inactive, stoichiometric proteinase inhibitor complex.[15,16] We know that in normal wound healing the spatial and temporal control of proteolysis is of critical importance. Both MMPs and TIMPs are expressed by cells in the wound environment, and mounting evidence suggests that specific cell types may express these proteins differentially. Such seems to be the case in the remodeling cornea, where cell-specific and temporal expression of the two gelatinases varies during healing,[17] as does the synthesis of collagenase and stromelysin.[18] For example, it has been demonstrated that keratinocytes may play a different role in repair than do fibroblasts, producing *in vivo* more collagenase and less TIMP.[19] Similarly, it appears that gelatinase-A localizes to fibroblasts, whereas gelatinase-B localizes to epidermal and endothelial cells.[20,21]

Wound fluid reflects some of the temporal changes in the wound environment that occur during healing. Chronic wound fluid has been shown to contain degradation products (fibronectin and vitronectin) indicative of excess proteolytic activity.[22,23] Chronic wound fluid also contains elevated levels of gelatinase-A and gelatinase-B.[24] Both gelatinase-A and gelatinase-B degrade denatured collagens (gelatins), basement membrane collagens, and several other matrix proteins,[25,26] and are secreted by many cell types found in the wound, including endothelial cells, fibroblasts, keratinocytes, monocytes, and macrophages.[25-27] In addition, chronic wound fluid (obtained from venous ulcers) contains elevated levels of gelatinolytic enzymes (both activated and superactivated forms) coupled with lower levels of TIMP-1. Superactivated gelatinases are truncated by the loss of their carboxyl domains and are poorly inhibited by TIMPs.[28,29] The presence of an active, poorly inhibitable enzyme would be destructive to surrounding tissue and lead to the degradation of basement membrane components secreted by the migrating keratinocyte.

Chronic wounds also contain elevated levels of inflammatory cytokines such as tumor necrosis factor α (TNFα) and the interleukins (IL-1, IL-6).[30] Cells secreting these factors respond to the presence of bacteria and their endotoxins. Chronic wounds provide a home to many bacteria and a battlefield for colonization of aerobes and anaerobes. Chronic wounds share a bacterial burden that triggers prolonged inflammation (proteolytic imbalance), which also affects epithelial migration.[31]

Cellular senescense is the aging of cells that results in reduced growth capacity of cells, morphologic changes, and overexpression of certain matrix proteins such as cellular fibronectin. It can be detected by enhanced activity of beta-galactosidase (senescence-associated beta-Gal).[32] Cellular senescense may also be induced by the presence of chronic wound fluid.[33] Senescent cells in general are less responsive to growth factor stimuli and are uniformly less active. Senescent keratinocytes are less migratory and may have limited replicative potential. It is likely that in chronic wounds an overabundance of senescent cells is present, making it harder for the wound to respond to healing stimuli.

In this chapter we will focus on two key issues that govern epidermal dermal communication during wound repair:

1. Keratinocyte function (regulation, adhesion, keratin synthesis)
2. The adaptive interaction created with the extracellular matrix

Since little *in vivo* information exists describing epidermal migration (or the lack thereof) in chronic wounds, we have incorporated the lessons learned from acute wound reepithelialization into this section. In addition, we summarize recent research providing valuable information about the chronic wound environment and chronic inflammation.

2.2 KERATINOCYTE FUNCTION AND WOUND HEALING

Skin integrity and its normal functioning directly depend on keratinocytes' awareness of their position in the structure of the epidermal tissue.[34–40] This means that keratinocytes have a defined "understanding" of the epidermal geography. Keratinocytes recognize exactly where the top, bottom, and sides are; who their neighbors are; and what function to perform at any particular time. In healthy epidermis, keratinocytes slowly proliferate in the basal layer and differentiate in the suprabasal layers. Mitotically active keratinocytes are located in the basal layer of epidermis, where they are in direct contact with basal lamina and dermal connective tissue. By leaving the basal layer, they become committed to terminal differentiation, a process that will lead them toward their death and toward the surface of the skin. During this upward movement (differentiation), keratinocytes undergo numerous biochemical and morphological changes including keratin synthesis, protein crosslinking and loss of nuclei. This perpetual process provides the essential epidermal function of self-renewing. It takes approximately 2 to 4 weeks to complete the differentiation cycle, and the ratio of cells produced by the basal keratinocytes to cells lost to desquamation is proportional. The signals that coordinate this process are not well understood.

The self-renewing property of epidermis plays a major role during wound healing. Because they are exposed to the surroundings, keratinocytes must be prepared to respond very quickly to injury. Given that so much depends on them, keratinocytes have developed strong "communication skills," i.e., they not only communicate with each other, but also communicate with dermis and the local immune system, thus creating a constant flow of information.[34,37–39] One of the best examples of epidermal communication is the wound healing process. Within moments of wounding, keratinocytes must inform each other that the barrier has been broken, and they must communicate the urgent need to repair the gap. They must also alert the defense mechanisms of the host that the barrier has been broken and that pathogens may be coming in. There are two major "languages" that keratinocytes use to communicate:

1. Production, secretion, and response to hormones/growth factors/cytokines.
2. Changes of adhesion molecules at their membrane, which subsequently alter the cytoskeleton keratinocytes at the wound edge release pre-stored inter-leukin-1 (IL-1), which is the first signal released upon wounding. This signal initiates the activation of keratinocytes and also alerts the surrounding tissues. Eventually, activated keratinocytes repair the epidermis and become deactivated, reverting to normal differentiation. This process, termed the keratinocyte activation cycle, is governed by extracellular signals, and is characterized by changes in expression of keratin proteins. Keratinocytes produce, secrete and respond to the tumor necrosis factor-α (TNFα), transforming growth factor α (TGFα), heparin-binding epidermal growth factor (HB-EGF), among others.[38] Keratinocytes also respond to polypeptide factors produced by lymphocytes and dermal fibroblasts.[41] In response to these signals a large group of transcription factors, such as activator protein-1 (AP-1), nuclear factor kappa B (NFκB), and CCAAT enhancer-binding protein (C/EBP), are translocated to the nuclei where they regulate the expression of target genes.

The transcriptional changes that occur at wounding trigger keratinocyte migration and proliferation. These changes are accompanied and paralleled by changes in keratinocyte adhesion and the cytoskeleton. To close the wound, keratinocytes need to "let go their anchor," i.e., loosen the adhesion to each other and to the basal lamina, and they need to obtain the flexibility and ability to "grasp, hold, and crawl" over on the provisional matrix freshly deposited by repairing cells.[34] This requires rearrangement of the integrin receptors, reassembly of the associated actin cytoskeleton, and changes in the keratin filament network. Lastly, once the wound surface is covered by a keratinocyte monolayer, the proliferation signals cease and a new stratification process begins again. The signals that "reset" the program from keratinocyte proliferation to differentiation during healing are not well understood.

2.3 KERATINS AS MARKERS OF EPIDERMAL PHYSIOLOGY AND WOUND HEALING

Epidermal keratinocytes have two alternative pathways open to them: differentiation and activation. Keratins, which form the intermediate filament network in all epithelial cells, are phenotypic markers of both pathways.[42] There are approximately 30 keratin proteins divided in two families, each encoded by its own gene whose expression follows specific rules: basal cells are mitotically active and express keratins K5 and K14; "spinous" cells express keratins K1 and K10.[43,44] Nonepidermal cells express specific keratin pairs, such as K3 and K12 in differentiating corneal epithelium and K4 and K13 in noncornified stratified epithelia. In addition, some physiological and pathological changes of epithelial cells are also reflected in specific keratin expression. During the activation cycle in wound healing, K6 and K16 keratins are expressed.[45,46] During epidermal inflammation, K17 keratin is expressed.[47] Keratin gene expression is regulated primarily at the transcriptional level in response to a specific combination of transcription factors targeted to a specific keratin promoter.[48,49] Keratin gene promoters have intrinsic epithelial specificity.[50] Factors such as signal protein (Sp-1), AP-1, and AP-2,[51–53] in addition to less known factors, are involved in the regulation of keratin gene expression.[54,55] Furthermore, retinoic acid, thyroid hormone, and glucocorticoids suppress keratin gene expression through their nuclear receptors.[56–60]

Keratin K6 has been a research focus because of its two unique properties: it is a hallmark of the wound-healing keratinocyte, and it is encoded by multiple functional genes (humans may have seven active K6 genes).[61,62] In mice, targeted deletion of the K6a gene resulted in a delay in reepithelialization from the hair follicle after superficial wounding, but full-thickness wounds healed normally. The lack of MK6a affects both proliferation and migration of the follicular keratinocytes *in vivo* but not *in vitro*.[61] Whenever in nature multiple genes encode a single product, it implies an important function and necessity for redundancy and compensation. Therefore, elimination of one out of seven K6 genes does not completely establish the role K6 plays in wound-healing keratinocytes. Furthermore, overexpression of K16 (the K6 dimerization partner) directly impacts properties such as adhesion, differentiation, and migration of keratinocytes.[63] EGF specifically induces both K6 and K16 in keratinocytes *in vitro*.[46] In contrast, corticosteroids repress K6 and K16 expression through specific molecular mechanisms.[60]

2.4 GROWTH FACTORS/CYTOKINES AS REGULATORS OF WOUND HEALING

The purpose of such complex signaling cascades in keratinocytes during wound healing is to regulate target genes, thus controlling the keratinocyte activation cycle. Previous studies have identified stimuli that trigger other stimuli and the endpoint phenotypic changes produced as a consequence. For example, among the genes induced by IL-1 are growth factors and cytokines that transmit the signals of the specific type of injury to the surrounding cells. These include granulocyte–macrophage colony stimulating factor (GM-CSF), TNFα, TGFβ, amphiregulin, and IL-1.[38] Activated keratinocytes also produce cell surface markers, such as intercellular adhesion molecule-1 (ICAM1) and integrins as well as fibronectin, a component of the basement membrane that promotes keratinocyte migration.[64-66] Once activated, keratinocytes synthesize additional signaling growth factors and cytokines including TGFβ, IL-3, IL-6, IL-8, granulocyte colony stimulating factor (G-CSF), GM-CSF, and macrophage colony stimulating factor (M-CSF).[41,67] The effects of these signaling molecules produced by keratinocytes are chemotactic for white blood cells and paracrine for lymphocytes, fibroblasts, and endothelial cells. Interestingly, these signaling molecules are also autocrine for keratinocytes themselves. They lead to secondary effects of keratinocyte activation. Several extracellular markers are specifically expressed by the activated keratinocytes. These include cell surface proteins, integrins, and components of the extracellular matrix, as well as receptors for both the autocrine factors and factors produced by the infiltrating immune cells.[68-70] In a feedback loop, the increase in the expression of cell surface receptors may augment the initial activation signal. The various signaling molecules may be synergistic or antagonistic with each other. This allows the activated phenotype to be specifically modified, which can lead to different activated phenotypes. Put simply, keratinocytes activated during wound healing, in psoriasis, or in other pathological conditions can have different variants of the activated keratinocyte phenotype.

2.4.1 INTERLEUKIN–1 (IL-1)

The most common initiator of keratinocyte activation is IL-1. Both the α and β forms of this cytokine are present unprocessed in the cytoplasm of keratinocytes, ready to respond to injury. They are unavailable for binding to the cell surface receptors because they are sequestered in the cytoplasm.[37,71,72] Injured keratinocytes process and release IL-1, allowing the surrounding cells to perceive it.[38,72,73] IL-1 is an autocrine signal that activates keratinocytes, i.e., makes them proliferate, become migratory, and express an activation-specific set of genes.[37,41] The released IL-1 also serves as a paracrine signal to dermal endothelial cells, as a chemoattractant for lymphocytes, and as an activator of dermal fibroblasts.[2,38] The epidermal responses to IL-1 are exquisitely finely tuned; keratinocytes must be ready to respond quickly to injury via IL-1 and at the same time, must be able to attenuate and shut off the IL-1 signals after the initial response. Signal transduction in response to IL-1 starts at the cell surface with the Type I receptor. The intracellular domain of this receptor associates with several proteins, e.g., TNF receptor associated factor 6 (TRAF 6), which recruits protein kinases such as IL-1 receptor associated kinase-1 (IRAK) and TGFβ activated kinase 1 (TAK1). Downstream from the kinases, the signal trifurcates and at least three transcription factor systems are activated: NFκB, C/EBPβ and AP-1.[74-76] These transcription factors then induce expression of the activation-specific proteins.

2.4.2 TUMOR NECROSIS FACTOR α (TNFα)

Whereas IL-1 initiates keratinocyte activation, other signals are used to maintain keratinocyte activation. One such signal induced by IL-1 is TNFα. TNFα can maintain keratinocytes in an activated state.[77,78] TNFα induces many inflammatory effects, such as fever and shock. In response to infection or injury, a wide variety of cells, primarily macrophages and monocytes but also epithelial cells including keratinocytes, produce TNFα.[79,80] TNFα activates immune responses by inducing production of additional signaling molecules, cytokines, growth factors, their receptors, and adhesion proteins (e.g., amphiregulin, TGFα, IL-1α, IL-1 receptor antagonist, epidermal growth factor receptor (EGF-R), and ICAM1.[64] The signaling cascades mediating cellular responses to TNFα have been partly elucidated.[38,81] There are two TNFα receptors, but keratinocytes express mainly the 55 kDa receptor, Type 1.[82] Three major intracellular effects are caused by TNFα. The first is the induction of apoptosis, the second involves production of ceramides, and the third, activation of transcription factors NFκB, C/EBPβ, and members of the AP-1 family.

2.4.3 Nuclear Factor kappa B (NFκB)

Transcription factors NFκB and C/EBPβ respond to IL-1 and TNFα. The NFκB family includes the proteins p65, p50 and c/rel, which both homo- and heterodimerize among themselves.[83] These proteins are stored latent in the cytoplasm, bound to the inhibitory protein, IκB. TNFα causes activation of IκB kinase (IKKs) — kinases that phosphorylate IκB and induce its degradation. The degradation of IκB results in activation and nuclear translocation of the NFκB protein.[84,85] NFκB proteins can interact with C/EBPβ, AP1, and other transcription factors to regulate gene expression.[86,87] In keratinocytes, *in vitro* overexpression of NFκB inhibits proliferation. It also protects normal epithelial cells from apoptosis-induced TNFα.[88] In epidermis *in vivo* NFκB is present in all layers but is nuclear only in the suprabasal ones.[89] On the other hand, constitutive activation of NFκB in IκB-knockout mice results in normal epidermal development and differentiation but a widespread and lethal dermatitis in the first few days of life.[90] It has recently been shown that NFκB and Ras initiate cell-cycle arrest. IκB-mediated inhibition of NFκB can circumvent this growth arrest, which may generate malignant human epidermal tissue.[91]

2.4.4 CCAAT/Enhancer Binding Protein β(C/EBPβ)

TNFα and other extracellular stimuli activate transcription factor C/EBPβ (a.k.a. nuclear factor interleukin 6 [NF-IL6] or leucine aminopeptidate [LAP]).[92] The mechanisms that activate C/EBPβ have not been fully characterized. C/EBPβ interacts with many other transcription factors, such as the retinoblastoma (Rb) protein, glucocorticoid receptor (GR), *c-Myc*, NFκB and AP1.[38,93] In epidermis, the C/EBP proteins are differentially expressed during differentiation.[94,95] While knockout mice lacking C/EBPβ have no cutaneous phenotype,[96] overexpression of C/EBPβ in keratinocytes causes growth arrest and induction of early differentiation markers.[97]

2.4.5 Epidermal Growth Factor (EGF/TGFα)

Whereas IL-1 and TNFα are proinflammatory signals with overlapping intracellular molecular pathways, under certain conditions keratinocytes need additional and different stimuli, which direct them to proliferate. In epidermis, several members of the EGF family can be produced, including TGFα, amphiregulin, HB-EGF, and heregulin. All are ligands of the receptor EGF-R, and all convey proliferative signals to keratinocytes.[38] Arguably the most extensively studied cellular receptor signaling pathways are those proceeding through EGF-R.[98] In adult epidermis, EGF-R is primarily expressed in the basal layer and to a lesser degree, the first suprabasal layers.[99] Binding of the appropriate ligands to the EGF-R can activate keratinocytes.[100] The signals activate nuclear proteins that regulate both gene expression and cell division. Among the regulated genes are those encoding additional regulators, leading to major morphological changes, developmental changes, and differentiation. In response to the activation of the EGF-R, keratinocytes proliferate, degrade components of the extracellular matrix, and become migratory.[67,101] The binding of a ligand to EGF-R causes the receptor to dimerize, with concomitant activation of its intracellular protein tyrosine kinase. A substrate for this kinase is the receptor itself; the two monomers phosphorylate each other. The phosphotyrosines serve as docking sites for Src homology domain 2 (SH2) domain-containing proteins (such as growth factor receptor-bound protein-2 [Grb2] or Src homology domain-containing [SHC]) that interact with proteins capable of activating Ras. Several growth factor receptors, via different adaptor molecules, activate Ras, which makes Ras a turning point for various signal transduction pathways. Activated Ras, in turn, activates a cascade of three protein kinases, Raf1, Mitogen-activated protein kinase/ERK Kinase (MEK), and extracellular signal-regulated protein kinase (ERK). The last one, ERK, translocates to the nucleus where it phosphorylates and thus activates transcription factors, such as Elk1 and SRF accessory protein-1 (SAP1).[98]

2.4.6 Activator Protein–1 (AP-1)

Perhaps the best-characterized EGF/TGFα-responsive transcription factors are those belonging to the AP-1 family. AP-1 is a nuclear transcription complex composed of dimers encoded by the *fos* and *jun* families of proto-oncogenes.[102,103] Whereas Fos proteins only heterodimerize with members of the Jun family, Jun proteins can dimerize with both Fos and other Jun proteins. In the epidermis, AP-1 regulates cell growth, differentiation, and transformation.[51,104] The expression of individual AP-1 proteins in epidermal layers is a controversial issue that awaits resolution. The AP-1 proteins in keratinocytes can regulate the expression of differentiation markers[49,105] and may convey the calcium- and PKC-dependent signals.[106,107] Functional AP-1 sites have been found in many keratin genes[51,108,109] including "migratory" K6 and K16 keratins.[46] Recent findings demonstrate that lack of c-Jun prevents EGF-induced expression of HB-EGF. This implies that c-Jun may participate in the formation of the epidermal leading edge through its control of an EGF receptor autocrine loop.[109a]

2.4.7 Transforming Growth Factor β (TGFβ)

TGFβ is an important regulator of epidermal keratinocyte function because it represses cell proliferation while it induces synthesis of extracellular matrix proteins and their cell surface receptors.[110] Many reports in the literature define the important role that TGFβ plays in wound healing. For example, TGFβ-1 and 2 may cause scarring whereas TGFβ-3 acts in the opposite way, improving the architecture of the new epidermis.[111,112]

TGFβ induces expression of fibronectin, laminin, collagen IV and VII, and extracellular proteases and their inhibitors, as well as cell surface proteins including integrins α5, αv, β1, β4, and β5, and bullous pemphigoid antigens (BPAGs) BPAG1 and BPAG2.[34,35,113] We have shown that TGFβ specifically induces synthesis of basal cell–specific keratins K5 and K14.[114] Mice with a knocked-out TGFβ gene develop normally, because of the maternally supplied TGFβ, only to succumb to exuberant multifocal inflammation due to unrestrained activation of the immune system. Skin-targeted overexpression of TGFβ causes hypoplasia, while loss of TGFβ expression, or resistance to TGFβ causes increased susceptibility to malignant conversion.[115–117] Interestingly, knockout of Smad 3 (one of the molecules of the TGFβ signaling cascade) accelerated wound healing, suggesting an inhibitory effect during normal wound healing.[118,119] It seems that that TGFβ promotes the synthesis of basal cell-specific proteins and therefore, promotes the basal phenotype.[81] This happens at the expense of both the activated phenotype and the differentiating phenotype. Our conclusion is strengthened by studies showing that keratinocyte growth arrest by TGFβ is reversible, does not result in terminal differentiation, and can be modulated by regulators of keratinocyte differentiation, such as retinoic acid or calcium.[120] These data suggest that the effects of TGFβ on keratinocytes are not antiproliferative, but antihyperproliferative.

2.4.8 KERATINOCYTE GROWTH FACTOR (KGF)

Keratinocyte growth factors, although not synthesized by keratinocytes, have a major impact on keratinocyte physiology and pathogenesis. KGF-1 and KGF-2 bind with high affinity to the same receptor, the keratinocyte growth factor receptor (KGFR) isoform of fibroblast growth factor receptor 2 (FGFR 2), which is exclusively expressed by epithelial cells.[121,122] KGF is expressed at a low level in human skin, but it becomes strongly induced in dermal fibroblasts after skin injury. Its binding to a transmembrane receptor on keratinocytes induces proliferation and migration of these cells and protects epithelial cells from the toxic effects of reactive oxygen species.[122] Keratinocyte growth factor-2 (KGF-2), also described as fibroblast growth factor-10 (FGF-10), is a member of the fibroblast growth factor family.[123] KGF-2 shares ~50% homology with KGF-1 and is 96% identical to the FGF-10. KGF-2 specifically stimulates growth of normal human epidermal keratinocytes and has been shown to increase mechanical strength and wound collagen content.

2.4.9 GROWTH FACTORS/CYTOKINES AS THERAPEUTIC AGENTS FOR CHRONIC WOUNDS

Exogenous and endogenous therapeutic use of growth factors and cytokines in wound healing is currently being developed. The role of these factors in normal wound healing (see above) is not completely understood and therefore, to date, clinical trials to evaluate their use in chronic wounds have not had positive results.[124] EGF did not significantly improve wound healing of skin graft donor sites.[125] Similarly, fibroblast growth factor (FGF) failed to improve angiogenesis in cryo-injured skin grafts in the rat model.[126] In pressure ulcers, recombinant (basic) bFGF demonstrated only marginal efficacy.[127] Platelet-Derived Growth Factor (PDGF) has been shown to decrease ulcer volume, and (recombinant human) rh-PDGF (topical gel (beclapermin) is available for use in diabetic neuropathic ulcers.[128] Topical IL-1b showed no significant effect in similar trials.[124] More encouraging results were observed in a pilot study where TGFβ-2 (delivered in a collagen sponge) improved the healing of chronic venous ulcers.[129] It is evident that our knowledge of how these factors operate during wound healing is developing. A better understanding of the wound healing process, the resolution of inflammation, and the chronic wound environment will lead to improved therapies with these active agents.

2.5 KERATINOCYTE ADHESION AND REEPITHELIALIZATION

The integrity of the skin depends on specific attachments of its keratinocytes to the extracellular matrix and to each other. However, little is known about movement of epidermal cells that keep contact with one another during wound healing. These cells have contact with the neighboring cells as well as the underlying extracellular matrix, requiring coordinated cell movement for correct wound closure.

The epidermis consists of two major keratinocyte phenotypes, basal and differentiating, each with subtypes. One of the major differences between the phenotypes is in their specific adhesion molecules.[9] Basal keratinocytes are held in a spatio-temporal orientation by their membrane molecules. They are attached to the basal lamina through hemidesmosomes, anchorages formed by laminin and integrin that are intracellularly linked to the keratin cytoskeleton.[130–132] During wound healing, in order to allow keratinocytes to migrate, hemidesmosome attachments have to be dissolved. The migrating keratinocytes produce a different set of membrane molecules such as integrin $\alpha5\beta1$, vitronectin (previously known as epibolin), and fibronectin receptors and they replace the collagen receptor.[35,133–135] Rearrangement of the integrins and the linked filament networks allows keratinocytes to migrate. Many growth factors active during wound healing, such as EGF, KGF, and TGFβ, are potential regulators of these processes.[136–139] Furthermore, it has been shown that the $\alpha6\beta4$ integrin, a major component of hemidesmosomes, is able to transduce signals from the extracellular matrix to the interior of the cell. These signals critically modulate the organization of the cytoskeleton, proliferation, apoptosis, and differentiation.[140–143]

Differentiating (suprabasal) keratinocytes are characterized by two types of cell adhesions: desmosomes and adherens junctions (AJs). Desmosomes are one of the principal types of cell–cell junctions in epithelia and are particularly abundant in epidermis. These are multimolecular complexes containing, as major components, two glycoproteins, desmocollin and desmoglein, two armadillo proteins, plakoglobin and plakophilin, and the plakin family protein desmoplakin.[144] The glycoproteins are involved in desmosomal adhesion, probably by heterophilic interaction.[145] Desmoplakin provides linkage between the desmosomal plaque and the keratin intermediate filament cytoskeleton. Plakoglobin is essential for the adhesive function of the glycoproteins and in linking the glycoproteins to desmoplakin.[145] A similar role may be inferred for plakophilin from studies of human mutations leading to an epidermal dysplasia/skin fragility syndrome.[146] Mutation of desmoglein 1 and haploinsufficiency of desmoplakin also give rise to epidermal disease.[147,148] The isoform of PKC is involved in a signaling pathway that results in modulation of desmosomal adhesions.[149]

Although it is not yet clear how, evidence exists that suprabasal keratinocytes also participate in wound healing. They begin expressing integrins normally restricted only to basal keratinocytes. Also, they show that desmosomal adhesion may be rapidly modulated in response to wounding and that a modulating signal generated at the wound edge can be propagated through the epidermal sheet.

Adherens junctions (AJ) are characterized by the presence of E-cadherin, α- and β-catenins, and γ-catenin (plakoglobin) at the membrane.[150] At AJs, E-cadherin molecules bind homotypically at their extracellular domain in a Ca^{2+}-dependent manner, and their cytoplasmic domain is linked indirectly to actin filaments via catenins.[151,152] Both the homotypic interactions of their extracellular domains and their association with actin filaments at their cytoplasmic domains through catenins are required for cadherins to function as adhesion molecules.[153,154] There is a controversy regarding the E-cadherin localization during wound healing.[155–157]

2.6 KERATINOCYTE BEHAVIOR IN CHRONIC WOUNDS

While many studies have focused on factors that stimulate keratinocyte migration and proliferation and on the molecular mechanisms and processes involved, keratinocytes from actual chronic wounds have not been extensively studied.[158–163] During impaired wound healing, the keratinocyte activation cycle does not proceed in expected fashion, and the migrating keratinocyte produces significantly more collagenase. In addition, stromelysin-1 and 2 are also expressed in the epidermis of chronic wounds but by functionally distinct subpopulations of basal keratinocytes.[14,20] Interestingly, normal keratinocytes (in the form of cell therapy delivered by tissue-engineered skin) has been shown to be effective for the treatment of chronic venous ulcers and chronic diabetic foot ulcers.[164,165] Is keratinocyte behavior at the edge of a chronic wound a consequence of inhibitory signals of some kind, lack of sufficient numbers of adequate multi-signals, or perhaps an overwhelming number of signals causing a "standstill?" Both molecular and clinical studies have shown that replacement therapy with specific growth factors lacks the ability to fully restore the keratinocyte activation cycle. Studies using human skin equivalent also show that it is the appropriate mixture of factors released by fibroblasts and keratinocytes rather than one or two major factors that is important in activating keratinocytes on the wound edge to undergo migration and proliferation. Furthermore, many studies in transgenic mouse models have identified several important molecules that may play a role in impaired epithelialization. For example, *c-Myc* has been shown to cause impaired wound healing due to lack of keratinocyte migration if expressed in basal keratinocytes[166] and affects the epidermal stem cell compartment.[167] Also, if overexpressed in suprabasal layers, it causes hyper- and para-keratosis, typically in the epithelium of a chronic wound.[168] Similarly, several additional studies have demonstrated the importance of keratins K6, K16, and K17 as cytoskeletal molecules during epidermal migration.[61,62,169]

In chronic wounds, keratinocytes proliferate normally but fail to move over the ulcer bed.[170–172] Perhaps the chronic wound edge keratinocytes do not receive signals or lack receptors for the signals for conversion into a migratory phenotype. Or perhaps the basement membrane proteins secreted by the migrating keratinocyte are rapidly destroyed by the abundant gelatinases and MMPs found in the chronic wound. Migrating keratinocytes require basement membrane components such as bullous pemphigoid, laminin, and collagens type IV and VII.[131] Other possibilities may be the overproduction of collagenase by chronic wound keratinocytes[14] and/or the expression of stromelysins by nonmigrating basal cells.[20] Such an abnormality could cause the degradation of basement membrane components as they are expressed by the migrating epidermis.

2.7 ENDOGENOUS PROTEINASES IN THE ECM

2.7.1 PROTEINASES IN NORMALLY HEALING WOUNDS

Proteinases are traditionally thought to facilitate keratinocyte movement by remodeling ECM proteins. But other important biological effects of proteinases are increasingly becoming evident. For example, proteinases modulate intracellular signaling as well as secretion, bioactivation, and stability of cytokines and growth factors important for epidermal healing.[173]

Four classes of mammalian proteinases exist:

1. Aspartic proteinases, which require aspartate residues for activity
2. Cysteine proteinases, which require cysteine residues for activity
3. Matrix metalloproteinases including the MMPs, which require zinc for activity
4. Serine proteinases, which require serine residues for activity

The proteinases most pertinent to repair processes of skin wounds are the serine proteinases and the MMPs.

2.7.2 SERINE PROTEINASES

The most studied serine proteinases in wound healing are plasmin/plasminogen, urokinase plaminogen activator (uPA), cathepsin G, and neutrophil elastase.

Plasmin is generated from plasminogen on the cell surface by uPA. Plasmin has broad trypsin-like substrate specificity; it degrades fibrin matrices, plays an important role in the maintenance of hemostatic balance, and contributes to tissue remodeling and cell migration. Plasmin can also activate MMP.[174] In plasminogen-deficient mice, Rømer et al.[175] demonstrated delayed epithelialization. Excessive accumulation of fibrin on the wound surface was observed, and the fibrin probably obstructed the moving keratinocytes in the mice lacking plasmin. In an *ex vivo* human wound model for studies on epithelialization, no effect of the plasmin and serine proteinase inhibitor aprotinin was found.[176] This finding suggests that serine proteinases are not required per se for keratinocyte locomotion in the absence of fibrin.

The function of the neutrophil-derived cathepsin G was examined in cathepsin G-deficient mice.[177] Lack of cathepsin G resulted in augmented neutrophil infiltration and early decreased wound-breaking strength.[177]

The effect of the endogenous inhibitor of serine proteinases SLPI (secretory leukocyte protease inhibitor) was studied in SLPI-deficient mice.[173] Wound healing was delayed compared with control mice. A pronounced increased inflammatory cell infiltration and neutrophil elastase activity was found. The investigators also demonstrated that neutrophil elastase was capable of converting latent TGFβ-1 into active TGFβ-1. Active TGFβ-1 could provide a chemotactic stimulus for invading neutrophils (a source of neutrophil elastase). From this study we can conclude that increased levels of neutrophil elastase activity impair normal wound healing.

MMPs are a family of zinc-dependent endopeptidases with 23 human members known to date.[178] Substrate specificities, chromosomal locations, and three-dimensional structures are available at http://www.circresaha.org. (supplement to reference 178).

The interstitial collagenases (MMP-1, MMP-8, MMP-13), gelatinases (MMP-2, MMP-9), stromelysins (MMP-3, MMP-10), macrophage elastase (MMP-12), matrilysin (MMP-7), epilysin (MMP-28), and membrane-type 1 MMP (MMP-14) have been studied in human wounds. MMPs can degrade most of the extracellular matrix components *in vitro*. The expression and activity of MMPs generally increase after tissue injury, although the temporal and spatial pattern varies among the different MMPs.[179–183] Inflammatory cells appear to be the predominant source of MMPs (MMP-8 and MMP-9) in the early acute phase of the wound-repair process.[184,185] Wound-edge epithelium also expresses specific MMPs.[183,186,187] As the acute inflammatory response resolves and healing commences, MMP activities drop (with the exception of MMP-2) to the low basal levels of uninjured skin (completely covered with epithelium).[179,180] The activity of MMPs in wounds is largely antagonized by naturally occurring tissue inhibitors of metalloproteinases (TIMPs), which exist in four subtypes (TIMP-1, TIMP-2, TIMP-3, and TIMP-4).

The obligatory role of MMPs in normal wound healing and specifically epithelialization has been shown with the use of synthetic broad-spectrum inhibitors that block MMP activities during healing of experimental skin wound in animals and humans.[176,183,188,189] The importance of individual MMP in the epithelialization process has not been delineated fully. The knowledge we have is largely based on the localization rather than the functionality of individual MMPs acquired by detailed immunohistochemical and *in situ* hybridization studies. Studies on knockout mice have supplemented this knowledge.[190]

MMP-1 or interstitial collagenase-1 appears to be particularly important for keratinocyte migration and is abundantly expressed at the wound edges.[183,186,191] In contrast, overexpression of MMP-1 is associated with impaired reepithelialization in mice.[192] Delayed epithelialization and elevation of collagenase 1 levels in granulation tissue have been observed in collagenase-resistant mouse wounds.[193] Interstitial collagenase-3 (MMP-13) shows no hybridization signal in either the epidermis or the granulation tissue of acute wounds in humans.[194] The gelatinase MMP-9 (92-kDa gelatinase or gelatinase B) is consistently expressed in the advancing epithelium.[183,195] Interestingly, MMP-9 does not appear to be necessary for epithelialization because healing rates were similar in mice lacking the MMP-9 gene and mice with the MMP-9 gene.[196] The other gelatinase, MMP-2 (72-k Da gelatinase or gelatinase A), has been detected in normal human epidermis by zymography[183] and wound epithelium by immunohistochemistry.[187] MMP-14, which activates MMP-2, is present in wound stroma but not in advancing epithelium.[195] On the other hand, human keratinocytes transfected with a sense MMP-14 construct exhibit increased migration and reduced apoptosis.[197] Although the stromelysins MMP-3 (stromelysin 1) and MMP-10 (stromelysin 2) have about the same substrate specificities, they are expressed in different locations.[186] MMP-3 is expressed more distally than MMP-10 in the epidermal tongue.[186] In MMP-3-deficient mice, wound contraction was impaired, whereas reepithelialization proceeded at a normal rate.[198] Although information on the role of the novel MMP-28 is limited, it appears to be expressed in a proliferative epidermal compartment different from that of MMP-1, MMP-10, and MMP-9.[199] MMP-7 does not appear to be linked to cutaneous wounds, and MMP-12 is expressed occasionally by macrophages in cutaneous wounds.

In normal healing skin wounds, TIMP-2 is localized at the epidermal tip, whereas TIMP-1 and TIMP-3 are expressed more distally in the proliferating keratinocyte compartment.[200]

2.7.3 PROTEINASES IN CHRONIC WOUNDS

The role of proteinases in the pathogenesis and maintenance of chronic wounds is less clear than in acute wounds. Most studies have been conducted on wound fluids collected from chronic wounds of different stages and etiologies. It should be kept in mind that wound fluid measurements reflect the net results of local cellular and biochemical reactions. There are also age-dependent changes in the rate of reepithelialization[201] and levels of endogenous proteinases in the skin,[187] which need to be taken into account when interpreting the results from chronic wound patients. Furthermore, ratios of MMPs and TIMPs are also altered in normal skin with intrinsic aging, favoring catabolic processes with increased age.[187,202]

The stromal architecture and the immunostaining for the extracellular matrix molecules collagen types I and III, laminin, and tenascin appear rather normal in venous leg ulcers.[203] The glycoprotein fibronectin is virtually deficient in the margin and base of venous ulcers in contrast to the prominent reaction to fibronectin in normal skin. Fibronectin is an essential component of the provisional matrix deposited during early wound repair and serves as a substrate for migrating keratinocytes.[2,204] Fibronectin reappears as the ulcers heal, which implies excessive degradation of fibronectin in chronic wounds.[203,205] Degradation products of fibronectin have also been found in wound fluid from venous leg ulcers.[22,23,206,207]

2.7.4 NEUTROPHIL ELASTASE

Grinnell and Zhu[207] were able to prevent degradation of fibronectin by wound fluid from chronic venous ulcers by the addition of specific inhibitors of neutrophil elastase *in vitro*. Neutrophils containing neutrophil elastase have been observed in chronic venous leg ulcers using immunostaining techniques.[208] In addition to elastin, neutrophil elastase cleaves a variety of matrix components such as collagens and fibronectin.[209] Neutrophil elastase activity is complexed and neutralized by α1-proteinase inhibitor and α2-macroglobulin. Neutrophil elastase activities decrease as the ulcer heals. However, Weckroth et al.[210] found no difference in the activity of neutrophil elastase in wound fluids from chronic venous ulcers and acute cutaneous wounds. This discrepancy might be due to degradation of the synthetic peptide substrate despite being bound to the inhibitor α2-macroglobulin.[207] Furthermore, extensive degradation of the inhibitors occurs in chronic venous leg ulcers.[5,207] Interestingly, the major proteinase upregulated in the skin of older women, in particular, is neutrophil elastase.[211] Thus, there may also be superimposed an age and gender dependency of the neutrophil elastase activity in chronic wounds.

2.7.5 MATRIX METALLOPROTEINASES (MMPS)

Overall enzymatic activity, measured with the substrate Azocoll, in wound fluid from chronic wounds was blocked by 90% by adding the metal chelator ethylenediamine tetra acetic acid (EDTA) or 100 μM of the hydroxamate synthetic MMP inhibitor GM 6001, also known as ilomastat or N-(2R)-2 hydroxyamolo-carbonyl-4-methyl pentanoyl-L-tryptophan methylamide, indicating that the majority of enzymes belong to the MMP family.[212] The Azocoll assay does not discriminate among the MMPs, and therefore it is not possible to deduce which of the MMPs contributed to the total enzymatic activity.

In a clinical study involving surgical patients, MMP-9 was found to be closely associated with the progression of wound healing. Therefore, MMP-9 appears to be an accurate prognostic marker of wound repair.[184] MM-9 levels are persistently elevated in nonhealing venous ulcers. In contrast, in acute (healing) wounds, the levels of MMP-9 are elevated at first and then significantly decrease as the wound closes.[195,213,214] Interestingly, the absolute levels or activity of MMP-9 in wound fluid and wound tissue do not differ significantly between acute and chronic wounds.[195,214] Endogenous activities of the gelatinases MMP-9 and MMP-2 in wound margin biopsies from acute and chronic wounds are shown in Figure 2.1.

Despite the similar MMP-9 (Figure 2.1) activities, a distinct difference between acute and chronic wounds is the absence of MMP-9 in chronic wound epithelium. In chronic wounds, MMP-9 is concentrated in the inflammatory cell infiltrate, indicating a disproportionate distribution of this particular gelatinase in chronic wounds.[195] Commonly, many MMP-9 immunopositive neutrophils are observed in close proximity to the MMP-9 immunonegative epithelium.[195] Excess MMP-9 in the ulcer may deprive the keratinocytes of signals by ECM molecules and may inhibit or delay wound healing.[215] In addition, MMP-9 is capable of degrading α1-proteinase inhibitor, which can result in elevated local neutrophil elastase activity.[216] Thus, MMP-9 can contribute to unfavorable conditions in several ways leading to delayed epithelialization.

Although no differences in MMP-2 levels were found between acute and chronic wounds (Figure 2.1), MMP-2 levels are elevated in lipodermatosclerotic skin from patients with chronic venous insufficiency.[217] This increased activity of MMP-2 may contribute to venous ulcer development.

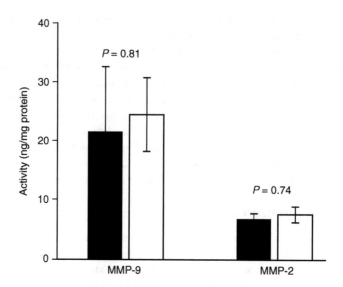

FIGURE 2.1 Endogenous activities of the gelatinases MMP-9 and MMP-2 in wound margin biopsies from 7-day-old dermatome acute wounds in healthy volunteers (black bars; n = 6) and chronic wounds (open bars; n = 13) of different etiologies measured by enzyme-linked immunosorbent assay (ELISA)-based activity assay. Neither the MMP-9 nor the MMP-2 activities were significantly different between the acute and chronic wounds (From Mirastschijski, U., Impola, U., Jahkola, T., Karlsmark, T., Ågren, M.S., and Saarialho-Kere, U., *Hum. Pathol.,* 33, 355–364, 2002.)

With respect to the three collagenases, neutrophil-derived collagenase-2 (MMP-8) activity is higher in chronic compared with acute wounds.[185] Furthermore, proportionally more basal keratinocytes are MMP-1 positive in chronic than in normally healing wounds.[186,218] While MMP-13 does not appear to be expressed in acute wounds, it is expressed in granulation tissue and in the areas of neoangiogenesis of chronic venous leg ulcers.[194] The MMP-14 expression pattern in chronic wounds resembles that of acute wounds.[195]

In sharp contrast to acute wounds, the expressions of TIMP-1, TIMP-2, and TIMP-3 are virtually absent in the epidermis of chronic venous ulcers.[200] Furthermore, TIMP levels are reduced in many chronic wounds, resulting in an imbalance of the proteolytic microenvironment.[212,219,221]

2.8 SUMMARY

Reepithelialization is the reconstitution of the cells of the epidermis into an organized, keratinized, stratified squamous epithelium, which covers the wound and restores the barrier properties of skin, decreasing morbidity and mortality after cutaneous injury. The process occurs rapidly in acute wounds, beginning within hours of the initial insult to the tissue and continuing throughout the proliferative phase of repair,[2] with the migration of intact keratinocytes from the free edge of the cut epidermis across the defect. The rate of migration is dependent on the tissue oxygen tension; it is highest in hyperbaric conditions, where the rate of cell movement is approximately 12 to 21 μm/h and on the humidity of the environment, with migration occurring at a faster rate in moist conditions.[222] Migration is made possible by a marked phenotypic alteration of the epithelial cells, involving the retraction of intracellular tonofilaments and temporary dissolution of intercellular attachments (desmosomes) and basement membrane attachments (hemi-desmosomes) freeing the cells, and the formation of peripherally located cytoplasmic actin filaments[223] and the projection of pseudopodia,[224] enabling cells to move.

The signals for epidermal cell phenotype switching are not entirely understood, but calcium is thought to be involved in the process.[2] More recently, gallium nitrate (GN, which has been shown to repress MMP activity in wounds) was shown to enhance partial thickness wound reepithelialization in the porcine wound model. The increased epidermal resurfacing was associated with alterations in expression of several keratinocyte integrin subunits. GN induced significant increase in α5 expression (α5β1 switching is a characteristic of the mobile phenotype in the setting of cutaneous injury). GN treatment also induced a significant (70%) decrease in the expression of the α subunit (α3β1 binds laminin 5 and is associated with hemidesmosome formation and reestablishment of a nonmotile phenotype).[225]

The exact pattern of epidermal migration is unknown but possibilities include:

1. Single cell migration ("leap-frogging," where cells superficial to the stratum basale at the edges of the wound migrate into the wound bed, while the cells above and behind migrate over the first cells to lie on the wound bed ahead of them)[226]
2. Movement of cells using a "tractor tread" mechanism (where integrin receptors are synthesized on the keratinocyte surface and bind to fibronectin on the wound bed)[227]

If the basement membrane is damaged by injury or enzymatic degradation, it is not reformed until migration ceases and the epidermal cells migrate over a provisional matrix of fibronectin fibrin and type V collagen produced partly by keratinocytes.[2,228] The migrating keratinocytes are phagocytes, and if they come across small foreign bodies on their route to closure they will ingest them.[224] If the foreign body is too large, the epidermal cells will migrate around them, dissecting viable tissue from nonviable tissue. This process involves the secretion on serine proteases and MMPs.

We are only beginning to comprehend the mechanisms responsible for keratinocyte migration on the extracellular matrix. The complexity of the chronic wound will continue to challenge clinicians for alternative therapies to improve the hostile environments that impede repair. The classical theory that correcting or improving the underlying pathology (causing the wound) will result in closure of the chronic wound is simplistic and only half of the challenge. Understanding the cellular and biochemical differences between acute and chronic wound environments should provide answers that will lead to better therapeutic interventions for the wound that refuses to heal.

REFERENCES

1. Trinkaus, J.P., *Cells into Organs: The Forces that Shape the Embryo,* Prentice Hall, Englewood Cliffs, NJ, 1984.
2. Clark, R.A.F., Wound repair: overview and general considerations, in *The Molecular and Cellular Biology of Wound Repair,* Clark, R.A.F., Ed., Plenum Press, New York, 1996, pp. 3–35.
3. Haslett, C. and Henson, P., Resolution of inflammation, in *The Molecular and Cellular Biology of Wound Repair,* Clark, R.A.F., Ed., Plenum Press, New York, 1996, pp. 143–168.
4. Grinnell, F. and Zhu, M., Identification of neutrophil elastase as the proteinase in burn wound responsible for degradation of fibronectin, *J. Invest. Dermatol.,* 103, 155–161, 1994.
5. Rao, C.N., Ladin, D.A., Liu, Y.Y., Chilukuri, K. et al., α1-Antitrypsin is degraded and nonfunctional in chronic wounds but intact and functional in acute wounds: the inhibitor protects fibronectin from degradation by chronic wound fluid enzymes, *J. Invest. Dermatol.,* 105, 572–578, 1995.
6. Carp, H., Miller, F., Hoidal, J.R., and Janoff, A., Potential mechanism of emphysema: α1-proteinase inhibitor recovered from lungs of cigarette smokers contains oxidized methionine and has decreased elastase inhibitory capacity, *Proc. Natl. Acad. Sci. U.S.A.,* 79, 2041–2045, 1982.
7. Zhang, G., Farrell, A.J., Blake, D.R., Chidwik, K., and Winyard, P., Inactivation of synovial fluid α1-antitrypsin by exercise of the inflamed rheumatoid joint, *FEBS Lett.,* 321, 274–278, 1993.
8. Desrochers, P.E. and Weiss, S.J., Proteolytic inactivation of α1-proteinase inhibitor by neutrophil metalloproteinase, *J. Clin. Invest.,* 81, 1646–1650, 1988.
9. Desrochers, P.E., Jeffrey, J.J., and Weiss, S.J., Interstitial collagenase (MMP-1) expresses serpinase activity, *J. Clin. Invest.,* 87, 2258–2265, 1991.
10. Desrochers, P.E., Mookthiar, K., Van Wart, H.E., Hasty, K.A., and Weiss, S.J., Proteolytic deactivation of α1-protease inhibitor and α1-antichymotrypsin by oxydatively activated human neutrophil metalloproteinases, *J. Biol. Chem.,* 267, 5005–5012, 1992.
11. Zhang, G., Winyard, P.G., Chidwik, K., Murphy, G., Wardell, M. et al., Proteolysis of human native and oxidized α1-protease inhibitor by matrilysin and stromelysin, *Biochim. Biophys. Acta,* 1199, 224–228, 1994.
12. Wysocki, A.B., Staiano-Coico, L., and Grinnell, F., Wound fluid from chronic leg ulcers contains elevated levels of metalloproteinases MMP-2 and MMP-9, *J. Invest. Dermatol.,* 101, 64–68, 1993.
13. Docherty, A.J.P. et al., The matrix metalloproteinases and their natural inhibitors: prospects for treating degenerative tissue diseases, *Tib. Tech.,* 10, 200–207, 1992.
14. Birkedal-Hansen, H., Moore, W.G., Bodden, M.K. et al,, Matrix metalloproteinases: a review, *Crit. Rev. Oral Biol. Med.,* 4, 197–250, 1993.
15. Cawston, T.E. et al., The interaction of purified rabbit bone collagenase with purified rabbit bone metalloproteinase inhibitor, *Biochem. J.,* 211, 313–318, 1993.
16. Howard, E.W. and Banda, M.J., Binding of tissue inhibitor metalloproteinase 2 to two distinct sites on human 72-kDa gelatinase: identification of a stabilization site, *J. Biol. Chem.,* 266, 17,972–17,977, 1991.
17. Matsubara, M., Girard, M.T., Kublin, C.L., Cintron, C., and Fini, M.E., Differential roles for two gelatinolytic enzymes of the matrix metalloproteinase family in the remodeling cornea, *Devel. Biol.,* 147, 425–439, 1991.

18. Girard, M.T. et al., Stromal fibroblasts synthesize collagenase and stromelysin during long-term tissue remodeling, *J. Cell Sci.,* 104, 1001–1011, 1993.
19. Saarialho-Kere, U.K. et al., Distinct localization of collagenase and tissue inhibitor of metalloproteinases in wound healing associated with ulcerative pyogenic granuloma, *J. Clin. Invest.,* 90, 152–157, 1992.
20. Oikarinen, A. et al., Demonstration of 72-kDa and 92-kDa type IV collagenase in human skin: variable expression in various blistering diseases, induction during reepithelialization and decrease by topical glucocorticoids, *J. Invest. Dermatol.,* 101, 205–210, 1993.
21. Salo, T., et al., Expression of matrix metalloproteinase-2 and 9 during early human wound healing, *Lab. Invest.,* 70, 176–182, 1994.
22. Wysocki, A.B. and Grinnell, F., Fibronectin profiles in normal and chronic wound fluid, *Lab. Invest.,* 63, 825–831, 1990.
23. Grinnell, F., Ho, C.H., and Wysocki, A.B., Degradation of fibronectin and vitronectin in chronic wound fluid: analysis by cell blotting, immunoblotting and cell adhesion assays, *J. Invest. Dermatol.,* 98, 410–416, 1992.
24. Wysocki, A.B., Staiano-Coico, L., and Grinnell, F., Wound fluid from chronic leg ulcers contains elevated levels of metalloproteinases MMP-2 and MMP-9, *J. Invest. Dermatol.,* 101, 64–68, 1993.
25. Collier, I.E. et al., H-ras oncogene-transformed human bronchial epithelial cells (TBE-1) secrete a single metalloprotease capable of degrading basement membrane collagen, *J. Biol. Chem.,* 263, 6579–6587, 1988.
26. Wilhelm, S.M., Collier, I.E., Marmer, B.L. et al., SV40-transformed human lung fibroblasts secrete a 92-kDa type IV collagenase, which is identical to that secreted by normal human macrophages, *J. Biol. Chem.,* 264, 17,213–17,221, 1989.
27. Borregaard, N., Lollike, K., Kjeldsen, L. et al., Human neutrophil granules and secretory vesicles, *Eur. J. Haematol.,* 51, 187–198, 1993.
28. Howard, E.W., Bullen, E.C., and Banda, M.J., Regulation of the autoactivation of human 72-kDa progelatinase by tissue inhibitor of metalloproteinases-2, *J. Biol. Chem.,* 266, 13,064–13,069, 1991.
29. Kjeldsen, L., Sengelov, H., Lollike, K. et al., Isolation and characterization of gelatinase granules from human neutrophils, *Blood,* 83, 1640–1649, 1994.
30. Staiano-Coico, L., Higgins, P.J., Schwartz, S.B. et al., Wound fluids: a reflection of the state of healing, *Ost./Wound Manag.,* 46, 85s–93s, 2000.
31. Robson, M.C., Stenberg, B.D., and Heggers, J.P., Wound healing alterations caused by infection, *Clin. Plast. Surg.,* 17, 484–492, 1990.
32. Mendez, M.V., Stanley, A., Park, H.Y., Shon, K. et al., Fibroblasts cultured from venous ulcers display cellular characteristics of senescence, *J. Vasc. Surg.,* 28, 876–883, 1998.
33. Agren, M.S., Steenfos, H.H., Dabelsteen, S., Hansen, J.B. et al., Proliferation and mitogenic response to PDGF-BB of fibroblasts isolated from chronic venous leg ulcers is ulcer age dependent, *J. Invest. Dermatol.,* 112, 463–469, 1999.
34. Martin, P., Wound healing: aiming for perfect skin regeneration, *Science,* 276, 75–81, 1997.
35. Singer, A.J. and Clark, R.A., Cutaneous wound healing, *N. Engl. J. Med.,* 341, 738–746, 1999.
36. O'Toole, E.A., Extracellular matrix and keratinocyte migration, *Clin. Exp. Dermatol.,* 26, 525–530, 2001.

37. Tomic-Canic, M., Komine, M., Freedberg, I.M., and Blumenberg, M., Epidermal signal transduction and transcription factor activation in activated keratinocytes, *J. Dermatol. Sci.,* 17, 167–181, 1998.
38. Freedberg, I.M., Tomic-Canic, M., Komine, M., and Blumenberg, M., Keratins and the keratinocyte activation cycle, *J. Invest. Dermatol.,* 116, 633–640, 2001.
39. Hackam, D.J. and Ford, H.R., Cellular, biochemical, and clinical aspects of wound healing, *Surg. Infect. (Larchmt.),* 3, S23–S35, 2002.
40. Coulombe, P.A., Towards a molecular definition of keratinocyte activation after acute injury to stratified epithelia, *Biochem. Biophys. Res. Commun.,* 236, 231–238, 1997.
41. Kupper, T.S., The activated keratinocyte: a model for inducible cytokine production by non-bone marrow-derived cells in cutaneous inflammatory and immune responses, *J. Invest. Dermatol.,* 94, 146S–150S, 1990.
42. Blumenberg, M., Keratinocytes: biology and differentiation, in *Cutaneous Medicine and Surgery,* Arndt, K.P., Ed., W.B. Saunders Company, Philadelphia, 1996, vol. 1, pp. 58–74.
43. Fuchs, E., Epidermal differentiation: the bare essentials, *J. Cell Biol.,* 111, 2807–2814, 1990.
44. Steinert, P.M. and Roop, D.R., Molecular and cellular biology of intermediate filaments, *Annu. Rev. Biochem.,* 57, 593–625, 1988.
45. Komine, M., Rao, L.S., Freedberg, I.M., Simon, M., Milisavljevic, V., and Blumenberg, M., Interleukin-1 induces transcription of keratin K6 in human epidermal keratinocytes, *J. Invest. Dermatol.,* 116, 330–338, 2001.
46. Jiang, C.K., Magnaldo, T., Ohtsuki, M., Freedberg, I.M., Bernerd, F., and Blumenberg, M., Epidermal growth factor and transforming growth factor alpha specifically induce the activation- and hyperproliferation-associated keratins 6 and 16, *Proc. Natl. Acad. Sci. U.S.A.,* 90, 6786–6790, 1993.
47. Jiang, C.K., Flanagan, S., Ohtsuki, M., Shuai, K., Freedberg, I.M., and Blumenberg, M., Disease-activated transcription factor: allergic reactions in human skin cause nuclear translocation of STAT-91 and induce synthesis of keratin K17, *Mol. Cell Biol.,* 14, 4759–4769, 1994.
48. Lersch, R., Stellmach, V., Stocks, C., Giudice, G., and Fuchs, E., Isolation, sequence, and expression of a human keratin K5 gene: transcriptional regulation of keratins and insights into pairwise control, *Mol. Cell Biol.,* 9, 3685–3697, 1989.
49. Lu, B., Rothnagel, J.A., Longley, M.A., Tsai, S.Y., Roop, D.R., Differentiation-specific expression of human keratin 1 is mediated by a composite AP-1/steroid hormone element, *J. Biol. Chem.,* 269, 7443–7449, 1994.
50. Jiang, C.K., Epstein, H.S., Tomic, M., Freedberg, I.M., and Blumenberg, M., Functional comparison of the upstream regulatory DNA sequences of four human epidermal keratin genes, *J. Invest. Dermatol.,* 96, 162–167, 1991.
51. Bernerd, F., Magnaldo, T., Freedberg, I.M., and Blumenberg, M., Expression of the carcinoma-associated keratin K6 and the role of AP-1 proto-oncoproteins, *Gene Expr.,* 3, 187–199, 1993.
52. Magnaldo, T., Vidal, R.G., Ohtsuki, M., Freedberg, I.M., and Blumenberg, M., On the role of AP2 in epithelial-specific gene expression, *Gene Expr.,* 3, 307–315, 1993.
53. Leask, A., Byrne, C., and Fuchs, E., Transcription factor AP2 and its role in epidermal-specific gene expression, *Proc. Natl. Acad. Sci. U.S.A.,* 88, 7948–7952, 1991.
54. Ohtsuki, M., Tomic-Canic, M., Freedberg, I.M., and Blumenberg, M., Nuclear proteins involved in transcription of the human K5 keratin gene, *J. Invest. Dermatol.,* 99, 206–215, 1992.

55. Ohtsuki, M., Flanagan, S., Freedberg, I.M., and Blumenberg, M., A cluster of five nuclear proteins regulates keratin gene transcription, *Gene Expr.,* 3, 201–213, 1993.

56. Tomic, M., Jiang, C.K., Epstein, H.S., Freedberg, I.M., Samuels, H.H., and Blumenberg, M., Nuclear receptors for retinoic acid and thyroid hormone regulate transcription of keratin genes, *Cell Regul.,* 1, 965–973, 1990.

57. Tomic-Canic, M., Sunjevaric, I., Freedberg, I.M., and Blumenberg, M., Identification of the retinoic acid and thyroid hormone receptor-responsive element in the human K14 keratin gene, *J. Invest. Dermatol.,* 99, 842–847, 1992.

58. Tomic-Canic, M., Day, D., Samuels, H.H., Freedberg, I.M., and Blumenberg, M., Novel regulation of keratin gene expression by thyroid hormone and retinoid receptors, *J. Biol. Chem.,* 271, 1416–1423, 1996.

59. Radoja, N., Diaz, D.V., Minars, T.J., Freedberg, I.M., Blumenberg, M., and Tomic-Canic, M, Specific organization of the negative response elements for retinoic acid and thyroid hormone receptors in keratin gene family, *J. Invest. Dermatol.,* 109, 566–572, 1997.

60. Radoja, N., Komine, M., Jho, S.H., Blumenberg, M., and Tomic-Canic, M., Novel mechanism of steroid action in skin through glucocorticoid receptor monomers, *Mol. Cell Biol.,* 20, 4328–4339, 2000.

61. Wojcik, S.M., Bundman, D.S., and Roop, D.R., Delayed wound healing in keratin 6a knockout mice, *Mol. Cell Biol.,* 20, 5248–5255, 2000.

62. McGowan, K. and Coulombe, P.A., The wound repair-associated keratins 6, 16, and 17. Insights into the role of intermediate filaments in specifying keratinocyte cytoarchitecture, *Subcell. Biochem.,* 31, 173–204, 1998.

63. Wawersik, M. and Coulombe, P.A., Forced expression of keratin 16 alters the adhesion, differentiation, and migration of mouse skin keratinocytes, *Mol. Biol. Cell,* 11, 3315–3327, 2000.

64. Griffiths, C.E., Voorhees, J.J., and Nickoloff, B.J., Characterization of intercellular adhesion molecule-1 and HLA-DR expression in normal and inflamed skin: modulation by recombinant gamma interferon and tumor necrosis factor, *J. Am. Acad. Dermatol.,* 20, 617–629, 1989.

65. Gailit, J., Welch, M.P., and Clark, R.A., TGF-beta 1 stimulates expression of keratinocyte integrins during reepithelialization of cutaneous wounds, *J. Invest. Dermatol.,* 103, 221–227, 1994.

66. Middleton, M.H. and Norris, D.A., Cytokine-induced ICAM-1 expression in human keratinocytes is highly variable in keratinocyte strains from different donors, *J. Invest. Dermatol.,* 104, 489–496, 1995.

67. Nickoloff, B.J., Griffiths, C.E., and Barker, J.N., The role of adhesion molecules, chemotactic factors, and cytokines in inflammatory and neoplastic skin disease — 1990 update, *J. Invest. Dermatol.,* 94, 151S–157S, 1990.

68. Marinkovich, M.P., Lunstrum, G.P., Keene, D.R., and Burgeson, R.E., The dermal–epidermal junction of human skin contains a novel laminin variant, *J. Cell Biol.,* 119, 695–703, 1992.

69. O'Keefe, E.J., Woodley, D.T., Falk, R.J., Gammon, W.R., and Briggaman, R.A., Production of fibronectin by epithelium in a skin equivalent, *J. Invest. Dermatol.,* 88, 634–639, 1987,

70. Wysocki, A.B., Staiano-Coico, L., and Grinnell, F., Wound fluid from chronic leg ulcers contains elevated levels of metalloproteinases MMP-2 and MMP-9, *J. Invest. Dermatol.,* 101, 64–68, 1993.

71. Hauser, C., Saurat, J.H., Schmitt, A., Jaunin, F., and Dayer, J.M., Interleukin 1 is present in normal human epidermis, *J. Immunol.,* 136, 3317–3323, 1986.

72. Kupper, T.S., Deitch, E.A., Baker, C.C., and Wong, W.C., The human burn wound as a primary source of interleukin-1 activity, *Surgery,* 100, 409–415, 1986.

73. Murphy, J.E., Robert, C., and Kupper, T.S., Interleukin-1 and cutaneous inflammation: a crucial link between innate and acquired immunity, *J. Invest. Dermatol.,* 114, 602–608, 2000.

74. Ling, L. and Goeddel, D.V., T6BP, a TRAF6-interacting protein involved in IL-1 signaling, *Proc. Natl. Acad. Sci. U.S.A.,* 97, 9567–9572, 2000.

75. Ninomiya-Tsuji, J., Kishimoto, K., Hiyama, A., Inoue, J., Cao, Z., and Matsumoto, K., The kinase TAK1 can activate the NIK-I kappaB as well as the MAP kinase cascade in the IL-1 signalling pathway, *Nature,* 398, 252–256, 1999.

76. Cao, Z., Xiong, J., Takeuchi, M., Kurama, T., and Goeddel, D.V., TRAF6 is a signal transducer for interleukin-1, *Nature,* 383, 443–446, 1996.

77. Nickoloff, B.J. and Turka, L.A., Keratinocytes: key immunocytes of the integument, *Am. J. Pathol.,* 143, 325–331, 1993.

78. LaDuca, J.R. and Gaspari, A.A., Targeting tumor necrosis factor alpha. New drugs used to modulate inflammatory diseases, *Dermatol. Clin.,* 19, 617–635, 2001.

79. Kolde, G., Schulze-Osthoff, K., Meyer, H., and Knop, J., Immunohistological and immunoelectron microscopic identification of TNF alpha in normal human and murine epidermis, *Arch. Dermatol. Res.,* 284, 154–158, 1992.

80. Nickoloff, B.J., Karabin, G.D., Barker, J.N., Griffiths, C.E., Sarma, V., Mitra, R.S., Elder, J.T., Kunkel, S.L., and Dixit, V.M., Cellular localization of interleukin-8 and its inducer, tumor necrosis factor-alpha, in psoriasis, *Am. J. Pathol.,* 138, 129–140, 1991.

81. Idriss, H.T. and Naismith, J.H., TNF alpha and the TNF receptor superfamily: structure–function relationship(s), *Microsc. Res. Tech.,* 50, 184–195, 2000.

82. Kondo, S. and Sauder, D.N., Tumor necrosis factor (TNF) receptor type 1 (p55) is a main mediator for TNF-alpha-induced skin inflammation, *Eur. J. Immunol.,* 27, 1713–1718, 1997.

83. Miyamoto, S. and Verma, I.M., Rel/NF-kappa B/I kappa B story. *Adv. Cancer Res.,* 66, 255–292, 1995.

84. Beg, A.A., Finco, T.S., Nantermet, P.V., and Baldwin, A.S., Tumor necrosis factor and interleukin-1 lead to phosphorylation and loss of I kappa B alpha: a mechanism for NF-kappa B activation, *Mol. Cell Biol.,* 13, 3301–3310, 1993.

85. Zandi, E., Chen, Y., and Karin, M., Direct phosphorylation of IkappaB by IKKalpha and IKKbeta: discrimination between free and NF-kappaB-bound substrate, *Science,* 281, 1360–1363, 1998.

86. Stein, B., Cogswell, P.C., and Baldwin, A.S., Functional and physical associations between NF-kappa B and C/EBP family members: a Rel domain-bZIP interaction, *Mol. Cell Biol.,* 13, 3964–3974, 1993.

87. Matsusaka, T., Fujikawa, K., Nishio, Y., Mukaida, N., Matsushima, K., Kishimoto, T., and Akira, S., Transcription factors NF-IL6 and NF-kappa B synergistically activate transcription of the inflammatory cytokines, interleukin 6 and interleukin 8, *Proc. Natl. Acad. Sci. U.S.A.,* 90, 10,193–10,197, 1993.

88. Seitz, C.S., Freiberg, R.A., Hinata, K., and Khavari, P.A., NF-kappaB determines localization and features of cell death in epidermis, *J. Clin. Invest.,* 105, 253–260, 2000.

89. Seitz, C.S., Lin, Q., Deng, H., and Khavari, P.A., Alterations in NF-kappaB function in transgenic epithelial tissue demonstrate a growth inhibitory role for NF-kappaB, *Proc. Natl. Acad. Sci. U.S.A.,* 95, 2307–2312, 1998.

90. Klement, J.F., Rice, N.R., Car, B.D., Abbondanzo, S.J., Powers, G.D., Bhatt, P.H., Chen, C.H., Rosen, C.A., and Stewart, C.L., IkappaBalpha deficiency results in a sustained NF-kappaB response and severe widespread dermatitis in mice, *Mol. Cell Biol.*, 16, 2341–2349, 1996.

91. Dajee, M., Lazarov, M., Zhang, J.Y., Cai, T., Green, C.L., Russell, A.J., Marinkovich, M.P., Tao, S., Lin, Q., Kubo, Y. et al., NF-kappaB blockade and oncogenic Ras trigger invasive human epidermal neoplasia, *Nature*, 421, 639–643, 2003.

92. Akira, S., Isshiki, H., Sugita, T., Tanabe, O., Kinoshita, S., Nishio, Y., Nakajima, T., Hirano, T., and Kishimoto, T., A nuclear factor for IL-6 expression (NF-IL6) is a member of a C/EBP family, *EMBO J.*, 9, 1897–1906, 1990.

93. Nishio, Y., Isshiki, H., Kishimoto, T., and Akira, S., A nuclear factor for interleukin-6 expression (NF-IL6) and the glucocorticoid receptor synergistically activate transcription of the rat alpha 1-acid glycoprotein gene via direct protein–protein interaction, *Mol. Cell Biol.*, 13, 1854–1862, 1993.

94. Maytin, E.V. and Habener, J.F., Transcription factors C/EBP alpha, C/EBP beta, and CHOP (Gadd153) expressed during the differentiation program of keratinocytes *in vitro* and *in vivo*, *J. Invest. Dermatol.*, 110, 238–246, 1998.

95. Oh, H.S. and Smart, R.C., Expression of CCAAT/enhancer binding proteins (C/EBP) is associated with squamous differentiation in epidermis and isolated primary keratinocytes and is altered in skin neoplasms, *J. Invest. Dermatol.*, 110, 939–945, 1998.

96. Tanaka, T., Akira, S., Yoshida, K., Umemoto, M., Yoneda, Y., Shirafuji, N., Fujiwara, H., Suematsu, S., Yoshida, N. and Kishimoto, T., Targeted disruption of the NF-IL6 gene discloses its essential role in bacteria killing and tumor cytotoxicity by macrophages, *Cell*, 80, 353–361, 1995.

97. Zhu, S., Oh, H.S., Shim, M., Sterneck, E., Johnson, P.F., and Smart, R.C., C/EBPbeta modulates the early events of keratinocyte differentiation involving growth arrest and keratin 1 and keratin 10 expression, *Mol. Cell Biol.*, 19, 7181–7190, 1999.

98. Ullrich, A. and Schlessinger, J., Signal transduction by receptors with tyrosine kinase activity, *Cell*, 61, 203–212, 1990.

99. Nanney, L.B., Stoscheck, C.M., King, L.E., Underwood, R.A., and Holbrook, K.A., Immunolocalization of epidermal growth factor receptors in normal developing human skin, *J. Invest. Dermatol.*, 94, 742–748, 1990.

100. Coffey, R.J., Derynck, R., Wilcox, J.N., Bringman, T.S., Goustin, A.S., Moses, H.L., and Pittelkow, M.R., Production and auto-induction of transforming growth factor-alpha in human keratinocytes, *Nature*, 328, 817–820, 1987.

101. Vasioukhin, V., Bauer, C., Yin, M., and Fuchs, E., Directed actin polymerization is the driving force for epithelial cell–cell adhesion, *Cell*, 100, 209–219, 2000.

102. Kallunki, T., Deng, T., Hibi, M., and Karin, M., c-Jun can recruit JNK to phosphorylate dimerization partners via specific docking interactions, *Cell*, 87, 929–939, 1996.

103. Hill, C.S. and Treisman, R., Differential activation of c-fos promoter elements by serum, lysophosphatidic acid, G proteins and polypeptide growth factors, *EMBO J.*, 14, 5037–5047, 1995.

104. Saez, E., Oppenheim, H., Smoluk, J., Andersen, J.W., Van Etten, R.A., and Spiegelman, B.M., c-Fos is not essential for v-abl-induced lymphomagenesis, *Cancer Res.*, 55, 6196–6199, 1995.

105. Lohman, F.P., Medema, J.K., Gibbs, S., Ponec, M., van de Putte, P., and Backendorf, C., Expression of the SPRR cornification genes is differentially affected by carcinogenic transformation, *Exp. Cell Res.*, 231, 141–148, 1997.

106. Welter, J.F., Crish, J.F., Agarwal, C., and Eckert, R.L., Fos-related antigen (Fra-1), junB, and junD activate human involucrin promoter transcription by binding to proximal and distal AP1 sites to mediate phorbol ester effects on promoter activity, *J. Biol. Chem.,* 270, 12,614–12,622, 1995.

107. Rutberg, S.E., Saez, E., Glick, A., Dlugosz, A.A., Spiegelman, B.M., and Yuspa, S.H., Differentiation of mouse keratinocytes is accompanied by PKC-dependent changes in AP-1 proteins, *Oncogene,* 13, 167–176, 1996.

108. Umezawa, A., Yamamoto, H., Rhodes, K., Klemsz, M.J., Maki, R.A., and Oshima, R.G., Methylation of an ETS site in the intron enhancer of the keratin 18 gene participates in tissue-specific repression, *Mol. Cell Biol.,* 17, 4885–4894, 1997.

109. Ma, S., Rao, L., Freedberg, I.M., and Blumenberg, M., Transcriptional control of K5, K6, K14, and K17 keratin genes by AP-1 and NF-kappaB family members, *Gene Expr.,* 6, 361–370, 1997.

109a. Li, G., Gustavson, M., Brown, C., Hans, S.K., Nason, K. et al., c-Jun is essential for organization of the epidermal leading edge, *Dev. Cell,* 4, 865–877, 2003.

110. Verrecchia, F. and Mauviel, A., Transforming growth factor-beta signaling through the Smad pathway: role in extracellular matrix gene expression and regulation, *J. Invest. Dermatol.,* 118, 211–215, 2002.

111. Shah, M., Foreman, D.M., and Ferguson, M.W., Neutralisation of TGF-beta 1 and TGF-beta 2 or exogenous addition of TGF-beta 3 to cutaneous rat wounds reduces scarring, *J. Cell Sci.,* 108, 985–1002, 1995.

112. Frank, S., Madlener, M., and Werner, S., Transforming growth factors beta1, beta2, and beta3 and their receptors are differentially regulated during normal and impaired wound healing, *J. Biol. Chem.,* 271, 10,188–10,193, 1996.

113. O'Kane, S. and Ferguson, M.W., Transforming growth factor beta s and wound healing, *Int. J. Biochem. Cell Biol.,* 29, 63–78, 1997.

114. Jiang, C.K., Tomic-Canic, M., Lucas, D.J., Simon, M., and Blumenberg, M., TGF beta promotes the basal phenotype of epidermal keratinocytes: transcriptional induction of Kœ5 and Kœ14 keratin genes, *Growth Factors,* 12, 87–97, 1995.

115. Jhappan, C., Geiser, A.G., Kordon, E.C., Bagheri, D., Hennighausen, L., Roberts, A.B., Smith, G.H., and Merlino, G., Targeting expression of a transforming growth factor beta 1 transgene to the pregnant mammary gland inhibits alveolar development and lactation, *EMBO J.,* 12, 1835–1845, 1993.

116. Sellheyer, K., Bickenbach, J.R., Rothnagel, J.A., Bundman, D., Longley, M.A., Krieg, T., Roche, N.S., Roberts, A.B., and Roop, D.R., Inhibition of skin development by overexpression of transforming growth factor beta 1 in the epidermis of transgenic mice, *Proc. Natl. Acad. Sci. U.S.A.,* 90, 5237–5241, 1993.

117. Glick, A.B., Kulkarni, A.B., Tennenbaum, T., Hennings, H., Flanders, K.C., O'Reilly, M., Sporn, M.B., Karlsson, S., and Yuspa, S.H., Loss of expression of transforming growth factor beta in skin and skin tumors is associated with hyperproliferation and a high risk for malignant conversion, *Proc. Natl. Acad. Sci. U.S.A.,* 90, 6076–6080, 1993.

118. Ashcroft, G.S., Yang, X., Glick, A.B., Weinstein, M., Letterio, J.L., Mizel, D.E., Anzano, M., Greenwell-Wild, T., Wahl, S.M., Deng, C. et al., Mice lacking Smad3 show accelerated wound healing and an impaired local inflammatory response, *Nat. Cell Biol.,* 1, 260–266, 1999.

119. Ashcroft, G.S. and Roberts, A.B., Loss of Smad3 modulates wound healing, *Cytokine Growth Factor Rev.,* 11, 125–131, 2000.

120. Choi, Y. and Fuchs, E., TGF-beta and retinoic acid: regulators of growth and modifiers of differentiation in human epidermal cells, *Cell Regul.,* 1, 791–809, 1990.

121. Xia, Y.P., Zhao, Y., Marcus, J., Jimenez, P.A., Ruben, S.M., Moore, P.A., Khan, F., and Mustoe, T.A., Effects of keratinocyte growth factor-2 (KGF-2) on wound healing in an ischaemia-impaired rabbit ear model and on scar formation, *J. Pathol.*, 188, 431–438, 1999.

122. Beer, H.D., Gassmann, M.G., Munz, B., Steiling, H., Engelhardt, F., Bleuel, K., and Werner, S., Expression and function of keratinocyte growth factor and activin in skin morphogenesis and cutaneous wound repair, *J. Invest. Dermatol. Symp. Proc.*, 5, 34–39, 2000.

123. Jimenez, P.A. and Rampy, M.A., Keratinocyte growth factor-2 accelerates wound healing in incisional wounds, *J. Surg. Res.*, 81, 238–242, 1999.

124. Karukonda, S.R., Flynn, T.C., Boh, E.E., McBurney, E.I., Russo, G.G., and Millikan, L.E., The effects of drugs on wound healing: part 1, *Int. J. Dermatol.*, 39, 250–257, 2000.

125. Limat, A. and French, L.E., Therapy with growth factors, *Curr. Probl. Dermatol.*, 27, 49–56, 1999.

126. Lees, V.C. and Fan, T.P., A freeze-injured skin graft model for the quantitative study of basic fibroblast growth factor and other promoters of angiogenesis in wound healing, *Br. J. Plast. Surg.*, 47, 349–359, 1994.

127. Greenhalgh, D.G. and Reiman, M., The effect of bFGF on the healing of partial thickness skin graft donor sites. A prospective, randomized, double blind study, *Wound Repair Regul.*, 2, 113–121, 1994.

128. Steed, D.L., Clinical evaluation of recombinant human platelet-derived growth factor for the treatment of lower extremity diabetic ulcers. Diabetic Ulcer Study Group, *J. Vasc. Surg.*, 21, 71–78, discussion 79–81, 1995.

129. Robson, M.C., Phillips, L.G., and Cooper, M.D., The safety and effect of transforming factor -B2 for the treatment of venous stasis ulcers, *Wound Repair Regen.*, 3, 227–283, 1995.

130. Nguyen, B.P., Ryan, M.C., Gil, S.G., and Carter, W.G., Deposition of laminin 5 in epidermal wounds regulates integrin signaling and adhesion, *Curr. Opin. Cell Biol.*, 12, 554–562, 2000.

131. Burgeson, R.E. and Christiano, A,M., The dermal–epidermal junction, *Curr. Opin. Cell Biol.*, 9, 651–658, 1997.

132. Borradori, L. and Sonnenberg, A., Structure and function of hemidesmosomes: more than simple adhesion complexes, *J. Invest. Dermatol.*, 112, 411–418, 1999.

133. Cavani, A., Zambruno, G., Marconi, A., Manca, V., Marchetti, M., and Giannetti, A., Distinctive integrin expression in the newly forming epidermis during wound healing in humans, *J. Invest. Dermatol.*, 101, 600–604, 1993.

134. Breuss, J.M., Gallo, J., DeLisser, H.M., Klimanskaya, I.V., Folkesson, H.G., Pittet, J.F., Nishimura, S.L., Aldape, K., Landers, D.V., Carpenter, W. et al., Expression of the beta 6 integrin subunit in development, neoplasia and tissue repair suggests a role in epithelial remodeling, *J. Cell Sci.*, 108, 2241–2251, 1995.

135. Haapasalmi, K., Zhang, K., Tonnesen, M., Olerud, J., Sheppard, D., Salo, T., Kramer, R., Clark, R.A., Uitto, V.J., and Larjava, H., Keratinocytes in human wounds express alpha v beta 6 integrin, *J. Invest. Dermatol.*, 106, 42–48, 1996.

136. Nanney, L.B. and King, L.E.J., Epidermal growth factor and transforming growth factor alpha, in *The Molecular and Cellular Biology of Wound Repair*, 2nd ed., Clark, R.A.F., Ed., Plenum Press, New York, 1996, pp. 171–194.

137. Werner, S., Smola, H., Liao, X., Longaker, M.T., Krieg, T., Hofschneider, P.H., and Williams, L.T., The function of KGF in morphogenesis of epithelium and reepithelialization of wounds, *Science*, 266, 819–822, 1994.

138. Abraham, J.A. and Klagsburn, M., Modulation of wound repair by members of the fibroblast growth factor family, in *The Molecular and Cellular Biology of Wound Repair,* 2nd ed., Clark, R.A.F., Ed., Plenum Press, New York, 1996, pp. 195–248.

139. Zambruno, G., Marchisio, P.C., Marconi, A., Vaschieri, C., Melchiori, A., Giannetti, A., and De Luca, M., Transforming growth factor-beta 1 modulates beta 1 and beta 5 integrin receptors and induces the de novo expression of the alpha v beta 6 heterodimer in normal human keratinocytes: implications for wound healing, *J. Cell Biol.,* 129, 853–865, 1995.

140. Fuchs, E., Dowling, J., Segre, J., Lo, S.H., and Yu, Q.C., Integrators of epidermal growth and differentiation: distinct functions for beta 1 and beta 4 integrins, *Curr. Opin. Genet. Dev.,* 7, 672–682, 1997.

141. Mainiero, F., Pepe, A., Yeon, M., Ren, Y., and Giancotti, F.G., The intracellular functions of alpha6beta4 integrin are regulated by EGF, *J. Cell Biol.,* 134, 241–253, 1996.

142. Kim, L.T., Wu, J., Bier-Laning, C., Dollar, B.T., and Turnage, R.H., Focal adhesion kinase up-regulation and signaling in activated keratinocytes, *J. Surg. Res.,* 91, 65–69, 2000.

143. Goldfinger, L.E., Hopkinson, S.B., deHart, G.W., Collawn, S., Couchman, J.R., and Jones J.C., The alpha3 laminin subunit, alpha6beta4 and alpha3beta1 integrin coordinately regulate wound healing in cultured epithelial cells and in the skin, *J. Cell Sci.,* 112, 2615–2629, 1999.

144. Green, K.J. and Gaudry, C.A., Are desmosomes more than tethers for intermediate filaments? *Nat. Rev. Mol. Cell Biol.,* 1, 208–216, 2000.

145. Green, K.J. and Jones, J.C., Desmosomes and hemidesmosomes: structure and function of molecular components, *FASEB J.,* 10, 871–881, 1996.

146. McGrath, J.A., McMillan, J.R., Shemanko, C.S., Runswick, S.K., Leigh, I.M., Lane, E.B., Garrod, D.R., and Eady, R.A., Mutations in the plakophilin 1 gene result in ectodermal dysplasia/skin fragility syndrome, *Nat. Genet.,* 17, 240–244, 1997.

147. Armstrong, D.K., McKenna, K.E., Purkis, P.E., Green, K.J., Eady, R.A., Leigh, I.M., and Hughes, A.E., Haploinsufficiency of desmoplakin causes a striate subtype of palmoplantar keratoderma, *Hum. Mol. Genet.,* 8, 143–148, 1999.

148. Rickman, L., Simrak, D., Stevens, H.P., Hunt, D.M., King, I.A., Bryant, S.P., Eady, R.A., Leigh, I.M., Arnemann, J., Magee, A.I. et al., N-terminal deletion in a desmosomal cadherin causes the autosomal dominant skin disease striate palmoplantar keratoderma, *Hum. Mol. Genet.,* 8, 971–976, 1999.

149. Wallis, S., Lloyd, S., Wise, I., Ireland, G., Fleming, T.P., and Garrod, D., The alpha isoform of protein kinase C is involved in signaling the response of desmosomes to wounding in cultured epithelial cells, *Mol. Biol. Cell,* 11, 1077–1092, 2000.

150. Geiger, B. and Ginsberg, D., The cytoplasmic domain of adherens-type junctions, *Cell Motil. Cytoskeleton,* 20, 1–6, 1991.

151. Geiger, B. and Ayalon, O., Cadherins, *Annu. Rev. Cell Biol.,* 8, 307–332, 1992.

152. Kemler, R., From cadherins to catenins: cytoplasmic protein interactions and regulation of cell adhesion, *Trends Genet.,* 9, 317–321, 1993.

153. Nagafuchi, A. and Takeichi, M., Cell binding function of E-cadherin is regulated by the cytoplasmic domain, *EMBO J.,* 7, 3679–3684, 1988.

154. Ozawa, M., Identification of the region of alpha-catenin that plays an essential role in cadherin-mediated cell adhesion, *J. Biol. Chem.,* 273, 29, 524–529, 1998

155. Brock, J., Midwinter, K., Lewis, J., and Martin, P., Healing of incisional wounds in the embryonic chick wing bud: characterization of the actin purse-string and demonstration of a requirement for Rho activation, *J. Cell Biol.,* 135, 1097–1107, 1996.

156. Takahashi, M., Fujimoto, T., Honda, Y., and Ogawa, K., Distributional change of fodrin in the wound healing process of the corneal epithelium, *Invest. Ophthalmol. Vis. Sci.,* 33, 280–285, 1992.

157. Danjo, Y. and Gipson, I.K., Actin "purse string" filaments are anchored by E-cadherin-mediated adherens junctions at the leading edge of the epithelial wound, providing coordinated cell movement, *J. Cell Sci.,* 111, 3323–3332, 1998.

158. Sharma, G.D., He, J., and Bazan, H.E., p38 and ERK1/2 coordinate cellular migration and proliferation in epithelial wound healing: evidence of cross-talk activation between MAP-kinase cascades, *J. Biol. Chem.,* 26, 26–31, 2003.

159. Kim, L.T., Wu, J., and Turnage, R.H., FAK induction in keratinocytes in an *in vitro* model of reepithelialization, *J. Surg. Res.,* 96, 167–172, 2001.

160. Li, W., Nadelman, C., Henry, G., Fan, J., Muellenhoff, M., Medina, E., Gratch, N.S., Chen, M., Han, J., and Woodley, D., The p38-MAPK/SAPK pathway is required for human keratinocyte migration on dermal collagen, *J. Invest. Dermatol.,* 117, 1601–1611, 2001.

161. Nagaoka, T., Kaburagi, Y., Hamaguchi, Y., Hasegawa, M., Takehara, K., Steeber, D.A., Tedder, T.F., and Sato, S., Delayed wound healing in the absence of intercellular adhesion molecule-1 or L-selectin expression, *Am. J. Pathol.,* 157, 237–247, 2000.

162. Garlick, J.A. and Taichman, L.B., Effect of TGF-beta 1 on re-epithelialization of human keratinocytes in vitro: an organotypic model, *J. Invest. Dermatol.,* 103, 554–559, 1994.

163. Pullar, C.E., Chen, J., and Isseroff, R., PP2A activation by {beta}2-adrenerigic receptor agonists: novel regulatory mechanism of keratinocyte migration, *J. Biol. Chem.,* 14, 14–18, 2003.

164. Brem, H., Balledux, J., Bloom, T., Kerstein, M.D., and Hollier, L., Healing of diabetic foot ulcers and pressure ulcers with human skin equivalent: a new paradigm in wound healing, *Arch. Surg.,* 135, 627–634, 2000.

165. Khachemoune, A., Bello, Y.M., and Phillips, T.J., Factors that influence healing in chronic venous ulcers treated with cryopreserved human epidermal cultures, *Dermatol. Surg.,* 28, 274–280, 2002.

166. Waikel, R.L., Kawachi, Y., Waikel, P.A., Wang, X.J., and Roop, D.R., Deregulated expression of c-Myc depletes epidermal stem cells, *Nat. Genet.,* 28, 165–168, 2001.

167. Arnold, I. and Watt, F.M., c-Myc activation in transgenic mouse epidermis results in mobilization of stem cells and differentiation of their progeny, *Curr. Biol.,* 11, 558–568, 2001.

168. Waikel, R.L., Wang, X.J., and Roop, D.R., Targeted expression of c-Myc in the epidermis alters normal proliferation, differentiation and UV-B induced apoptosis, *Oncogene,* 18, 4870–4878, 1999.

169. Mazzalupo, S., Wong, P., Martin, P., and Coulombe, P.A., Role for keratins 6 and 17 during wound closure in embryonic mouse skin, *Dev. Dyn.,* 226, 356–365, 2003.

170. Adair, H.M., Epidermal repair in chronic venous ulcers, *Br. J. Surg.,* 64, 800–804, 1977.

171. Seiler, W.O., Stahelin, H.B., Zolliker, R., Kallenberger, A., and Luscher, N.J., Impaired migration of epidermal cells from decubitus ulcers in cell cultures. A cause of protracted wound healing? *Am. J. Clin. Pathol.,* 92, 430–434, 1989.

172. Adriessen, M.P.M., van Bergen, B., Spruijt, K.I.J., Go, I.H., Schalkwijk, J., and van de Kerkhof, P.C.M., Epidermal proliferation is not impaired in chronic venous ulcers, *Acta. Derm. Venereol. (Stockh.),* 75, 459–462, 1995

173. Ashcroft, G.S., Lei, K., Longnecker, G., Kulkarni, A.B. et al., Secretory leukocyte protease inhibitor mediates nonredundant functions necessary for normal wound healing, *Nat. Med.,* 6, 1114–1153, 2000.

174. Netzel-Arnett, S., Mitola, D.J., Yamada, S.S., Chrysovergis, K. et al., Collagen dissolution by keratinocytes requires cell surface plasminogen activation and matrix metalloproteinase activity, *J. Biol. Chem.,* 277, 154–161, 2002.

175. Rømer, J., Bugge, T.H., Pyke, C., Lund, L.R., Flick, M.J., Degen, J.L., and Danø, K., Impaired wound healing in mice with a disrupted plasminogen gene, *Nat. Med.,* 2, 287–292, 1996.

176. Mirastschijski, U., Impola, U., Karsdal, M.A., Saarialho-Kere, U., and Ågren, M.S., Matrix metalloproteinase inhibitor BB-3103, unlike the serine proteinase inhibitor aprotinin, abrogates epidermal healing of human skin wounds *ex vivo, J. Invest. Dermatol.,* 118, 55–64, 2002.

177. Abbott, R.E., Corral, C.J., MacIvor, D.M., Lin, X., Ley, T.J., Mustoe, T.A., Augmented inflammatory responses and altered wound healing in cathepsin G-deficient mice, *Arch. Surg.,* 133, 1002–1006, 1998.

178. Visse, R. and Nagase, H, Matrix metalloproteinases and tissue inhibitors of metalloproteinases: structure, function, and biochemistry, *Circ. Res.,* 92, 827–839, 2003.

179. Ågren, M.S., Taplin, C.J., Woessner, J.F., Jr., Eaglstein, W.H., and Mertz, P.M., Collagenase in wound healing: effect of wound age and type, *J. Invest. Dermatol.,* 99, 709–714, 1992.

180. Ågren, M.S., Gelatinase activity during wound healing, *Br. J. Dermatol.,* 131, 634–640, 1994.

181. Madlener, M., Parks, W.C., and Werner, S., Matrix metalloproteinases (MMPs) and their physiological inhibitors (TIMPs) are differentially expressed during excisional skin wound repair, *Exp. Cell Res.,* 242, 201–210, 1998.

182. Soo, C., Shaw, W.W., Zhang, X., Longaker, M.T., Howard, E.W., and Ting, K., Differential expression of matrix metalloproteinases and their tissue-derived inhibitors in cutaneous wound repair, *Plast. Reconstr. Surg.,* 105, 638–647, 2000.

183. Ågren, M.S., Mirastschijski, U., Karlsmark, T., and Saarialho-Kere, U.K., Topical synthetic inhibitor of matrix metalloproteinases delays epidermal regeneration of human wounds, *Exp. Dermatol.,* 10, 337–348, 2001.

184. Ågren, M.S., Jorgensen, L.N., Andersen, M., Viljanto, J., and Gottrup. F., Matrix metalloproteinase 9 level predicts optimal collagen deposition during early wound repair in humans, *Br. J. Surg.,* 85, 68–71, 1998.

185. Nwomeh, B.C., Liang, H.X., Cohen, I.K., and Yager, D.R., MMP-8 is the predominant collagenase in healing wounds and nonhealing ulcers, *J. Surg. Res.,* 81, 189–195, 1999.

186. Vaalamo, M., Weckroth, M., Puolakkainen, P., Kere, J., Saarinen, P., Lauharanta, J., and Saarialho-Kere, U.K., Patterns of matrix metalloproteinase and TIMP-1 expression in chronic and normally healing human cutaneous wounds, *Br. J. Dermatol.,* 135, 52–59, 1996.

187. Ashcroft, G.S., Horan, M.A., Herrick, S.E., Tarnuzzer, R.W., Schultz, G.S., and Ferguson, M.W.J., Age-related differences in the temporal and spatial regulation of matrix metalloproteinases (MMPs) in normal skin and acute cutaneous wounds of healthy humans, *Cell Tissue Res.,* 290, 581–591, 1997.

188. Ågren, M.S., Matrix metalloproteinases (MMPs) are required for re-epithelialization of cutaneous wounds, *Arch. Dermatol. Res.,* 291, 583–590, 1999.

189. Lund, L.R., Rømer, J., Bugge, T.H., Nielsen, B.S., Frandsen, T.L., Degen, J.L., Stephens, R.W., and Danø, K., Functional overlap between two classes of matrix-degrading proteases in wound healing, *EMBO J.*, 18, 4645–4656, 1999.
190. Parks, W.C., Matrix metalloproteinases in repair, *Wound Repair Regen.*, 7, 423–432, 1999.
191. Inoue, M., Kratz, G., Haegerstrand, A., and Ståhle-Bäckdahl, M., Collagenase expression is rapidly induced in wound-edge keratinocytes after acute injury in human skin, persists during healing, and stops at re-epithelialization, *J. Invest. Dermatol.*, 104, 479–483, 1995.
192. Di Colandrea, T., Wang, L., Wille, J., D'Armiento, J., and Chada, K.K., Epidermal expression of collagenase delays wound-healing in transgenic mice, *J. Invest. Dermatol.*, 111, 1029–1033, 1998.
193. Beare. A.H., O'Kane, S., Krane, S.M., and Ferguson, M.W.J., Severely impaired wound healing in the collagenase-resistant mouse, *J. Invest. Dermatol.*, 120, 153–163, 2003.
194. Vaalamo, M., Mattila, L., Johansson, N., Kariniemi, A.L., Karjalainen-Lindsberg, M.L., Kähäri, V.M., and Saarialho-Kere, U., Distinct populations of stromal cells express collagenase-3 (MMP-13) and collagenase-1 (MMP-1) in chronic ulcers but not in normally healing wounds, *J. Invest. Dermatol.*, 109, 96–101, 1997.
195. Mirastschijski, U., Impola, U., Jahkola, T., Karlsmark, T., Ågren, M.S., and Saarialho-Kere, U., Ectopic localization of matrix metalloproteinase-9 in chronic cutaneous wounds, *Hum. Pathol.*, 33, 355–364, 2002.
196. Mohan, R., Chintala, S.K., Jung, J.C., Villar, W.V., McCabe, F., Russo, L.A., Lee, Y., McCarthy, B.E., Wollenberg, K.R., Jester, J.V., Wang, M., Welgus, H.G., Shipley, J.M., Senior, R.M., and Fini, M.E., Matrix metalloproteinase gelatinase B (MMP-9) coordinates and effects epithelial regeneration, *J. Biol. Chem.*, 277, 2065–2072, 2002.
197. Nagavarapu, U., Relloma, K., and Herron, G.S., Membrane type 1 matrix metalloproteinase regulates cellular invasiveness and survival in cutaneous epidermal cells, *J. Invest. Dermatol.*, 118, 573–581, 2002.
198. Bullard, K.M., Lund, L., Mudgett, J.S., Melin, T.N., Hunt, T.K., Murphy, B., Ronan, J., Werb, Z., and Banda, M.J., Impaired wound contraction in stromelysin-1-deficient mice, *Ann. Surg.*, 230, 260–265, 1999.
199. Saarialho-Kere, U., Kerkela, E., Jahkola, T., Suomela, S., Keski-Oja, J., and Lohi, J., Epilysin (MMP-28) expression is associated with cell proliferation during epithelial repair, *J. Invest. Dermatol.*, 119, 14–21, 2002.
200. Vaalamo, M., Leivo, T., and Saarialho-Kere, U., Differential expression of tissue inhibitors of metalloproteinases (TIMP-1, -2, -3, and -4) in normal and aberrant wound healing, *Hum. Pathol.*, 30, 795–802, 1999.
201. Holt, D.R., Kirk, S.J., Regan, M.C., Hurson, M., Lindblad, W.J., and Barbul, A., Effect of age on wound healing in healthy human beings, *Surgery*, 112, 293–297, 1992.
202. Ashcroft, G.S, Herrick, S.E., Tarnuzzer, R.W., Horan, M.A., Schultz, G.S., and Ferguson M.W., Human ageing impairs injury-induced *in vivo* expression of tissue inhibitor of matrix metalloproteinases (TIMP)-1 and -2 proteins and mRNA, *J. Pathol.*, 183, 169–176, 1997.
203. Herrick, S.E., Sloan, P., McGurk, M., Freak, L., McCollum, C.N., and Ferguson, M.W., Sequential changes in histologic pattern and extracellular matrix deposition during the healing of chronic venous ulcers, *Am. J. Pathol.*, 141, 1085–1095, 1992.
204. Clark, R.A., Lanigan, J.M., DellaPelle, P., Manseau, E., Dvorak, H.F., and Colvin, R.B., Fibronectin and fibrin provide a provisional matrix for epidermal cell migration during wound reepithelialization, *J. Invest. Dermatol.*, 79, 264–269, 1982.

205. Herrick, S.E., Ireland, G.W., Simon, D., McCollum, C.N., and Ferguson, M.W., Venous ulcer fibroblasts compared with normal fibroblasts show differences in collagen but not fibronectin production under both normal and hypoxic conditions, *J. Invest. Dermatol.,* 106, 187–193, 1996.

206. Wysocki, A.B. and Grinnell, F., Fibronectin profiles in normal and chronic wound fluid, *Lab. Invest.,* 63, 825–831, 1990.

207. Grinnell, F. and Zhu, M., Fibronectin degradation in chronic wounds depends on the relative levels of elastase, α1-proteinase inhibitor, and α2-macroglobulin, *J. Invest. Dermatol.,* 106, 335–341, 1996.

208. Claudy, A.L., Mirshahi, M., Soria, C., and Soria, J., Detection of undegraded fibrin and tumor necrosis factor-alpha in venous leg ulcers, *J. Am. Acad. Dermatol.,* 25, 623–627, 1991.

209. Kafienah, W., Buttle, D.J., Burnett, D., and Hollander, A.P., Cleavage of native type I collagen by human neutrophil elastase, *Biochem. J.,* 330, 897–902, 1998.

210. Weckroth, M., Vaheri, A., Lauharanta, J., Sorsa, T., and Konttinen, Y.T., Matrix metalloproteinases, gelatinase and collagenase, in chronic leg ulcers, *J. Invest. Dermatol.,* 106, 1119–1124, 1996.

211. Herrick, S., Ashcroft, G., Ireland, G., Horan, M., McCollum, C., and Ferguson, M., Up-regulation of elastase in acute wounds of healthy aged humans and chronic venous leg ulcers is associated with matrix degradation, *Lab. Invest.,* 77, 281–288, 1997.

212. Trengove, N.J., Stacey, M.C., MacAuley, S., Bennett, N., Gibson, J., Burslem, F., Murphy, G., and Schultz, G., Analysis of the acute and chronic wound environments: the role of proteases and their inhibitors, *Wound Repair Regen.,* 7, 442–452, 1999.

213. Wysocki, A.B., Kusakabe, A.O., Chang, S., and Tuan, T.L., Temporal expression of urokinase plasminogen activator, plasminogen activator inhibitor and gelatinase-B in chronic wound fluid switches from a chronic to acute wound profile with progression to healing, *Wound Repair Regen.,* 7, 154–165, 1999.

214. Ågren, M.S., Eaglstein, W.H., Ferguson, M.W.J., Harding, K.G., Moore, K., Saarialho-Kere, U., and Schultz, G.S., Causes and effects of the chronic inflammation in venous leg ulcers, *Acta Derm. Venereol. (Stockh.) Suppl.,* 210, 3–17, 2000.

215. Dovi, J.V., He, L.K., and DiPietro, L.A., Accelerated wound closure in neutrophil-depleted mice, *J. Leukoc. Biol.,* 73, 448–455, 2003.

216. Liu, Z., Zhou, X., Shapiro, S.D., Shipley, J.M., Twining, S.S., Diaz, L.A., Senior, R.M., and Werb, Z., The serpin alpha1-proteinase inhibitor is a critical substrate for gelatinase B/MMP-9 *in vivo, Cell,* 102, 647–655, 2000.

217. Herouy, Y., May, A.E., Pornschlegel, G., Stetter, C., Grenz, H., Preissner, K.T., Schöpf, E., Norgauer, J., and Vanscheidt, W., Lipodermatosclerosis is characterized by elevated expression and activation of matrix metalloproteinases: implications for venous ulcer formation, *J. Invest. Dermatol.,* 111, 822–827, 1998.

218. Saarialho-Kere, U.K., Patterns of matrix metalloproteinase and TIMP expression in chronic ulcers, *Arch. Dermatol. Res. (Suppl.),* 290, S47–S54, 1998

219. Bullen, E.C., Longaker, M.T., Updike, D.L., Benton, R., Ladin, D., Hou, Z., and Howard E.W., Tissue inhibitor of metalloproteinases-1 is decreased and activated gelatinases are increased in chronic wounds, *J. Invest. Dermatol.,* 104, 236–240, 1995.

220. Ladwig, G.P., Robson, M.C., Liu, R., Kuhn, M.A., Muir, D.F., and Schultz, G.S., Ratios of activated matrix metalloproteinase-9 to tissue inhibitor of matrix metallo-proteinase-1 in wound fluids are inversely correlated with healing of pressure ulcers, *Wound Repair Regen.,* 10, 26–37, 2002.

221. Lobmann, R., Ambrosch, A., Schultz, G., Waldmann, K., Schiweck, S., and Lehnert, H., Expression of matrix-metalloproteinases and their inhibitors in the wounds of diabetic and non-diabetic patients, *Diabetologia,* 45, 1011–1016, 2002.

222. Alvarez, O.M., Goslen, J.B., Eaglstein, W.H., Welgus, H.G., and Strickiln, G.P., Wound healing, in *Dermatology in General Medicine,* 3rd ed., Eisen, A., Freedberg, I., and Fitzpatrick, T., Eds., McGraw-Hill Book Co., New York, 1987.

223. Gabbiani, G., Chapponier, C., and Hunter, I., Cytoplasmic filaments and gap junctions in epithelial cells and myofibroblasts during wound healing, *J. Cell Biol.,* 76, 561–568, 1978.

224. Odland, G. and Ross, R., Human wound repair I. Epidermal regeneration, *J. Cell Biol.,* 39, 135–151, 1968.

225. Goncalves, J., Wasif, N., Esposito, D., Coiso, J.M., Higgins, P.J. et al., Gallium nitrate accelerates partial thickness wound repair and alters keratinocyte integrin expression to favor a motile phenotype, *J. Surg. Res.,* 103, 134–140, 2002.

226. Winter, G.D., Epidermal regeneration studied in the domestic pig, in *Epidermal Wound Healing*, Maibach H.I., and Rovee, D.T., Eds., Yearbook Medical Publishers, Chicago, 1972, pp. 71–112.

227. Waldorf, H., and Fewkes, J., Wound healing, *Adv. Dermatol.,* 10, 77–96, 1995.

228. Kubo, M., Norris, D.A., Howell, S.E. et al., Human keratinocytes synthesize, secrete and deposit fibronectin in the pericellular matrix, *J. Invest. Dermatol.,* 82, 580–586, 1984.

3 The Biochemistry of Epidermal Healing

Patricia A. Hebda and Vlad C. Sandulache

CONTENTS

0-8493-1561-1/04/$0.00+$1.50
© 2004 by CRC Press LLC

59

INTRODUCTION

This chapter will provide an overview of biochemical signals and pathways associated with the epidermal response to injury, as they are normally thought to occur. The biochemistry of epidermal healing has been and continues to be a burgeoning area of research; thus, it is not possible in a single chapter to discuss or even to mention in passing all of the published papers that contribute to our current understanding. Therefore, this chapter will focus on key biochemical signals associated with normal wound healing of the epidermis, as studied in human and other vertebrate skin. It is intended to provide an updated overview of relatively recent discoveries, within the mainstream of the field and confirmed if possible by independent investigators, and using selected citations to guide the reader to other resources for more extensive study. The successful exploration of this area of research has led to novel approaches for wound management directed toward employing and enhancing these biochemical events, some of which are further discussed in other chapters in this book.

3.1 INJURY AND THE ONSET OF BIOCHEMICAL SIGNALING

Coordination of degradative and regenerative processes requires a delicate balance of biochemical signaling and cellular responsiveness, which is mediated by locally released growth factors, cytokines and chemokines, which may act in an autocrine or paracrine manner. All phases of wound healing are either directly or indirectly controlled by these molecules, and it is the balance of these mediators rather than the mere presence or absence of one or more cytokines that plays a decisive role in regulating the initiation, progression, and resolution of wound healing.

Cells from different layers of the skin respond to injury according to their specific phenotypes. In the epidermis, only basal keratinocytes are continually renewing under normal conditions, while the suprabasal cells become postmitotic once they lose contact with the basement membrane and commit to terminal differentiation. In response to injury, basal keratinocytes at the skin surface and in hair follicles and sweat ducts regenerate by a regulated migration, mitosis, maturation sequence. This ability to respond depends on biochemical signaling — the molecular communication among cells of the same type (autocrine and juxtacrine induction) and between cells of different types (paracrine induction). Injured keratinocytes send out signals that recruit inflammatory cells, mainly neutrophils and macrophages, to the site of injury. The participating cells reconfigure their extracellular environment by regulation of the activities of proteases and by secreting extracellular matrix molecules. See Figure 3.1.

Biochemical Signals for Epidermal Wound Healing

Regulatory genes and signal transduction

Growth factors, cytokines, and chemokines

Blood coagulation products — complement cascade, platelet aggregation, fibrin formation

Extracellular matrix components — collagens, glycoproteins, proteoglycans

Cell adhesion molecules — cadherins and integrins

Protease activity — protease activators and inhibitors

Inorganic molecules — nitric oxide and reactive oxygen species

FIGURE 3.1 Biochemical signals for epidermal wound healing.

3.1.1 MIGRATION

Cells use mechanisms that depend on chemotaxis (directed movement in a chemical gradient) and pathway guidance (movement along or within a specific extracellular environment). Because they are anchorage-dependent cells, keratinocytes depend upon their cell–cell and cell–matrix attachments. Epidermal cells at the wound edges undergo structural changes, allowing them to reduce their tight connections to other epidermal cells, through decreased cadherins (cell–cell adherence junctions), and to their basement membrane, through altered expression of integrins (cell–matrix adherence junctions).[1] At the same time, they increase gap junctions (cell–cell communication junctions), and soluble signals (growth factors, cytokines, chemokines, and proteases) are locally activated and released to induce and support epidermal migration.[2,3,4] All of these processes combine to enable basal keratinocytes to switch from a stationary/resting to a migratory/activated phenotype — the cells change shape from cuboidal to squamous with lamellipodia and filopodia (cellular projections), become less firmly attached to neighboring cells, and move from the basement membrane, a substratum rich in laminin and collagen type IV, onto and across the wound bed, a substratum rich in fibrin, fibronectin, and collagen type I.[3,4]

Change in cell shape is controlled by reorganization of the cytoskeleton. In the cytoplasm, intracellular actin microfilaments are formed, which are attached to the cell membrane through focal adhesions. Focal adhesions are formed by a chain of proteins linked together that connect to the ends of actin filaments in the cytoplasm on one side and to integrin receptors in the cell membrane on the other side. The integrin receptors in turn attach to extracellular matrix molecules, thus allowing the epidermal cells to move across the wound surface through the directional formation of focal adhesions.[5,6] Calpains are a large family of intracellular proteases whose precise and limited cleavage of specific proteins might be an integral regulatory aspect of keratinocyte migration. They have been implicated in enabling cell spreading by modifying adhesion sites and in promoting locomotion of adherent cells by facilitating rear-end detachment of focal adhesions.[7]

Cells are enticed to migrate directionally, by a process called chemotaxis, which involves the movement of cells through a chemical gradient of a molecular stimulus or chemoattractant.[3,4] Numerous cytokines and growth factors can function in this role, and recently a new class of small proteins called chemokines has been described that appears to be specifically dedicated to this function.[8]

As cells migrate, they dissect the wound and separate the overlying fibrinous crust from the underlying viable tissue by localized release and activation of proteases, including collagenase-1, also called matrix metalloproteinase-1 (MMP-1), and plasmin. Epidermal cells secrete collagenases and other MMPs (gelatinases), which break down collagen, and plasminogen activator (PA), which stimulates production of plasmin. Plasmin promotes clot dissolution along the path of epithelial cell migration. Keratinocytes synthesize and secrete urokinase-type PA (uPA) bound in an autocrine manner to a specific receptor (uPA-R) at the keratinocyte surface. Plasminogen that is also bound to keratinocytes is readily activated by uPA-receptor–bound uPA. Thus, plasmin is provided for proteolysis of pericellular glycoproteins. Expression of uPA and the uPA receptor is limited to migrating keratinocytes during epidermal wound healing, rather than to keratinocytes of the normal epidermis.[9,10] The importance of plasminogen and plasmin in the wound healing cascade has been underscored by studies in transgenic mice missing or overexpressing the gene for PA inhibitor (PAI). These genetic knockout animals demonstrate a deficient wound healing phenotype, with severely delayed reepithelialization.[11] The importance of PAI activity for normal basal keratinocyte function has been confirmed by an independent group.[12]

The extracellular wound matrix over which epithelial cells migrate has received increased emphasis in wound healing research. Migrating epithelial cells interact with a provisional matrix of fibrin crosslinked to fibronectin and collagen. The matrix components may be a source of cell signals to facilitate epithelial cell proliferation and migration. In particular, fibronectin seems to promote keratinocyte adhesion to guide these cells across the wound bed.

During cutaneous wound repair, migrating keratinocytes were found to avoid the fibrin-rich clot, migrating instead along the collagen-rich dermal wound margin and over fibronectin-rich granulation tissue. The mechanism underlying keratinocyte movement in this precise pathway is attributed to the lack of expression of functional integrin receptors for fibrinogen/fibrin, specifically the αv-$\beta 3$ integrin. The investigators interpret these findings to mean that fibrinogen and fibrin are authentic antiadhesives for keratinocytes, and they further postulate that this attribute may explain why the migrating epidermis dissects the fibrin crust from wounds.[13]

Epithelial cell migration also may be facilitated in wound beds containing critical water content. Wounds with adequate tissue hydration demonstrate a faster and more direct course of epithelialization. Occlusive and semiocclusive dressings applied within a few hours after injury maintain tissue humidity and optimize epithelialization.[14,15]

The biochemical signals for these migratory events include:

1. Early genes, c-fos, c-jun, and other signal transduction molecules
2. Growth factors, cytokines, and chemokines, including transforming growth factor beta (TGF-β), interleukin (IL)-1, IL-6, IL-8, scatter factor/hepatocyte growth factor, epidermal growth factor (EGF), TGF-α, fibroblast growth factor (FGF)-2, keratinocyte growth factor (KGF)/FGF-7
3. Products of blood coagulation including fibrin-split peptides
4. Extracellular matrix components
5. Cell adhesion molecules — cadherins and integrins
6. Proteases, their activators and inhibitors
7. Nitric oxide (NO) and reactive oxygen species (ROS)

Most of these factors have complex interactions with epidermal cells during wound healing. For example, TGF-β, a potent inhibitor of epithelial cell proliferation, is present in the leading migrating edge and absent from the mitotically active compartment of regenerating epidermis.[16] TGF-β has been shown to increase epidermal outgrowth in skin explant cultures independent of mitosis;[17] this enhancement of migration may be due to the early induction of integrins for fibronectin.[18]

As migration progresses, some of the cells cease to migrate and commit to re-formation of the basement membrane. Other cells commit to mitosis to replace tissue volume lost during wounding. The stop signals for epidermal migration are not well characterized as yet, but it is clear that contact inhibition occurs as the migratory keratinocyte sheets converge within the wound. As keratinocytes re-form their basement membrane including the deposition of bullous pemphigoid antigen, collagen type IV, and laminins, keratinocytes re-express integrins specific for these basement membrane components.[19] In animal studies, laminin does not appear consistently until the migratory epithelium becomes stationary, suggesting that laminin inhibits migration *in vivo*.[20] Laminin also has been shown to inhibit keratinocyte migration *in vitro*.[21] Recent evidence indicates that molecules secreted by fibroblasts in the dermal compartment inhibit keratinocyte motility.[22] Deactivation may also occur as short-lived biochemical signals for migration diminish with the progression of healing.

3.1.2 MITOSIS

It is helpful and appropriate to consider the mitotic phase of epidermal wound healing as an ongoing process occurring in a specialized compartment, or microenvironment, within the newly forming epidermis rather than as a temporally distinct event. The biochemical components of this microenvironment provide the signals that regulate mitotic activity. Mitogenic growth factors for the epidermis include EGF, TGF-α, tumor necrosis factor alpha (TNF-α), FGF-2, and KGF/FGF-7, acting through signal transduction pathways.[3,4,23,24] Keratinocytes respond to these signals only if they are expressing the appropriate receptors. Within the mitotic compartment, cells are protected from antimitotic signals, such as TGF-β, which is absent from the mitotic region in epidermal wound healing,[16] and from apoptotic induction, by the protective signaling of the EGF receptor.[25] As mitosis proceeds, the keratinocytes become stratified and increase desmosomes (cell–cell attachments) with neighboring cells. Within the mitotic compartment, keratinocytes in the basal layer begin synthesizing and secreting bullous pemphigoid antigen and collagen type IV to reestablish the basement membrane.

Recently, plasminogen activator (PA) expression has been implicated in epidermal proliferation. Urokinase-PA (uPA), but not PA-inhibitor (PA-I), was found to be consistently elevated in the proliferative population of keratinocytes in a diverse range of hyperproliferative states, including wound healing. The investigators offered two hypotheses: either uPA plays a regulatory role in the activation of epidermal proliferation or uPA is involved in the vertical migration of keratinocytes that must accompany increased cell proliferation.[26] The second alternative would presumably involve u-PA activating interstitial plasminogen to form plasmin, which would cleave cell–cell attachments, thus permitting individual cell motility.

3.1.3 MATURATION

The completion of reepithelialization occurs with the regeneration of a stratified epidermis and restoration of a barrier in the stratum corneum. Much of this stage involves the normal ongoing process of terminal differentiation, but a few significant biochemical features should be noted. A transient hypertrophic phenotype is assumed by some of the cells accompanied by the expression of keratins 6 and 16.[24] Laminin synthesis is upregulated to complete the re-formation of the basement membrane, and keratinocytes in the basal layer increase expression of the laminin-specific integrin.[21] The cytoskeleton is reorganized to return to a resting, nonmigratory state. Actin reassembly is regulated by the Rho/ROCK signal transduction pathway.[27] The basement membrane zone is stabilized by minor matrix components including collagen type XVI[28] and laminin-5.[29]

3.1.4 SIGNAL TRANSDUCTION AND TRANSCRIPTION FACTORS IN REEPITHELIALIZATION

Signal transduction is the transmission of activation signals from outside to inside the cell, often through transmembrane receptors, some of which have enzymatically active cytoplasmic segments, e.g., kinase activity. The signal is propagated along a pathway of induction of cytoplasmic mediators and reaches the nucleus to affect selective gene expression. Transcription factors are regulatory proteins that mediate changes in gene expression in response to extracellular stimuli. Transcription factor activation in response to wounding is largely unexplored despite the potential of these factors to regulate the expression of key genes required during reepithelialization and other events of wound healing. Some features of growth factor–induced signal transduction relevant to wound healing are discussed below. The reader is directed to recent references in the literature for a more comprehensive treatment.

Members of the EGF growth factor family, including EGF and TGF-α, bind to the EGF receptor and activate mitogen activated protein kinase (MAPK), a tyrosine kinase, and its signaling pathway. The integrated biological responses to receptor signaling are pleiotropic and include mitogenesis or apoptosis, enhanced cell motility, protein secretion, and differentiation or dedifferentiation.[30]

The TGF-β family has several membrane receptors, each possessing a serine–threonine kinase activity within its cytoplasmic domain involved in signal transduction.[31] Recently, a novel group of proteins, Smads, has been shown to be specifically activated in response to TGF-β superfamily members.[32] Upon ligand binding, activation of serine–threonine kinase receptors of TGF-β induces phosphorylation of receptor-regulated Smads. Given the diverse and variable cellular responses elicited by TGF-β, it is not surprising that its signal transduction is rich in diversity. There are several members of the Smad family of cytoplasmic proteins, which combine during signal transduction and translocate to the nucleus where they activate gene expression directly or recruit nuclear transcription factors to participate in gene activation. At least one of the Smads, Smad7, is inhibitory to signal transduction, thus being implicated in some of the inconsistent cellular responses to TGF-β.[33]

FGF and vascular endothelial cell growth factor (VEGF) cell surface receptors have tyrosine kinase activity. These two related growth factor families exhibit high affinities for proteoglycans, and heparan sulfate proteoglycans help to regulate their signaling by direct molecular association with the growth factor and its receptor. The receptors for FGF and VEGF are tyrosine kinase-type receptors requiring the formation of a threshold number of phosphorylated cytoplasmic domains to initiate a specific signaling cascade; therefore, heparan sulfate proteoglycans may serve as co-activators of the receptor, or they may help to retain a critical number of growth factor ligands by limiting diffusion.[34]

Members of the activator protein-1 (AP-1) family, in particular c-fos and c-jun, are among the most widely studied wound-induced transcription factors. The signal transduction pathways linking cellular injury to AP-1 stimulation appear to involve an increase in intracellular Ca^{2+} and activation of MAPKs.[35] Wound-induced AP-1 activation has the potential to coordinate epidermal wound healing by regulating expression of genes involved in migration and differentiation in suprabasal epidermal layers and stimulating expression of proliferation genes in the basal layer. Additionally, cooperation with other transcription factors, including signal transducer and activator of transcription (STAT) and NF-κB, can broaden the range of downstream genes that are regulated.

E2F factors are involved in proliferation and apoptosis, and have been extensively studied.[36] A recent study using transgenic mice lacking E2F-1 gene expression revealed that this transcription factor is apparently essential for normal epidermal wound healing. E2F-1(–/–) keratinocytes showed impaired migration, attachment to extracellular matrix (ECM) proteins, and an impaired chemotactic response. Furthermore, E2F-1(–/–) keratinocytes, but not dermal fibroblasts, exhibit altered patterns of proliferation, including significant delays in transit through both G(1) and S phases of the cell cycle. In a subsequent experiment *in vivo,* E2F-1(–/–) mice had impaired cutaneous wound healing, with substantially reduced local inflammatory responses and rates of reepithelialization.[37]

Braun et al.[38] discuss a novel downstream target of KGF, transcription factor NF-E$_2$ related factor 2 (NRF2). NRF2 belongs to a family of transcription factors that bind to promoters of target genes using an antioxidant response element. Genes that are targeted by the NRF proteins include glutathione S-transferase, heme oxy-genase, and other detoxifying enzymes such as catalase and superoxide dismutase 1. By upregulating the expression of these genes, KGF can reduce the reactive oxygen species (ROS) load within the newly forming wound bed, while at the same time stimulating wound reepithelialization.

Peroxisome proliferator-activated receptors (PPARs) are transcription factors belonging to the family of ligand-inducible nuclear receptors. They control many cellular and metabolic processes including lipid metabolism and energy homeostasis. Three isotypes called PPARα, PPARβ/δ and PPARγ have been identified. PPARα and PPARγ control energy homoeostasis and inflammatory responses. Little is known about the main function of PPARβ/δ, but it is believed to play a role in skin wound healing; specifically, PPARβ/δ may be involved in keratinocyte maturation during wound healing.[119]

It will be very exciting to follow future development in this active area of research. Intracellular signaling molecules present another level of complexity in the wound healing arena but also provide numerous potential targets for therapeutic interventions.

3.2 KERATINOCYTES TALK (AND LISTEN)

The cutaneous wound healing process is a complex phenomenon characterized by the onset of a series of molecular events with a great degree of cross-talk. In order to restore the epithelial barrier, keratinocytes must migrate, proliferate, and differentiate into the normal epithelial structures. The course of these processes post-wounding is quite complex and relies not only upon normal keratinocyte properties, but also on interactions with the underlying mesenchymal layers as well as the immune system brought to bear on the wound by the adjacent circulation. Thus, epidermal wound healing becomes a process involving numerous cellular components and processes. The cells involved communicate with one another via physical interactions, but mostly through chemical signaling via growth factors and chemokines. Some signaling loops are direct, such as keratinocyte stimulation of fibroblast activity; others are indirect, such as keratinocyte stimulation of fibroblast release of keratinocyte-stimulating factors.

3.2.1 EPIDERMAL–DERMAL COMMUNICATION

In the skin, the interplay among keratinocytes, fibroblasts, resident and infiltrating leukocytes, endothelial cells, and stem cells is complex and contributes greatly to the maintenance of normal epidermal function and to the epidermal response to injury. Keratinocytes and fibroblasts are two of the most prominent players in epidermal wound healing.[40] Due to the complexity of the epidermis as a whole, several *in vitro* models have been developed to study the interactions between fibroblasts and keratinocytes. Keratinocytes and fibroblasts can be co-cultured in multiwell plates, with the fibroblasts forming a confluent monolayer on the bottom of each well. Keratinocytes are seeded and grown on inserts that are suspended above the fibroblast layer, thus allowing chemical signaling between the two cell populations. Keratinocytes can also be seeded directly onto a feeder layer of terminally irradiated fibroblasts. The underlying fibroblasts cannot divide, but they continue to secrete growth factors and cytokines that support keratinocyte growth. This methodology has been used to show *in vitro* that fibroblast feeder layers secrete insulin-like growth factors (IGFs) that can regulate keratinocyte growth.[41] Organotypic cultures, such as skin explants, maintain more of the epidermal and dermal organization found *in vivo*. These *in vitro* models have been used to evaluate effects of growth factors and other biochemical mediators on epithelialization within the presence of dermal components.[17] In other cases, *in vivo* wound healing has been studied using animal wound healing models and human tissues and wounds. Each model provides insight into certain aspects of wound healing within a complex environment. However, results must be interpreted accordingly; *in vitro* models afford more control and simplification to focus on isolated features, whereas *in vivo* models are more complex and provide for systemic as well as local interactions.

3.2.2 KEY GROWTH FACTORS AND OTHER WOUND MEDIATORS

3.2.2.1 Epidermal Growth Factor, a Classic Epidermal Mitogen

Epidermal growth factor (EGF) was one of the first growth factors to be identified, and it was quickly shown to have wound-healing properties. Another member of the EGF family is transforming growth factor alpha (TGF-α); both act on cells by binding to the EGF receptor. One of EGF's major functions is to stimulate mitosis in epithelial cells, but like other factors, it can contribute to additional aspects of wound healing. EGF may play a dominant early role in wound healing by stimulating keratinocyte proliferation and migration while keratinocyte growth factor (KGF) may play a role later in the repair process by stabilizing epidermal turnover and barrier function.[42]

3.2.2.2 Fibroblast Growth Factors, a Family of Epidermal Modulators

Fibroblast growth factor-2 (FGF-2) and keratinocyte growth factor (KGF), also named FGF-7, are produced by fibroblasts following stimulation from keratinocyte signaling. Although FGF-2 acts on both fibroblasts and keratinocytes, KGF acts exclusively on epidermal cells; both have been shown to stimulate epidermal wound healing.[43,44] To add to the complexity, keratinocytes release factors that act on fibroblasts to induce their secretion of KGF (see below).

KGF has a unique role as a mediator of mesenchymal–epithelial interactions. It originates from mesenchymal cells yet acts exclusively on epithelial cells. A good review of the history and functions of KGF can be found in Beer et al.[45] KGF has close homology to FGF-10, with both molecules signaling via the FGFR2-IIIb receptor. The activities of these two factors with respect to wound healing have been shown to be complementary and somewhat redundant. KGF is normally expressed at low levels by fibroblasts, among other cells. Upon injury, KGF is significantly upregulated. Exposure to KGF results in increased keratinocyte proliferation and migration. KGF is also thought to reduce toxicity in the wound bed by reducing exposure to reactive oxygen species (ROS), as discussed above.[38]

A signaling loop mechanism involving keratinocytes and fibroblasts has been described by Maas-Szabowski et al.[39] Upon stimulation by injury or other means, keratinocytes begin to secrete interleukin-1 (IL-1). IL-1 can, among other activities, stimulate production of KGF by the underlying layers of fibroblasts. KGF is then detected by the keratinocytes and upregulates various epidermal functions such as proliferation. Another example of this epidermal–dermal communication is parathyroid hormone-related protein (PTHrP). PTHrP is produced in keratinocytes, where its major function is thought to be the regulation of cell growth and differentiation including hair follicle development, but it is also a potential paracrine regulator of KGF expression by dermal fibroblasts *in vivo*.[46]

3.2.2.3 Transforming Growth Factor Beta, a Master Growth Factor

Transforming growth factor beta (TGF-β) is one of the more intriguing growth factors participating in epidermal wound healing, not only for its wide variety of activities, including the modulation of other growth factors, but also for its interesting temporal distribution.[47] TGF-β has been shown to induce epidermal migration and motility.[17] TGF-β1 expression appears to be well coordinated with increased integrin expression during the initial reepithelialization of the wound, facilitating epidermal migration during early wound healing.[48] In addition to this effect, TGF-β1 has been shown to inhibit keratinocyte proliferation of basal cells. At the same time, it inhibits normal keratinization in suprabasal cells and promotes differentiation.[49] TGF-β can affect the synthesis of keratinocyte proteins, especially those controlled by keratin promoters such as K5 and K14.[50] In turn, keratinocytes appear to be able to suppress TGF-β expression by fibroblasts.[51]

Inhibition of keratinocyte mitosis by factors such as TGF-β is important in the early stages of healing, when keratinocytes must be recruited for migration and reepithelialization. It is also important in later stages when the wound healing response must be downregulated to prevent hypertrophy and hyperproliferation. In these later stages of wound healing, TGF-β can alter the expression of metalloproteinases (MMPs) and their respective tissue inhibitors (TIMPs). This effect is a synergistic one, in which TGF-β acts as a modulator of the activities of other growth factors such as EGF and FGF-2.[52] TGF-β can also increase matrix incorporation of fibronectin and collagen.[53]

TGF-β offers an interesting insight into the importance of spatial and temporal regulation of the wound healing process. More importantly, it proves that the healing process depends to a large degree on the close cooperation of the epidermal and dermal layers. Initially, TGF-β secretion serves to promote keratinocyte migration and covering of the fresh wound bed. In the later stages, TGF-β serves to aid in the deposition of the new ECM. As the process winds down, fibroblasts and keratinocytes communicate with one another via TGF-β in order to downregulate the healing response and become differentiated and quiescent.

3.2.2.4 Hepatocyte Growth Factor

Hepatocyte growth factor (HGF) and macrophage-stimulating protein (MSP) are structurally related molecules that stimulate epithelial migration and proliferation. HGF is alternatively called scatter factor because it promotes the dissociation of epidermal cells, a necessary step in the migratory response, as previously discussed. MSP also acts directly as a chemoattractant for resident macrophages. All of these activities are integral to the wound healing processes of inflammation, reepithelialization, and tissue remodeling. HGF and its receptor are increased after wounding primarily in dermal fibroblasts.[54]

3.2.2.5 Cytokines and Chemokines, Signals for Inflammatory Responses

Proinflammatory cytokines, including TNF-α, IL-1, IL-6, and IL-8, are present in epidermal wounds and have been found to promote wound healing responses. It was reported that addition of either TNF-α or IL-1 induced the secretion of uPA and upregulation of the PA receptor in a human keratinocyte cell line (HaCaT). This induction caused detachment of HaCaT cells from the culture substratum. The overall effect of these activities supports a role for TNF-α and IL-1β in inducing keratinocyte motility.[10]

The chemokines IL-8 and growth-related oncogene-alpha (GRO-α) play a prominent part in wound healing as well as in inflammatory skin disorders, such as psoriasis. Both are involved in neutrophil recruitment and activation and also have the potential to stimulate keratinocyte proliferation *in vitro*. Their expression in keratinocytes is induced by IL-1 and they may be the primary means by which IL-1 stimulates keratinocyte proliferation, since antibodies against IL-8 greatly reduced IL-1 mitotic effects on keratinocytes in culture.[55] The recruitment of neutrophils by these chemokines also provides protection from bacterial growth in the wound.

3.2.2.6 Nitric Oxide Expression in Wound Healing

Another signaling pathway that has been implicated in epidermal–dermal communication during wound healing is the nitric oxide (NO) pathway. NO has long been categorized as a blood vessel relaxing factor. In addition to vasodilatory properties, NO has been shown to possess antimicrobial, immunoregulatory, and neurotransmitter properties. NO is synthesized by the enzyme nitric oxide synthase (NOS) via the oxidation of L-arginine with O_2 to form NO and L-citrulline. There are several isoforms of the enzyme, of which three are well characterized. Two isoforms depend on intracellular calcium concentrations and exogenous calmodulin. These isoforms are constitutively expressed (cNOS). The inducible NOS (iNOS) isoform is not dependent on intracellular calcium and has its own bound calmodulin unit. This isoform is upregulated under specific conditions, such as inflammation.

Production of NO has been identified in normal human keratinocytes. Keratinocytes possess the constitutively expressed cNOS enzyme,[56] and dermal fibroblasts express the cNOS isoform as well the iNOS isoform of the enzyme.[57] In fibroblasts, iNOS reacts to inflammatory cytokines such as ILs, TNF-α, interferon gamma (IFN-γ) or bacterial lipopolysaccharide (LPS). The expression of NOS during wound healing by both keratinocytes and fibroblasts leads to the speculation that NO may play an important role in the wound healing process.

It has not yet been established that keratinocytes and fibroblasts communicate with one another via NO. However, since both have the capacity to produce NO, it follows that this production would be coordinated under normal wound healing conditions. With strict cooperation, keratinocytes and fibroblasts can produce NO in such a quantity and with such a temporal expression as to ensure proper development of new blood vessels and thus coordinate angiogenesis in the newly forming wound bed.

Disregulation of NO signaling has been identified in abnormal wound healing responses as well as in aberrant epidermal conditions. In psoriasis, the iNOS isoform is upregulated in psoriatic plaques when compared to normal skin.[58] More importantly, cNOS is downregulated in hypertrophic wound-derived fibroblasts, whereas iNOS activity remains unaltered.[59] These alterations in the expression patterns of NOS isoforms in aberrant epidermal responses serve to further implicate NO as having a role in epidermal healing.

In addition to its angiogenic activity, NO has been implicated in other aspects of wound healing. Exogenous NO has a biphasic effect on keratinocyte proliferation and differentiation,[60] further indicating the need for coordinated regulation of NO synthesis and release.

3.2.2.7 Temporal Sequence of Growth Factor Release

Keratinocytes and fibroblasts can be perceived as having a dual role. Both cell types have an anabolic function: rebuilding the extracellular matrix (ECM). At the same time, both are secretory factories, releasing growth factors, chemokines, and cytokines. It is important to realize that this secretory process has a very important temporal component. A specific growth factor released at the beginning of the wound healing process can have a very different effect from the same factor released later in the process because the wound environment and responding cells have changed.

As described above, IL-1 secretion by keratinocytes alters keratinocyte properties via fibroblast mediation. In addition to this effect, IL-1α has been shown to have an important role in inhibiting connective tissue growth factor (CTGF) production in fibroblasts. CTGF is important in directing fibroblast proliferation and collagen synthesis, activities which occur relatively late in the wound healing response. Early induction of CTGF is inappropriate, as is delayed induction. Interestingly, CTGF activity is also controlled to a large degree by TGF-β. Dual control of CTGF by IL-1 and TGF-β must be properly timed and integrated, so that one signal does not nullify the action of the other. On a larger scale, fibroblast involvement in the wound healing process must be timed in such a manner so that it correlates with keratinocyte migration, infiltration of the wound by inflammatory cells, and other ongoing processes.[61]

The integration of the various growth factors in a coherent wound healing response is crucial to proper restoration of epidermal integrity and structure. Secretion of EGF and FGF, for example, must be precisely timed to take full advantage of their respective activities. Keratinocytes respond to EGF by increasing proliferation and migration, accompanied by keratin 6 and 16 expression.[42] These two molecules are involved in rearrangement of the cytoskeleton, which is crucial to keratinocyte migration. In contrast, KGF appears to act later in the wound healing process, contributing to reestablishment of the barrier function of the epidermis and restructuring events. A more detailed review of the process of keratinocyte activation is offered by Freedberg et al.[62]

3.2.2.8   Extracellular Matrix in Regulation of Epidermal Healing

The extracellular matrix (ECM) is of crucial importance in epidermal–dermal communication during wound healing. The ECM is synthesized and remodeled largely, though not exclusively, by fibroblasts. Fibroblasts migrate into the wound bed and secrete collagens, glycoproteins, proteoglycans, and other molecules, which are then remodeled into a permanent matrix. The composition of the provisional matrix that is available can significantly alter the behavior of the overlying keratinocyte population. In order to reepithelialize the wound, keratinocytes must migrate into the newly denuded area. This migration is a complex process of cytoskeletal rearrangement, coupled to attachment and detachment from the underlying surface. Studies *in vitro* have found enhanced attachment by activated keratinocytes to collagen types I and IV and to matrigel (a basement-membrane-derived ECM), but not to substrates having the RGD-cell attachment site, including vitronectin and fibronectin. (The term RGD refers to the tripeptide Arg-Gly-Asp, a cell attachment sequence in many ECM proteins.) The substrate can alter not only attachment but also proliferation.[63] It then becomes evident that ECM deposition must be coordinated through cross-talk between keratinocytes and fibroblasts. This cross-talk is accomplished via the numerous secreted biochemical signals, growth factors and cytokines, some of which have been discussed above.

Syndecan 1 is a membrane proteoglycan that contains both heparin and chondroitin sulfate side chains and is found mostly in epithelia. Syndecan 1 is upregulated at the messenger RNA (mRNA) and protein levels in wound edge keratinocytes. Syndecan 1 has been found to be activated by KGF, but in an ECM-dependent manner. For example, fibronectin enhances syndecan 1 induction.[64]

The role of laminin, primarily laminin-1, in signaling keratinocytes to stop migration is well known.[21] However, another member of the laminin family, laminin 5, has more recently been shown to play a related role in this signaling. Laminin 5 deposited by leading keratinocytes onto dermal collagen dominates over dermal ligands and changes the integrin expression from collagen dependent to laminin 5 dependent. Thus, deposition of laminin 5 is believed to direct keratinocytes to switch from an activated phenotype to a quiescent and integrated epithelial phenotype.[29]

Ruehl et al.[65] have reported that KGF binds collagen molecules using a consensus sequence of glycine–proline–hydroxyproline. The functional purpose of this binding is as yet unclear, but it is likely to increase the available concentration of KGF in a region-specific manner, increasing the specificity of the signals that are sent back and forth between keratinocytes and fibroblasts.

A possible role of collagen in regulating protease activation was recently reported. In this study, exposed interstitial collagens (collagen types I and III) were shown to selectively regulate expression of PA and PAI in keratinocytes in an *in vitro* model system. Activated keratinocytes were cultured in dishes coated with collagen or other ECM substrates. Then, tissue plasminogen activator (tPA), uPA, and PAI-1 mRNA and protein levels were measured. When activated keratinocytes were attached to fibronectin, vitronectin, collagen IV, or RGD peptide, there was no effect. In contrast, attachment to native collagen I, collagen III, or laminin completely suppressed expression of PAI-1 mRNA and protein and further increased tPA expression and activity; this effect was lost with denatured molecules. Thus, it would appear that interstitial collagens and laminin regulate the gene expression of molecules associated with plasminogen activation in favor of increased plasmin activation. This finding provides an additional dimension in the regulation of cell movement and matrix remodeling by the extracellular environment.[66]

In summary, the ECM must be deposited in a controlled manner, so as to support wound repair. Interactions between cells and the ECM are dependent on the growth factors available as well as the ECM itself. Finally, the secretion of growth factors is influenced by the surrounding matrix, which can either trap or release them and thus impact communication.

3.2.2.9 Matrix Metalloproteinases and Other Proteases

Matrix metalloproteinases (MMPs) are a family of at least 20 zinc-dependent endopeptidases activated by other proteinases, e.g., plasmin and other MMPs, as well as by autocatalysis.[67] MMP activity is antagonized by specific, naturally occurring tissue inhibitors of MMPs (TIMPs) and by synthetic inhibitors.[68] Several MMPs and serine proteinases are upregulated in migrating keratinocytes during cutaneous wound repair. Interstitial collagenase-1 (MMP-1) is involved in the activation of epithelial migration *in vitro*[69] and *in vivo* in early wound healing.[70,71]

The roles of the two gelatinases, MMP-2 and MMP-9, in epidermal healing are less well studied, possibly due to varying experimental circumstances producing disparate results.[72,73] *In vitro*, MMP-9, but not MMP-2, is induced when primary human keratinocytes are juxtaposed to type I collagen.[74] Furthermore, conversion to a migratory keratinocyte phenotype coincided with MMP-9 induction.[75] In contrast, Charvat et al.[76] found that repopulation of denuded human keratinocyte monolayers (HaCaT cells) on collagen type I was inhibited in a concentration-dependent manner by the synthetic MMP inhibitor BB-2516 (marimastat) and was associated with increased activity of MMP-2, but not of MMP-9. This finding that MMP-2 but not MMP-9 is upregulated in wound healing has recently been independently confirmed.[77] In other *in vitro* studies,

MMP-2 expression increased in keratinocytes co-cultured with dermal fibro-blasts.[74,78,79] These observations emphasize the complex cell–cell and cell–matrix interactions in MMP regulation.

Epilysin (MMP-28) is a recently identified member of the matrix metallopro-teinase enzyme family. It is produced by mitotic keratinocytes distal from the wound edge in both acute and chronic wounds and does not generally colocalize with other MMPs found in migrating keratinocytes. Its expression is upregulated by several early wound healing signals, including TNF-α. Epilysin expression is regulated spatially and temporally during epidermal healing. Although the *in vivo* substrates of epilysin are not presently known, its expression pattern suggests that it may be involved in restructuring the basement membrane and/or degrading cell–cell adhesive proteins for the recruitment of keratinocytes to the migrating front.[80]

Fibroblasts and keratinocytes have the ability to restructure the extracellular matrix using a variety of secreted MMPs and TIMPs. The overall activity of each enzyme thus depends on the relative ratio of the MMP to its specific TIMP. The aggregate ratio of all MMPs to all TIMPs can offer a global view of the status of the ECM. This process becomes particularly important during wound healing when the provisional ECM must be laid down quickly, only to be replaced later by the permanent ECM. MMP activity is largely controlled by multiple growth factors involved in the wound healing process. TGF-β1 in particular plays an important role in MMP regulation. In general, TGF-β stabilizes the extracellular matrix by coor-dinately decreasing MMPs and increasing TIMP levels.[47]

Proteinases are involved in several processes during wound healing. Serine proteinases, such as uPA and plasmin, and MMPs are the main proteinases implicated in epidermal repair.[9,81–83] In plasminogen-deficient mice, Rømer et al.[81] demonstrated impaired healing of wounds, although epithelialization was not totally blocked. Using the same plasminogen-deficient animal wound model, Lund et al.[84] were able to block healing completely by administering the synthetic MMP inhibitor GM 6001 systemically, thus demonstrating indirectly the importance of PAs and MMPs in epidermal healing.

These proteinases primarily facilitate keratinocyte movement by remodeling extracellular matrix proteins. MMP-1 has been ascribed a crucial role in keratinocyte migration.[69] In addition, proteinases modulate intracellular signaling, secretion, bio-activation, and stability of cytokines and growth factors important for epidermal healing.[85–89] In addition to other roles in wound healing, growth factors regulate MMP activities.[74,79,90]

3.2.3 COMMUNICATION WITH OTHER SYSTEMS

It is important to realize that since every cell present in the wound bed has some secretory capability, all the cells in this environment have the potential to cross-talk with one another in order to synchronize the overall response to injury. Therefore, attention must be paid to all cellular components in order to obtain a generalized, integrated picture of the wound healing response.

3.2.3.1   Inflammation and the Immune System

Epidermal activation and migration can take place in the absence of blood coagulation or any inflammatory events. In normal skin, suction and friction blisters, and pure epidermal wounds initiate healing almost immediately and rapidly proceed to complete reepithelialization, especially with occlusion. One is led to the conclusion that the biochemical signals necessary for epidermal healing are available within the epidermal compartment. In fetal wounds of the skin, the inflammatory response is absent or greatly attenuated, and in this scenario as well, healing progresses with no apparent need for mediators generated during inflammation.[91]

However, there is also evidence for biochemical communication between keratinocytes and inflammatory cells, including several cytokines and chemokines secreted by keratinocytes. IL-1, IL-6, IL-8, and GRO-α have all been found to be produced by keratinocytes in response to injury.[92–94] Macrophages release cytokines and growth factors that target the epidermis, including TGF-β and TNF-α.

It has been shown that gamma delta T cells play an important role in wound healing. Gamma delta T cells produce KGF and thus stimulate keratinocyte functions. Secretion of KGF is not constitutive, but rather it is upregulated upon activation via the T cell receptor (TCR). Mice that lack gamma delta T cells have a delayed wound healing response and exhibit decreased epidermal proliferation.[95]

There is also clear evidence that the wound healing process is influenced by the immune system and the overall immune status of the individual. Patients with keloids exhibit altered immune profiles, with decreased levels of IFN-α and IFN-γ as well as TGF-β; whereas IL-6, TGF-α, and IFN-β are upregulated systemically.[96]

These changes indicate an important role for the immune system, including T-lymphocytes, in regulation of the wound healing response. Conversely, it has been reported that epithelial coverage of dermal wounds downregulated inflammation and the expression of inflammatory mediators.

3.2.3.2   Angiogenesis

Both hydrogen peroxide and TNF-α induce keratinocytes to increase mRNA and protein levels of vascular endothelial cell growth factor (VEGF), a potent promoter of angiogenesis.[97,98] Keratinocytes during wound healing *in vivo* are also a source of placenta growth factor, another member of the VEGF family, which suggests a role for this factor in the neoangiogenesis process associated with cutaneous wound repair.[99]

Many of the growth factors, cytokines, and proteases that stimulate epidermal healing also induce similar responses in vascular endothelial cells (a type of epithelial tissue), promoting migration, mitosis, and maturation of new blood vessels in wound granulation tissue.

3.2.3.3   Innervation

Epidermal injury activates neural components in the epidermis. Various studies have suggested that the rate of healing may in some way be dependent on signals emanating from cutaneous nerves. Furthermore, wounds become hyperinnervated by sensory nerves during the process of healing. In a chick wound healing model, it was found that from the earliest stages of skin healing, the presence of nerves is beneficial to the healing process.[100]

Effects of local stimulation of sympathetic postganglionic neurons with 6-hydroxydopamine were studied in a rat wound healing model. The results showed a 35% increase in the rate of epidermal wound healing, as measured by increases in electrical resistance. The conclusion of the study was that pharmacological stimulation of sympathetic postganglionic neurons markedly accelerates skin wound healing at both the epidermal and dermal levels. This was the first study to show that peripheral nerve stimulation and specifically sympathetic stimulation accelerates cutaneous wound healing.[101]

3.3 KELOID KERATINOCYTES (DO THEY SEND DIFFERENT SIGNALS?)

Studies of normal epidermal–dermal interactions have been aided by analysis of aberrant epidermal healing responses, as in the case of keloid formation. Aberrant healing can shed light on normal communication between keratinocytes and the underlying fibroblasts.

Keloids represent an aberrant wound healing response in which the scar that is formed is unusually large and extends beyond the initial edges of the wound. The cause of keloids has yet to be identified, but both keratinocytes and fibroblasts are thought to play a role, as there appear to be alterations in the phenotypes of both types of cells. At the level of the fibroblast, levels of hyaluronic acid secretion by normal fibroblasts are higher than those of their keloid counterparts.[102] Collagen production by keloid fibroblasts is increased.[103] Keloid fibroblasts may also have a decreased dependence on growth factors present in the environment, which may allow for hyperproliferation and increased collagen synthesis, despite the lack of indications of activation in the surrounding epidermal tissuen.[104]

While fibroblasts have intrinsic properties that seem to be responsible for keloid response to injury, keratinocytes play a crucial role in influencing this process. Significantly, increased proliferation was seen in normal fibroblasts co-cultured with keloid keratinocytes, as compared with normal keratinocyte controls. Keloid keratinocytes increase the rate of keloid fibroblast proliferation even more than normal fibroblasts do.[105]

Normal keratinocytes can increase secretion of soluble collagen types I and III by normal and keloid fibroblasts. Keloid keratinocytes have the added effect of altering the ratios of soluble to insoluble collagen types I and III. They also alter the pattern of collagen fiber assembly, resulting in denser, more random-looking fibers.[106] Normal fibroblasts retain a fairly precise ratio of soluble to insoluble collagen, as well as a ratio between the various types of collagen produced; however, keloid fibroblasts appear to not be constrained in this manner. In keloids, the fibroblasts appear to be constitutively disregulated. The addition of keloid keratinocytes pushes this disregulation even further, exacerbating the abnormal rates of collagen production and deposition, presumably by means of the same epidermal–dermal communication pathways already discussed. In the case of hypertrophic scarring, another type of fibrotic healing, IL-1α and platelet-derived growth factor (PDGF) showed significant alterations compared to normal healing tissue.[107] TGF-β1 has been shown to have a significant impact on fibroblast collagen production.[108]

3.4 FETAL WOUND HEALING

Within a certain gestational window that is different for different mammalian species, cutaneous fetal wound healing occurs regeneratively and without scarring. The study of fetal wound healing is intriguing and may result in the discovery of an optimal wound therapy that would allow wounds to heal with little or no scar formation.

The fetal wound healing phenotype has several distinctive features. First, the cells involved exhibit a phenotype distinct from that of their adult counterparts. A significant body of research shows that fetal fibroblasts, particularly dermal fibroblasts, have ECM synthetic properties different from those of adult fibroblasts. Fetal keratinocytes, though less well studied, also appear to have different properties from adult keratinocytes. The response of fetal keratinocytes to retinoic acid, an important dermal and epidermal messenger, differs from that of neonatal keratinocytes with respect to morphology and various differentiation markers.[109] The expression patterns of differentiation-specific keratins, filaggrin, and retinoic acid-inducible K19 show that they are expressed in fetal skin, modulated by retinoic acid, but have an aberrant distribution compared with neonatal skin. Depending on their gestational stage, fetal keratinocytes have variable ability to form the fully differentiated stratum corneum.

A second distinguishing feature of fetal skin is altered cell–cell communication. Gap junction formation in the fetal epidermis increases with increasing gestational age, indicating that fetal epidermal tissue has relatively low cell–cell communication capability.[110] A third feature is the altered interaction between resident cells and the extracellular matrix in fetal tissue. Following injury, fetal skin exhibits increased expression of integrins at the wound edge, which continues until epithelialization is complete.[111] Since integrins are important in keratinocyte migration, it is possible that different rates of integrin expression translate into different rates of keratinocyte migration. The rate of integrin upregulation in the wound edge appears to be different in adult and fetal tissue. Increased keratinocyte migration leads to faster reepithelialization, which decreases exposure of the wound to the external environment, while at the same time reducing inflammation.

There is speculation that the differences in the wound biochemical environment in early gestational age fetal wounds, rather than the responding fetal cells, account for the absence of scar formation. One difference in the fetal wound environment is the greatly diminished inflammatory response with relatively fewer neutrophils and more monocytes. There are also differences in the expression of cytokines and growth factors, and a proportionately greater amount of collagen type III in contrast to adult wounds. TGF-β activity, believed to have a central role in scar formation, has been a focus of fetal wound healing research to date. A greater amount of EGF (a mitogen for epithelialization), a faster rate of wound healing, and a greater amount of hyaluronic acid in the extracellular matrix have been documented in fetal wound healing models and suggest a more efficient process of wound healing in the fetus.

In addition, fibronectin is more abundant in fetal wounds and was reported to accelerate wound healing in fetal rat models.[91,112] Being a very large molecule, fibronectin synthesis involves transcriptional splicing steps leading to the formation of several splicing isoforms of fibronectin. It is of interest to note that the pattern of fibronectin splicing during wound healing appears to revert to an embryonic pattern. This suggests that alternative splicing may be used to generate forms of this important matrix molecule that best promote cell migration and proliferation associated with tissue repair.[113]

In fetal wounds, TGF-β1 has been found to be decreased compared to adult wounds. Given the ability of TGF-β to stabilize ECM through its effects on MMP and TIMP activities (see above), one would predict that matrix turnover is accelerated in the presence of lower levels of TGF-β. Addition of exogenous TGF-β1 to fetal wounds results in adult-like scarring, mainly via regulation of the MMPs involved, such as collagenase.[114] Recently, it has been reported that expression levels of FGFs and their receptors are significantly lower in scarless fetal wound healing.[115] These findings are interesting and somewhat surprising given the importance of both TGF-βs and FGFs in development, yet they reflect the effective compartmentalization of metabolic activities by the organism.

The fetal wound healing phenotype is thus dependent on the various cellular components involved. Just as importantly, however, it is dependent on the cross-talk among these various components. Keratinocytes and fibroblasts interact with each other and with the surrounding matrix, as well as the various inflammatory components, to create an altered healing motif, with more structured ECM construction, increased epithelialization, and decreased inflammation. Embryonic dermis exercises a unique transient induction of the embryonic epidermis for generation of epidermal appendages (sweat glands and hair follicles), which occurs in a restricted stage of fetal development. Fetal tissue undergoes a switch to healing with scar formation concurrent with loss of epidermal inductive capacity manifested as a decreased ability to induce epidermal appendage formation, suggesting that epidermal–dermal interactions play an important role in scarless fetal repair.[112]

Little research has focused on fetal epidermal healing. However, it has been reported that epidermal wound closure is qualitatively different in fetal vs. adult skin. Studies in the chick embryo indicate that rather than cytoskeletal rearrangement to form lamellipodia and migrating keratinocytes, wound closure is achieved, at least in part, by the reorganization of actin filaments circumferentially in cells along the margin, after which the edges are pulled together by contraction of this actin network through the action of myosin, recruited to the site.[116,117] Healing of the epithelium depends on a combination of purse-string contraction and zipper-like closure of the gap between the cut edges of the epithelium.[117] Blocking studies indicate that actin assembly is essential for reepithelialization and that it occurs through a Rho-dependent signaling pathway.[117] However, a more recent study indicates that migration is also important for fetal reepithelialization. In this case, human fetal skin was transplanted onto immunodeficient mice and wounds created. In this model, grafts reepithelialized rapidly (within 24 to 36 h) and healed scarlessly. Within several hours, the grafts showed increased integrin expression at the epidermal wound edges, which persisted until healing was complete. This altered integrin expression in fetal wounds suggests that reepithelialization is occurring by keratinocyte migration over the wound substratum and may be important in limiting the induction of inflammatory mediators and scar.[111] The differential results in two different fetal wound healing models may be attributable to species differences, differences in gestational stage relative to the scarless fetal wound healing phenotype, or differences in the experimentally constructed wound environments.

While there is evidence that early fetal wound models heal more efficiently than adult wounds do, the explanation of how this more efficient process leads to the absence of scar formation remains elusive. The potential to control the formation of the scar may lie in alterations of the wound environment to mimic fetal wound models, but further study is required before such an endeavor is possible.

3.5 CONCLUSION

As the biochemical signaling pathways of epidermal healing become known, improved wound healing therapies should follow. Current wound care is designed to support and enhance this process. For example, the use of occlusive wound dressings for moist wound healing provides a favorable environment in which these molecules can function.[118] The application of exogenous proteases and growth factors to chronic wounds such as pressure ulcers and diabetic foot ulcers has had some success in improving impaired healing.[3] However, challenges still remain in achieving a comprehensive understanding of this complex process; knowing which factor is acting at what time on which population of responsive target cells is an ongoing vital quest in wound healing research.

ABBREVIATIONS

AP-1	Activator protein-1
ECM	Extracellular matrix
EGF	Epidermal growth factor
FGF	Fibroblast growth factor
GRO-α	Growth-related oncogene alpha
HGF	Hepatocyte growth factor (a.k.a. scatter factor)
IL	Interleukin
KGF	Keratinocyte growth factor (a.k.a. FGF-7)
MAPK	Mitogen activated protein kinase
MMP	Matrix metalloproteinase
MSP	Macrophage stimulating protein
NOS (iNOS or cNOS)	Nitric oxide synthase (inducible or constitutive)
PA (t or u)	Plasminogen activator (tissue or urokinase)
PAI	Plasminogen activator inhibitor
PDGF	Platelet-derived growth factor
PPAR	Peroxisome proliferator-activated receptor
RGD	Tripeptide Arg-Gly-Asp, a cell attachment sequence in many ECM proteins

ROS   Reactive oxygen species
TGF-(α and β)   Transforming growth factor alpha and beta
TNF-α Tumor necrosis factor alpha
VEGF   Vascular endothelial cell growth factor

REFERENCES

1. Larjava, H., Salo, T., Haapasalmi, K., Kramer, R.H., and Heino, J., Expression of integrins and basement membrane components by wound keratinocytes, *J. Clin. Invest.*, 92, 1425–1435, 1993.
2. Bennett, N.T. and Schultz, G.S., Growth factors and wound healing: part II. Role in normal and chronic wound healing. *Am. J. Surg.*, 166, 74–81, 1993.
3. Clark, R.A.F., Wound repair: overview and general considerations, in Clark. R.A.F., Ed., *The Molecular and Cellular Biology of Wound Repair*, Plenum Press, New York, 1996, pp. 3–50.
4. Falanga, V., Ed., *Cutaneous Wound Healing*, Martin Dunitz, London, 2001.
5. Petit, V. and Thiery, J.P., Focal adhesions: structure and dynamics, *Biol. Cell*, 92, 477–494, 2000.
6. Mostafavi-Pour, Z., Askari, J.A., Parkinson, S.J., Parker, P.J., Ng, T.T., and Humphries, M.J., Integrin-specific signaling pathways controlling focal adhesion formation and cell migration, *J. Cell Biol.*, 161, 155–167, 2003.
7. Glading, A., Lauffenburger, D.A., and Wells, A., Cutting to the chase: calpain proteases in cell motility, *Trends Cell Biol.*, 12, 46–54, 2002.
8. Gillitzer, R. and Goebeler, M., Chemokines in cutaneous wound healing, *J. Leukocyte Biol.*, 69, 513–521, 2001.
9. Grondahl-Hansen, J., Lund, L.R., Ralfkiaer, E., Ottevanger, V., and Dano, K., Urokinase- and tissue-type plasminogen activators in keratinocytes during wound reepithelialization *in vivo*, *J. Invest. Dermatol.*, 90, 790–795, 1988.
10. Bechtel, M.J., Reinartz, J., Rox, J.M., Inndorf, S., Schaefer, B.M., and Kramer, M.D., Upregulation of cell-surface-associated plasminogen activation in cultured keratinocytes by interleukin-1 beta and tumor necrosis factor-alpha, *Exp. Cell Res.*, 223, 395–404, 1996.
11. Eitzman, D.T. and Ginsburg, D., Of mice and men. The function of plasminogen activator inhibitors (PAIs) *in vivo*, *Adv. Exp. Med. Biol.*, 425, 131–141, 1997.
12. Li, F., Goncalves, J., Faughnan, K., Steiner, M.G., Pagan-Charry, I., Esposito, D., Chin, B., Providence, K.M., Higgins, P.J., and Staiano-Coico, L., Targeted inhibition of wound-induced PAI-1 expression alters migration and differentiation in human epidermal keratinocytes, *Exper. Cell Res.*, 258, 245–253, 2000.
13. Kubo, M., Van de Water, L., Plantefaber, L.C., Mosesson, M.W., Simon, M., Tonnesen, M.G., Taichman, L., and Clark, R.A., Fibrinogen and fibrin are antiadhesive for keratinocytes: a mechanism for fibrin eschar slough during wound repair, *J. Invest. Dermatol.*, 117, 1369–1381, 2001.
14. Fisher, L.B. and Maibach, H.I., The effect of occlusive and semipermeable dressings on the mitotic activity of normal and wounded human epidermis, *Br. J. Dermatol.*, 86, 593–600, 1972.
15. Eaglstein, W.H., Davis, S.C., Mehle, A.L., and Mertz, P.M., Optimal use of an occlusive dressing to enhance healing. Effect of delayed application and early removal on wound healing, *Arch. Dermatol.*, 124, 392–395, 1988.

16. Kane, C.J., Hebda, P.A., Mansbridge, J.N., and Hanawalt P.C., Direct evidence for spatial and temporal regulation of transforming growth factor beta 1 expression during cutaneous wound healing, *J. Cell Physiol.*, 148, 157–173, 1991.

17. Hebda, P.A., Stimulatory effects of transforming growth factor-beta and epidermal growth factor on epidermal cell outgrowth from porcine skin explant cultures. *J. Invest. Dermatol.* 91, 440–445, 1988.

18. Sung, C.C., O'Toole, E.A., Lannutti, B.J., Hunt, J., O'Gorman, M., Woodley, D.T., and Paller, A.S., Integrin alpha 5 beta 1 expression is required for inhibition of keratinocyte migration by ganglioside GT1b, *Exper. Cell Res.*, 239, 311–319, 1998.

19. O'Toole, E.A., Extracellular matrix and keratinocyte migration, *Clin. Exper. Dermatol.*, 26, 525–530, 2001.

20. Clark, R.A.F., Folkvord, J.M., and Wertz, R.L., Fibronectin as well as other extracellular matrix proteins mediate human keratinocyte adherence, *J. Invest. Dermatol.*, 85, 368–383, 1985.

21. Woodley, D.T., Bachmann, P.M., and O'Keefe, E.J., Laminin inhibits human keratinocyte migration, *J. Cell Physiol.*, 136, 140–146, 1988.

22. Shiraha, H., Glading, A., Gupta, K., and Wells, A., Chemokine transmodulation of EGF receptor signaling: IP-10 inhibits motility by decreasing EGF-induced calpain activity. *J. Cell Biol.*, 146, 243–253, 1999.

23. Klein, S.B., Fisher, G.J., Jensen, T., Mendelsohn, J., Voorhees, J.J., and Elder, J.T., Regulation of TGF-α expression in human keratinocytes: PKC-dependent and -independent pathways, *J. Cell Physiol.*, 151, 326–336, 1992.

24. Romo, T., III and McLaughlin, L.A., Wound Healing, Skin. http://www.emedicine.com/ent/topic13.htm 2001.

25. Stoll, S., Benedict, M., Mitra, R., Hiniker, A., Elder, J., and Nunez, G., EGF receptor signaling inhibits keratinocyte apoptosis: evidence for mediation by Bcl-XL, *Oncogene*, 16, 1493–1499, 1998.

26. Jensen, P.J., and Lavker, R.M., Modulation of the plasminogen activator cascade during enhanced epidermal proliferation *in vivo*, *Cell Growth Differen.*, 7, 1793–1804, 1996.

27. Vaezi, A., Bauer, C., Vasioukhin, V., and Fuchs, E., Actin cable dynamics and Rho/rock orchestrate a polarized cytoskeletal architecture in the early steps of assembling a stratified epithelium, *Dev. Cell*, 3, 367–381, 2002.

28. Grässel, S., Unsöld, C., Schäcke, H., Bruckner-Tuderman, L., and Bruckner, P.. Collagen XVI is expressed by human dermal fibroblasts and keratinocytes and is associated with the microfibrillar apparatus in the upper papillary dermis, *Matrix Biol.*, 18, 309–317, 1999.

29. Nguyen, B.P., Ryan, M.C., Gil, S.G., and Carter, W.G., Deposition of laminin 5 in epidermal wounds regulates integrin signaling and adhesion, *Curr. Opin. Cell Biol.*, 12, 554–562, 2000.

30. Wells, A., EGF receptor, *Int. J. Biochem. Cell Biol.*, 31, 637–643, 1999.

31. Wrana, J.L., Attisano, L., Carcamo, J., Zentella, A., Doody, J., Laiho, M., Wang, X.F., and Massague, J., TGF beta signals through a heteromeric protein kinase receptor complex, *Cell*, 71, 1003–1014, 1992.

32. Massague, J., How cells read TGF-β signals, *Nat. Rev. Mol. Cell. Biol.*, 1, 169–178, 2000.

33. Nakao, A., Afrakhte, M., Moren, A., et al., Identification of Smad7, a TGF-β-inducible antagonist of TGF-β signaling, *Nature*, 389, 631–635, 1997.

34. Iozzo, R.V. and San Antonio, J.D., Heparan sulfate proteoglycans: heavy hitters in the angiogenesis arena, *J. Clin. Invest.*, 108, 349–355, 2001.

35. Yates, S. and Rayner, T.E., Transcription factor activation in response to cutaneous injury: role of AP-1 in reepithelialization, *Wound Repair Regen.*, 10, 5–15, 2002.

36. Slansky, J.E. and Farnham, P.J., Introduction to the E2F family: protein structure and gene regulation, *Curr. Top. Microbiol. Immunol.*, 208, 1–30, 1996.

37. D'Souza, S.J., Vespa, A., Murkherjee, S., Maher, A., Pajak, A., and Dagnino, L., E2F-1 is essential for normal epidermal wound repair, *J. Biol. Chem.*, 277, 10626–10632, 2002.

38. Braun, S., Hanselmann, C., Gassmann, M.G., auf dem Keller, U., Born-Berclaz, C., Chan, K., Kan, Y.W., and Werner, S., Nrf2 transcription factor, a novel target of keratinocyte growth factor action which regulates gene expression and inflammation in the healing skin wound, *Mol. Cell. Biol.*, 22, 5492–5505, 2002.

39. Maas-Szabowski, N., Shimotoyodome, A., and Fusenig, N.E., Keratinocyte growth regulation in fibroblast cocultures via a double paracrine mechanism, *J. Cell Sci.*, 112, 1843–1853, 1999.

40. Babu, M. and Wells, A., Dermal–epidermal communication in wound healing, *Wounds*, 13, 183–189, 2002.

41. Barreca, A., De Luca, M., Del Monte, P., Bondanza, S., Damonte, G., Cariola, G., Di Marco, E., Giordano, G., Cancedda, R., and Minuto, F., *In vitro* paracrine regulation of human keratinocyte growth by fibroblast-derived insulin-like growth factors, *J. Cell. Physiol.*, 151, 262–268, 1992.

42. Gibbs, S., Silva Pinto, A.N., Murli, S., Huber, M., Hohl, D., and Ponec, M., Epidermal growth factor and keratinocyte growth factor differentially regulate epidermal migration, growth, and differentiation, *Wound Repair Regen.*, 8, 192–203, 2000.

43. Hebda, P.A., Klingbeil, C.K., Abraham, J.A., and Fiddes, J.C., Basic fibroblast growth factor stimulation of epidermal wound healing in pigs, *J. Invest. Dermatol.*, 95, 626–631, 1990.

44. Staiano-Coico, L., Krueger, J.G., Rubin, J.S., D'limi, S., Vallat, V.P., Valentino, L., Fahey, T., 3rd, Hawes, A., Kingston, G., Madden, M.R. et al., Human keratinocyte growth factor effects in a porcine model of epidermal wound healing, *J. Exper. Med.*, 178, 865–878, 1993.

45. Beer, H.D., Gassmann, M.G., Munz, B.. Steiling, H.. Engelhardt, F.. Bleuel, K.. and Werner, S., Expression and function of keratinocyte growth factor and activin in skin morphogenesis and cutaneous wound repair, *J. Invest. Dermatol., Symp. Proc.*, 5, 34–39, 2000.

46. Blomme, E.A., Sugimoto, Y., Lin, Y.C., Capen, C.C., and Rosol, T.J., Parathyroid hormone-related protein is a positive regulator of keratinocyte growth factor expression by normal dermal fibroblasts, *Mol. Cell. Endocrinol.*, 152, 189–197, 1999.

47. Border, W.A. and Noble, N.A., Transforming growth factor beta in tissue fibrosis, *N. Engl. J. Med.*, 331, 1286–1292, 1994.

48. Gailit, J., Welch, M.P., and Clark, R.A., TGF-beta 1 stimulates expression of keratinocyte integrins during reepithelialization of cutaneous wounds, *J. Invest. Dermatol.*, 103, 221–227, 1994.

49. Choi, Y. and Fuchs, E., TGF-beta and retinoic acid: regulators of growth and modifiers of differentiation in human epidermal cells, *Cell Regul.*, 1, 791–809, 1990.

50. Jiang, C.K., Tomic-Canic, M.. Lucas, D.J., Simon, M., and Blumenberg, M., TGF beta promotes the basal phenotype of epidermal keratinocytes: transcriptional induction of K#5 and K#14 keratin genes, *Growth Factors*, 12, 87–97, 1995.

51. Le Poole, I.C. and Boyce, S.T., Keratinocytes suppress transforming growth factor-beta 1 expression by fibroblasts in cultured skin substitutes, *Br. J. Dermatol.*, 140, 409–416, 1999.

52. Edwards, D.R., Murphy, G.. Reynolds, J.J., Whitham, S.E., Docherty, A.J., Angel, P., and Heath, J.K., Transforming growth factor beta modulates the expression of collagenase and metalloproteinase inhibitor, *EMBO J.,* 6, 1899–1904, 1987.

53. Ignotz, R.A. and Massague, J., Transforming growth factor-beta stimulates the expression of fibronectin and collagen and their incorporation into the extracellular matrix, *J. Biol. Chem.,* 261, 4337–4345, 1986.

54. Cowin, A.J., Kallincos, N., Hatzirodos, N., Robertson, J.G., Pickering, K.J., Couper, J., and Belford, D.A., Hepatocyte growth factor and macrophage-stimulating protein are upregulated during excisional wound repair in rats, *Cell Tissue Res.,* 306, 239–250, 2001.

55. Steude, J., Kulke, R., and Christophers, E., Interleukin-1-stimulated secretion of interleukin-8 and growth-related oncogene-alpha demonstrates greatly enhanced keratinocyte growth in human raft cultured epidermis, *J. Invest. Dermatol.,* 119, 1254–1260, 2002.

56. Baudouin, J.E. and Tachon, P., Constitutive nitric oxide synthase is present in normal human keratinocytes, *J. Invest. Dermatol.,* 106, 428–431, 1996.

57. Wang, R., Ghahary, A., Shen, Y.J., Scott, P.G., and Tredget, E.E., Human dermal fibroblasts produce nitric oxide and express both constitutive and inducible nitric oxide synthase isoforms, *J. Invest. Dermatol.,* 106, 419–427, 1996.

58. Sirsjo, A.. Karlsson, M., Gidlof, A., Rollman, O., and Torma, H., Increased expression of inducible nitric oxide synthase in psoriatic skin and cytokine-stimulated cultured keratinocytes, *Br. J. Dermatol.,* 134, 643–648, 1996.

59. Wang, R., Ghahary, A., Shen, Y.J., Scott, P.G., and Tredget, E.E., Nitric oxide synthase expression and nitric oxide production are reduced in hypertrophic scar tissue and fibroblasts, *J. Invest. Dermatol.,* 108, 438–444, 1997.

60. Krischel, V.. Bruch-Gerharz, D., Suschek, C., Kroncke, K.D., Ruzicka, T., and Kolb-Bachofen, V., Biphasic effect of exogenous nitric oxide on proliferation and differentiation in skin-derived keratinocytes but not fibroblasts, *J. Invest. Dermatol.,* 111, 286–291, 1998.

61. Nowinski, D., Hoijer, P., Engstrand, T., Rubin, K., Gerdin, B., and Ivarsson, M., Keratinocytes inhibit expression of connective tissue growth factor in fibroblasts *in vitro* by an interleukin-1 alpha-dependent mechanism, *J. Invest. Dermatol.,* 119, 449–455, 2002.

62. Freedberg, I.M., Tomic-Canic, M., Komine, M., and Blumenberg, M., Keratins and the keratinocyte activation cycle, *J. Invest. Dermatol.,* 116, 633–640, 2001.

63. Dawson, R.A., Goberdhan, N.J., Freedlander, E., and MacNeil, S., Influence of extracellular matrix proteins on human keratinocyte attachment, proliferation and transfer to a dermal wound model, *Burns,* 22, 93–100, 1996.

64. Maatta, A., Jaakkola, P., and Jalkanen, M., Extracellular matrix-dependent activation of syndecan-1 expression in keratinocyte growth factor-treated keratinocytes, *J. Biol. Chem.,* 274, 9891–9898, 1999.

65. Ruehl, M., Somasundaram, R., Schoenfelder, I., Farndale, R.W., Knight, C.G., Schmid, M., Ackermann, R., Riecken, E.O., Zeitz, M., and Schuppan, D., The epithelial mitogen keratinocyte growth factor binds to collagens via the consensus sequence glycine–proline–hydroxyproline, *J. Biol. Chem.,* 277, 872–878, 2002.

66. Jones, J.M., Cohen, R.L., and Chambers, D.A., Collagen modulates gene activation of plasminogen activator system molecules, *Exper. Cell Res.,* 280, 244–254, 2002.

67. Nagase, H. and Woessner, J.F. Jr., Matrix metalloproteinases, *J. Biol. Chem.,* 274, 21, 491–21,494, 1999.

68. Vaalamo, M., Leivo, T., and Saarialho-Kere, U., Differential expression of tissue inhibitors of metalloproteinases (TIMP-1, -2, -3, and -4) in normal and aberrant wound healing, *Hum. Pathol.*, 30, 795–802, 1999.

69. Pilcher, B.K., Dumin, J.A., Sudbeck, B.D., Krane, S.M., Welgus, H.G., and Parks, W.C., The activity of collagenase-1 is required for keratinocyte migration on a type I collagen matrix, *J. Cell Biol.*, 137, 1445–1457, 1997.

70. Saarialho-Kere, U.K., Kovacs, S.O., Pentland, A.P., Olerud, J.E., Welgus, H.G., and Parks, W.C., Cell–matrix interactions modulate interstitial collagenase expression by human keratinocytes actively involved in wound healing, *J. Clin. Invest.*, 92, 2858–2866, 1993.

71. Inoue, M., Kratz, G., Haegerstrand, A., and Ståhle-Bäckdahl, M., Collagenase expression is rapidly induced in wound-edge keratinocytes after acute injury in human skin, persists during healing, and stops at reepithelialization, *J. Invest. Dermatol.*, 104, 479–483, 1995.

72. Salo, T., Makela, M., Kylmaniemi, M., Autio-Harmainen, H., and Larjava, H., Expression of matrix metalloproteinase-2 and -9 during early human wound healing, *Lab. Invest.*, 70, 176–182, 1994.

73. Ashcroft, G.S., Horan, M.A., Herrick, S.E., Tarnuzzer, R.W., Schultz, G.S., and Ferguson, M.W., Age-related differences in the temporal and spatial regulation of matrix metalloproteinases (MMPs) in normal skin and acute cutaneous wounds of healthy humans, *Cell Tissue Res.*, 290, 581–591, 1997.

74. Sarret, Y., Woodley, D.T., Goldberg, G.S., Kronberger, A., and Wynn, K.C., Constitutive synthesis of a 92-kDa keratinocyte-derived type IV collagenase is enhanced by type I collagen and decreased by type IV collagen matrices, *J. Invest. Dermatol.*, 99, 836–841, 1992.

75. McCawley, L.J., O'Brien, P., and Hudson L.G., Epidermal growth factor (EGF)- and scatter factor/hepatocyte growth factor (SF/HGF) mediated keratinocyte migration is coincident with induction of matrix metalloproteinase (MMP)-9, *J. Cell Phys.*, 176, 255–265, 1998.

76. Charvat, S., Le Griel, C., Chignol, M.C., Schmitt, D., and Serres, M., Ras-transfection up-regulated HaCaT cell migration: inhibition by Marimastat, *Clin. Exp. Metastasis*, 17, 677–685, 1999.

77. Mirastschijski, U., Impola, U., Karsdal, M.A., Saarialho-Kere, U., and Agren, M.S., Matrix metalloproteinase inhibitor BB-3103 unlike the serine proteinase inhibitor aprotinin abrogates epidermal healing of human skin wounds *ex vivo, J. Invest. Dermatol.*, 118, 55–64, 2002.

78. Kratz, G., Jansson, K., Gidlund, M., and Hægerstrand, A., Keratinocyte conditioned medium stimulates type IV collagenase synthesis in cultured human keratinocytes and fibroblasts, *Br. J. Dermatol.*, 133, 842–846, 1995.

79. Zeigler, M.E., Dutcheshen, N.T., Gibbs, D.F., and Varani, J., Growth factor-induced epidermal invasion of the dermis in human skin organ culture: expression and role of matrix metalloproteinases, *Invasion Metastasis*, 16, 11–18, 1996.

80. Saarialho-Kere, U., Kerkela, E., Jahkola, T., Suomela, S., Keski-Oja, J., and Lohi, J., Epilysin (MMP-28) expression is associated with cell proliferation during epithelial repair, *J. Invest. Dermatol.*, 119, 14–21, 2002.

81. Romer, J., Lund, L.R., Eriksen, J. et al., Differential expression of urokinase-type plasminogen activator and its type-1 inhibitor during healing of mouse skin wounds, *J. Invest. Dermatol.*, 97, 803–811, 1991.

82. Madlener, M., Parks, W.C., and Werner, S., Matrix metalloproteinases (MMP) and their physiological inhibitors (TIMP) are differentially expressed during excisional skin wound repair, *Exp. Cell Res.,* 242, 201–210, 1998.
83. Ravanti, L. and Kähäri, V.M., Matrix metalloproteinases in wound repair, *Int. J. Mol. Med.,* 6, 391–407, 2000.
84. Lund, L.R., Rømer, J., Bugge, T.H. et al., Functional overlap between two classes of matrix degrading proteases in wound healing, *EMBO J.,* 18, 4645–4656, 1999.
85. Gak, E., Taylor, W.G., Chan, A.M., and Rubin, J.S., Processing of hepatocyte growth factor to the heterodimeric form is required for biological activity, *FEBS Lett.,* 311, 17–21, 1992.
86. Ito, A., Mukaiyama, A., Itoh, Y., Nagase, H., Thogersen, I.B., Enghild, J.J., Sasaguri, Y., Mori, Y., Degradation of interleukin 1B by matrix metalloproteinases, *J. Biol. Chem.,* 271, 14657–14660, 1996.
87. Gallea-Robache, S., Morand, V., Millet, S., Bruneau, J.M., Bhatnagar, N., Chouaib, S., and Roman-Roman, S., A metalloproteinase inhibitor blocks the shedding of soluble cytokine receptors and processing of transmembrane cytokine precursors in human monocytic cells, *Cytokine,* 9, 340–346, 1997.
88. Imai, K., Hiramatsu, A., Fukushima, D., Pierschbacher, M.D., and Okada, Y., Degradation of decorin by matrix metalloproteinases: identification of the cleavage sites, kinetic analyses and transforming growth factor-beta 1 release, *Biochem. J.,* 322, 809–814, 1997.
89. Wakita, H., Furukawa, F., and Takigawa, M., Thrombin and trypsin induce granulocyte-macrophage colony-stimulating factor and interleukin-6 gene expression in cultured normal human keratinocytes, *Proc. Assoc. Am. Phys.,* 109, 190–207, 1997.
90. Sato, C., Tsuboi, R., Shi, C.M., Rubin, J.S., and Ogawa, H., Comparative study of hepatocyte growth factor/scatter factor and keratinocyte growth factor effects on human keratinocytes, *J. Invest. Dermatol.,* 104, 958–963, 1995.
91. Bullard, K.M., Longaker, M.T., and Lorenz, H.P., Fetal wound healing: current biology, *World J. Surg.,* 27, 54–61, 2003.
92. Sauder, D.N., Mounessa, N.L., Katz, S.I., Dinarello, C.A., and Gallin, J.I., Chemotactic cytokines: the role of leukocytic pyrogen and epidermal cell thymocyte-activating factor in neutrophil chemotaxis, *J. Immunol.,* 132, 828–832, 1984.
93. Gallucci, R.M., Simeonova, P.P., Matheson, J.M., Kommineni, C., Guriel, J.L., Sugawara, T., and Luster, M.I., Impaired cutaneous wound healing in interleukin-6-deficient and immunosuppressed mice, *FASEB J.,* 14, 2525–2531, 2000.
94. Schröder, J.M., Gregory, H., Young, J., and Christophers, E., Neutrophil-activating proteins in psoriasis, *J. Invest. Dermatol.,* 98, 241–247, 1992.
95. Jameson, J., Ugarte, K., Chen, N., Yachi, P., Fuchs, E., Boismenu, R., and Havran, W.L., A role for skin gamma-delta T cells in wound repair, *Science,* 296, 747–749, 2002.
96. McCauley, R.L., Chopra, V.. Li, Y.Y., Herndon, D.N., and Robson, M.C., Altered cytokine production in black patients with keloids, *J. Clin. Immunol.,* 12, 300–308, 1992.
97. Brown, L., Yeo, K., Berse, B. et al., Expression of vascular permeability factor (vascular endothelial growth factor) by epidermal keratinocytes during wound healing, *J. Exp. Med.,* 176, 1375–1379, 1992.
98. Khanna, S., Roy, S., Bagchi, D., Bagchi, M., and Sen, C.K., Upregulation of oxidant-induced VEGF expression in cultured keratinocytes by a grape seed proanthocyanidin extract, *Free Rad. Biol. Med.,* 31, 38–42, 2001.

99. Failla, C.M., Odorisio, T., Cianfarani, F., Schietroma, C., Puddu, P., and Zambruno, G., Placenta growth factor is induced in human keratinocytes during wound healing, *J. Invest. Dermatol.*, 115, 388–395, 2000.

100. Harsum, S., Clarke, J.D., and Martin, P., A reciprocal relationship between cutaneous nerves and repairing skin wounds in the developing chick embryo, *Dev. Biol.*, 238, 27–39, 2001

101. Lincoln, R.K. and Pomeranz, B., The sympathomimetic agent, 6-hydroxydopamine, accelerates cutaneous wound healing, *Eur. J. Pharmacol.*, 376, 257–264, 1999.

102. Meyer, L.J., Russell, S.B., Russell, J.D., Trupin, J.S., Egbert, B.M., Shuster, S., and Stern, R., Reduced hyaluronan in keloid tissue and cultured keloid fibroblasts, *J. Invest. Dermatol.*, 114, 953–959, 2000.

103. Sato, M., Ishikawa, O., and Miyachi, Y., Distinct patterns of collagen gene expression are seen in normal and keloid fibroblasts grown in three-dimensional culture, *Br. J. Dermatol.*, 138, 938–943, 1998.

104. Russell, S.B., Trupin, K.M., Rodriguez-Eaton, S., Russell, J.D., and Trupin, J.S., Reduced growth-factor requirement of keloid-derived fibroblasts may account for tumor growth, *Proc. Natl. Acad. Sci. U.S.A.*, 85, 587–591, 1988.

105. Lim, I.J., Phan, T.T., Song, C., Tan, W.T., and Longaker, M.T., Investigation of the influence of keloid-derived keratinocytes on fibroblast growth and proliferation *in vitro*, *Plast. Reconstruct. Surg.*, 107, 797–808, 2001.

106. Lim, I.J., Phan, T.T., Bay, B.H., Qi, R., Huynh, H., Tan, W.T., Lee, S.T., and Longaker, M.T., Fibroblasts cocultured with keloid keratinocytes: normal fibroblasts secrete collagen in a keloidlike manner, *Am. J. Physiol. Cell Physiol.*, 283, C212–C222, 2002.

107. Niessen, F.B., Andriessen, M.P., Schalkwijk, J., Visser, L., and Timens, W., Keratinocyte-derived growth factors play a role in the formation of hypertrophic scars, *J. Pathol.*, 194, 207–216, 2001.

108. Ghahary, A., Tredget, E.E., Chang, L.J., Scott, P.G., and Shen, Q., Genetically modified dermal keratinocytes express high levels of transforming growth factor-beta 1, *J. Invest. Dermatol.*, 110, 800–805, 1998.

109. Haake, A.R. and Cooklis, M., Incomplete differentiation of fetal keratinocytes in the skin equivalent leads to the default pathway of apoptosis, *Exper. Cell Res.*, 231, 83–95, 1997.

110. Arita, K., Akiyama, M., Tsuji, Y., McMillan, J.R., Eady, R.A., and Shimizu, H., Changes in gap junction distribution and connexin expression pattern during human fetal skin development, *J. Histochem. Cytochem.*, 50, 1493–1500, 2002.

111. Cass, D.L., Bullard, K.M., Sylvester, K.G., Yang, E.Y., Sheppard, D., Herlyn, M., and Adzick, N.S., Epidermal integrin expression is upregulated rapidly in human fetal wound repair, *J. Pediatr. Surg.*, 33, 312–316, 1998.

112. Mackool, R.J., Gittes, G.K., and Longaker, M.T., Scarless healing. The fetal wound, *Clin. Plast. Surg.*, 25, 357–365, 1998.

113. Ffrench-Constant, C., Van de Water, L., Dvorak, H.F., and Hymes, R.O., Reappearance of an embryonic pattern of fibronectin splicing during wound healing in the adult rat, *J. Cell Biol.*, 109, 903–914, 1989.

114. Bullard, K.M., Cass, D.L., Banda, M.J., and Adzick, N.S., Transforming growth factor beta-1 decreases interstitial collagenase in healing human fetal skin, *J. Pediatr. Surg.*, 32, 1023–1027, 1997.

115. Dang, C.M., Beanes, S.R., Soo, C., Ting, K., Benhaim, P., Hedrick, M.H., and Lorenz, H.P., Decreased expression of fibroblast and keratinocyte growth factor isoforms and receptors during scarless repair, *Plast. Reconstruct. Surg.*, 111, 1969–1979, 2003.

116. Martin. P.. Mechanisms of wound healing in the embryo and fetus, *Curr. Top. Dev. Biol.,* 32, 175–203, 1996.

117. Brock, J., Midwinter, K, Lewis, J., and Martin, P., Healing of incisional wounds in the embryonic chick wing bud: characterization of the actin purse-string and demonstration of a requirement for Rho activation, *J. Cell Biol,* 135, 1097–1107, 1996.

118. Field, F.K. and Kerstein, M.D., Overview of wound healing in a moist environment, *Am. J. Surg.,* 167, 2S–6S, 1994.

119. Wahli,W., Peroxisome proliferator-activated receptors (PPARs): from metabolic control to epidermal wound healing, *Swiss Med. Weekly,* 132, 83–91, 2002.

Part II

Local Environment and Healing

4 Moist Wound Healing from Past to Present

Laura L. Bolton

CONTENTS

> Healing is a matter of time, but it is sometimes also a matter of opportunity.

> **Hippocrates *Precepts,* Chapter 1**

PERSPECTIVE

Modern practitioners may scoff at outdated medical practices, yet an objective look at the gaps between scientific knowledge and current practice gives us pause. One such gap occurs in the way we treat wounds. There is ample evidence on how to give wounds the opportunity to heal by providing a moist physiological environment for the cells that do the work of healing. Yet practitioners thoughtlessly expose wounded tissue to desert environments that desiccate and kill healing cells. This dried tissue, often with gauze remnants acting as foreign bodies,[1] is more prone to infection and pain, and heals more slowly than if it were kept physiologically moist, placing patients at risk of amputation or longer hospital stays. The medical profession eradicated smallpox but often ignores the most basic evidence on how to heal wounds. What caused this gap between science and practice? Perhaps by understanding it, we can close it. We review here the history of moist wound healing as it gained scientific credibility and explore why the scientific advances did not emerge into generally accepted clinical practice. In the context of current medical practice, we will explore clinical outcomes reported using moist wound healing and dispel the myths surrounding this term so that more medical professionals are enabled to reap its benefits for their patients.

4.1 HISTORIC ORIGINS OF MOIST WOUND HEALING

Egyptians may have been the first to apply an "adhesive" bandage, in the form of lint coated with resin, honey and/or grease, to close wounds. At least theirs is the only account to survive the centuries. It is found in the text of the Smith papyrus, remnants of which Mustapha Aga of Thebes sold to Dr. Edwin Smith, an American scholar, on January 20, 1862. Smith reassembled these remnants, which remained in the New York Historical Society as *The Smith Papyrus* until Dr. James Breasted of the Oriental Institute in Chicago translated them between 1920 and 1930. The text consists of a series of case descriptions of ailments, from head to waist, and the approach to each, as described by an Egyptian physician likely to have lived sometime between 2600 and 2200 B.C.[2] Though Breasted's use of the term "adhesive" has been questioned, this remains in literature as the historic landmark for the use of adhesive bandages to promote moist wound healing. Another form of moist wound healing practiced by the original author of *The Smith Papyrus* was to cover the wound with either fat or "meat of an ox so that the wound may rot." It is not clear if the purpose of this meat dressing was to initiate hemostasis,[2] to provide an early version of autolytic debridement, as suggested by the concept of allowing the wound to "rot," or simply to use flesh to mend flesh, as boxers do today for their bruises.[2] Poultices held in place with willow or sycamore leaves were also prescribed by this ancient physician for the purpose of keeping wounds moist while delivering a variety of medications.

Centuries passed. Egyptian civilization waned, and medical practice declined into a phase of mysticism and quackery, yet potentially occlusive poultices of resins such as frankincense or myrrh enjoyed continued use through 1500 B.C., as documented in the Ebers papyrus.[2]

Though it is likely that similar practices occurred in China, India, and Greece, no surviving written records exist of wound care that would be characterized as moist wound healing. The *Sushruta Samhita,* a collection of Ayurvedic oral verse and prose on surgery in India that originated between 1000 B.C. and A.D. 800, describes a potentially occlusive leg ulcer dressing. The wound was covered with an ointment of honey and clarified butter covered with a pad of leaves tied over the wound to hold the ointment in place and to generate heat or cold.[2]

Similar practices, especially use of resins such as myrrh, secreted by *Balsamodendron myrrha* following damage to its branches, and use of fig sap to clot blood were recorded by the Greek poet, Homer in the *Iliad* in the ninth century B.C. Hippocrates favored these saps and resins, along with bandages soaked in wine, in his medical teachings on the island of Cos, ca. 400 B.C. It is difficult to discern whether his intention was to prevent what we now realize is infection, to conserve or preserve wound moisture, or to set the stage for reducing wound exudate.[3]

Celsus, the first to differentiate slowly healing ulcers from normally healing wounds, continued Hippocrates's practices in the first century A.D., but added lead, antimony, mercury, or copper compounds to the dried pitch or pine resin poultices. Use of these topical poisons began a Dark Age of wound care, wherein causing inflammation was deemed beneficial. Celsus had frequent opportunity to observe the acute signs of inflammation that he coined: *"rubor et tumor cum calore et dolore."* Though the antiseptic value may have intermittently rewarded use of these inflammatory agents, their benefit to healing remains doubtful. These toxic prescriptions gave rise to Galen's opinion, ca. A.D. 180, that wound dressings should be designed to generate pus, a theory that survived in translation through the Middle Ages as "laudable pus."[4]

Ambroise Paré, a military wound-dresser in the Hotel Dieu in Paris, brought about the ending of the age of "laudable pus" and thus paved the way for the rediscovery that occlusive environments foster wound healing. The then-current theory was that "wounds not curable by iron are curable by fire," resulting in expert opinion that gunshot wounds should be first dressed with boiling oil. In his treatise *The Method of Treatment for Wounds Caused by Firearms,* published in 1545, Paré described increased survival rates and reduced pain in soldiers whose gunshot wounds he merely cleansed and dressed after exhausting his supply of oil.[5] Though Paré was not considered an expert within the medical community, his outcomes trumped expert opinion, and medical practice began to change. If boiling oil were still used today, the benefits of moist healing with occlusive dressings might have gone unnoticed.

In 1797, Thomas Baynton was first to apply occlusive adhesive tape to venous ulcers.[3] He tightly wrapped the leg 1-in. distal to 2- to 3-in. proximal to the ulcer, with overlapping layers of adhesive tape strips 2-in. wide, with the intention of drawing the edges of the ulcer closed. A layer of soft calico bandage surrounding the adhesive tape was moistened with cool water if the ulcer was inflamed. The ulcers healed despite failure to pull their edges together. In fact, Baynton discovered that ulcers remaining covered with tape healed more rapidly than those dressed with conventional gauze dressings.

4.2 THE DAWNING SCIENCE OF MOIST WOUND HEALING

One hundred fifty years passed before Norwegian dermatologist, Oscar Gilje, published scientific confirmation that ulcers covered with adhesive tape healed faster than those covered with gauze.[6] After noticing that portions of venous ulcers covered with adhesive tape epithelized faster, Dr. Gilje replicated the test under highly skeptical supervision at the Rigshospital in Copenhagen. He dressed 23 patients' venous ulcers with tightly applied adhesive tape strips 2.5-cm wide, separated by 2 to 3 mm, covering the ulcer. Over these he placed a pad of dry gauze to absorb exudate and then covered the gauze with an elastic compression bandage. Fifteen patients (65%) healed in 12 weeks, with the sixteenth healing by 92 d. He later published his dissertation on more than 268 patients, placing the tape over distal or proximal, dorsal or ventral, left or right sides of the ulcer, and found the same accelerated healing under the tape-covered sides each time.

These first scientifically controlled studies of moist wound healing beneath adhesive tape ushered in the age of scientific exploration of wound dressings. As with chemistry and physics, the knowledge base grew quickly under scientific scrutiny. Fourteen years after Gilje's discovery, George Winter, a British surgeon, showed that swine partial-thickness excision wounds kept moist with polyethylene film epithelized more rapidly than similar adjacent air-exposed excisions.[7] Less than a year later, Hinman and Maibach, two dermatologists from the University of California,[8] confirmed that human shave biopsies healed "twice as fast" when dressed with polyethylene film than when exposed to air. Since these early discoveries, hundreds of preclinical and clinical studies on thousands of full- and partial-thickness[9] acute[10] and chronic[11] wounds have confirmed the faster healing rates,[8,12] decreased pain[9,12] and scarring,[13,14] and reduced likelihood of infection[15] in wounds dressed with moisture-retentive dressings. Despite the growing foundation of evidence supporting moist wound healing, however, medical practice has lagged behind the science of wound dressings. Most wounds are dressed today much as the ancient Egyptians did, using gauze, but without moisture-retentive "resins, honey, or grease."

4.3 BARRIERS TO PRACTICING MOIST WOUND HEALING

4.3.1 OCCLUSION BABEL

One barrier to use of moisture-retentive dressings has been the lack of a common language to describe them. Terms such as "occlusion" or "moist healing" have been used to describe moisture retentive dressings without clear definition. "Moist healing" could be misinterpreted as applying saline gauze. "Occlusion" may raise unfounded fears of infection. Occlusive to what? Semi-permeable? Permeable to what? Impermeable to what? Moist wound healing? How moist? Understanding occlusive dressings should begin with a clear operational definition that all can apply.

A solution: For the purposes of this chapter, occlusive dressings will be defined as *dressings retaining sufficient moisture to maintain healing equivalent to that in a physiologically moist environment.* Some dressings also provide thermal,[16] gaseous,[17] bacterial,[18] or viral[19] barriers. These properties will not be addressed here. If we accept moisture retention as the criterion by which dressings are judged "occlusive," then water vapor transmission rate (WVTR) is an objective measure of a dressing's moisture barrier function; low WVTR is less permeable to water, and high WVTR is more permeable to water. The operational definition of the water vapor transmission rate[20] through a perfectly uniform film is the water vapor transmission rate:

$$\text{WVTR} \ (g \cdot m^2 \cdot h^{-1}) = (P \cdot \Delta p)/L$$

where the film's water vapor permeability, P $(g \cdot mm \cdot h^{-1} \cdot kPa^{-1})$ is the amount (g) of water vapor passing through each mm thickness of the film per unit surface area (m^2) per unit time (h^{-1}) induced per unit vapor pressure difference across the film (kPa). $\Delta p \cdot kPa$ is the water vapor pressure difference across the film and L is the thickness of the film.

Although dressings are not perfectly uniform films, dressing WVTR is a fairly robust predictor of wound healing. Dressing thickness varies as adhesives and films expand and increase in porosity with moisture or physical expansion of the adhesive. Dressing adhesives interact with skin and wounds in widely differing ways, adding variability to their effects on healing. To compensate for these sources of variability and increase clinical relevance, one may measure the WVTR through the dressing after it is in place for 24 h on a highly exuding wound. Under these circumstances, dressing WVTR values less than or equal to 35 g/m^2/h have reportedly maintained wound surfaces sufficiently moist to optimize healing outcomes.[21] Wet or impregnated gauze remains moist on most wounds for less than an 8-h shift, so it is not a moisture-retentive dressing. The reliability of this finding is sufficient to support construct validity of low dressing WVTR as a correlate controlling partial-thickness ($r^2 = 0.58$; $\alpha = 0.029$) and full-thickness ($r^2 = 0.66$; $\alpha < 0.05$) wound healing outcomes in swine. Moreover, clinical acute and chronic wounds with more moisture-retentive dressing environments experienced fewer days to healing (Wilcoxon: $\alpha = 0.016$) and were more likely to heal than properly applied impregnated gauze controls during fixed-duration controlled clinical studies on partial- and full-thickness venous ulcers, pressure ulcers, and neuropathic foot ulcers (Wilcoxon: $\alpha = 0.004$).[22]

4.3.2 MYTHS ABOUT MOIST WOUND HEALING

Myths about moist wound healing are a second barrier to its clinical use. Belief that wounds need dry environments originated from varying interpretations of Hippocrates' advice on wound care. The fact is that healing cells and the immunologically active cells triggering their activities thrive in moist environments.[23] This common knowledge for cell biologists is only beginning to be accepted into clinical practice.

Fear of infection arose from observations that microbes proliferate rapidly *in vitro* in moist culture plates isolated from the immunologically rich wound environment. General practitioners are often unaware that the compromised circulation and foreign matter-like gauze strands or necrotic tissue are more important potentiators of wound infection than numbers of bacteria.[24] Few realize that in clinical wounds, microbial populations are as frequent and as numerous under gauze dressings as under hydrocolloid or film dressings.[25] Furthermore, potential for cross-contamination may be limited through use of moisture-retentive dressings. Removing a gauze dressing may disperse more airborne bacteria into treatment room air than removing a hydrocolloid dressing for up to 30 minutes after dressing removal,[26] expanding opportunities for wound infection in hospitals and wound clinics.

Maceration is another phenomenon with little foundation in science, the fear of which deprives patients of the benefits of moist wound healing. Most clinicians are unaware that the range of WVTR values for dressings that provide moist wound healing is similar to that of human skin. The weight of clinical opinion suggests that maceration of callus permits penetration by microorganisms, which may invade tissue with compromised circulation. However, in clinical wounds, new epidermis is often mistaken for maceration until it becomes thick enough to acquire its familiar pink hue one to two days after appearing as a white border to the wound. We will never know how many wounds have lost delicate new epidermis to drying environments through fear of maceration. This would be a valuable area for definitive research. Literature searches failed to identify a single scientific study associating maceration with delayed wound healing.

4.3.3 VARYING DRESSING PROPERTIES

One source of confusion is the variability among the properties of moisture-retentive dressings. Moisture-retentive dressings are usually made of an outer film or film-foam backing with an adhesive facing the wound. Ideally, the outer backing matches the WVTR of the skin, while the adhesive absorbs and seals in wound exudate to preserve a moist wound environment. Within the major categories of dressings, WVTR of dressing backings varies widely (Table 4.1); not all film or hydrocolloid dressings are equally moisture retentive. Moreover, film dressings often form channels allowing leakage of wound exudate and entry of bacteria,[27] so their moisture retention is not completely reflected by WVTR.

Backings are not the only variables differentiating moisture-retentive wound dressings. Adhesives vary too. Some dressing backings absorb and hold wound fluid under pressure, while it is squeezed out of others under the same pressures.[28] Adhesives vary in aggressiveness, swelling, and capacity to absorb moisture. Some acrylic adhesives bond strongly to epidermis, requiring special care to remove the adhesive dressing without damaging new epidermis[29] with its incompletely formed rete ridges. Other adhesives swell or become slippery when moist, lifting or sliding off wounds instead of retaining wound moisture. Expansion of the adhesive is not always well matched to the expansion coefficient of the backing, so the film–foam backing of the dressing may split under tension as the adhesive swells, allowing leakage of wound fluid. All these variables in dressing construction and components cause differences in their capacity to preserve a moist environment as well as in clinical wear time and healing outcome.[30] In summary, complex interactions exist between widely varying dressing structures and wound fluid. Data describing isolated dressing features such as absorbency or WVTR do not always reflect in-use dressing performance. This suggests that wound-dressing decisions may be more clincally relevant if based on *bona fide* controlled evidence of outcomes or performance such as measured healing, wear time before leakage, or incidence of infection.

4.3.4 IMPROPER DRESSING USE

Moisture-retentive dressings were a new and unfamiliar technology for many years. Clinicians newly acquainted with their use required training for proper application and removal. To provide the desired moist wound environment, moisture-retentive dressings should be applied, smoothing out wrinkles, then pressed in place for 20 to 30 sec, allowing the adhesive to flow and conform to the skin surface. Adherence to the skin may increase for up to 2 d, then gradually decline, as moisture from the skin and wound interact with the adhesive to loosen its bond with the skin. Too

TABLE 4.1
Clinical Wound Healing as a Function of Dressing Moisture Retention

Clinical Wound	Hydrocolloid (WVTR = 11 ± 2)	Film (WVTR =14 ± 1) or Bioengineered Skin	Foam (WVTR =33 ± 4)	Gauze or Impregnated Gauze (WVTR = 67 ±4)
Venous ulcers (with adequate sustained graduated compression)	55% of >27-month-duration venous ulcers healed in 12 weeks (n = 164)[32] 38% in 13 weeks (n = 50)[33] 7 of 15 (48%) venous or arterial ulcers healed in 6 weeks[34] 51% of 530 venous ulcers healed in 12 weeks in a meta-analysis of literature[11] 54% of 72 full-thickness leg ulcers healed in 56 d[35]	61% of 127 venous ulcers of >1 month duration healed in 25 weeks managed with bioengineered skin + a nonadhering dressing[36] 45% of 130 venous ulcers healed in 12 weeks in a meta-analysis of literature[11] Granulation tissue replaced yellow slough as measured chromatically or clinically in 14 d without exogenous enzymes[37]	34% in 13 weeks (n = 50)[33]	2 of 15 (13%) venous or arterial ulcers healed in 6 weeks[34] 44% of 106 >1-month-duration venous ulcers managed with nonadhering gauze healed during 25 weeks[36] 39% of 223 venous ulcers healed in 12 weeks in a meta-analysis of literature[11]
Pressure ulcers (with pressure relief; Stage III or IV are full thickness; Stage II is partial thickness)	37% of Stage III, IV pressure ulcers healed in a mean of 8 weeks (n = 48)[38] 33% of Stage II, III healed in 6 weeks (n = 49)[33] Median time to healing for 16 Stage II pressure ulcers was 9 d[39] 42% of 19 Stage II, III pressure ulcers healed in a median of 17.5 d[40] 61% of 281 (or 48% of 136 with a different hydrocolloid dressing) Stage II–III pressure ulcers healed in 12 weeks in a meta-analysis of literature[11]		20% of Stage II, III healed in 6 weeks (n = 50)[33] 42% of 24 Stage II, III pressure ulcers healed in 12 weeks[41] 40% of 20 Stage II, III pressure ulcers healed in a median of 32 d[40]	23% of full-thickness pressure ulcers healed in 16 weeks with 100 μg/g rh PDGF-BB[a] (n = 31) vs. 0% healed in 16 weeks with placebo gel (n = 31)[42] Median time to healing for 18 Stage II pressure ulcers was 11 d[18] 14% of 14 Stage II, III pressure ulcers healed in 12 weeks[41]

TABLE 4.1 (CONTINUED)
Clinical Wound Healing as a Function of Dressing Moisture Retention

Clinical Wound	Hydrocolloid (WVTR = 11 ± 2)	Film (WVTR = 14 ± 1) or Bioengineered Skin	Foam (WVTR = 33 ± 4)	Gauze or Impregnated Gauze (WVTR = 67 ± 4)
Neuropathic ulcers (with appropriate off-loading)	80% of 36 diabetic and 10 Hansen's disease patients with neuropathic ulcers healed in 10 weeks with consistent off-loading with a total contact cast[43] 88.1% of 84 foot ulcers in 45 patients with insulin-dependent or non-insulin-dependent diabetes healed in a mean of 14 weeks; retrospectively measured probability of developing infection was 2.5%.[44]	51% of 100 patients with full-thickness ulcers healed in 12 weeks with weekly dermal replacement[45]		32% of 126 patients dressed with saline gauze healed in 12 weeks[45] 50% of 123 patients treated with 100 µg/g rHBB-PDGF healed in 20 weeks vs. 35% with gauze and placebo gel (n = 127)[46] 61% of 49 patients healed after 20 weeks with platelet releasate vs. 29% of 21 patients managed with saline gauze[47] Retrospectively measured probability of developing infection was 6.0%[44]
Acute biopsies	100% of full-thickness biopsies healed in 48 d for stressed caregivers versus 39 d for nonstressed[48] 100% of 7 shave biopsies healed in 2 weeks; 36% of full-thickness punch biopsies healed in 2 weeks[49]			63% of 16 shave biopsies healed in 2 weeks; 7% of 14 full-thickness punch biopsies healed in 2 weeks[49]

Acute burns	Hydrocolloid-dressed half of 10 partial-thickness burn wounds healed in 7.8 d[50] 22 partial thickness burns healed in 10.2 d[51]	Film-dressed half of 10 partial-thickness burns healed in 13.8 d[50]	20 partial thickness burns dressed with 1% silver sulfadiazine gauze healed in 15.6 d[51] 11 d for 20 second degree burns managed with film of *C. axillaris* extract vs. 17 d for 19 managed with saline gauze[52]
Acute split-thickness skin graft donor sites	100% healing of 15 patients with mirror image donor sites healed in 9 d[10] Mean healing time 9.54 d[53] Hydrocolloid-dressed half of 13 sites healed in 7.1 d[50]	Mean healing time 9.47 d[53] Film-dressed half of 13 sites healed in 14.3 d[50]	100% of the opposing mirror image control donor sites on 15 patients healed in 18 d[10] Mean healing time 11.07 to 12.79 d[53]

Note: Dressing average WVTR values ± standard error were recorded after 24 h *in situ* on fresh swine donor site wounds (Bolton, L.L., Monte, K., and Pirone, L.A., *Ostomy/Wound Manage.*, 46 (1A Suppl.), 51S–64S, 2000.

[a] Recombinant human platelet-derived growth factor BB.

frequent, vigorous, or abrupt removal without regard to the dynamic interaction between adhesive and skin may cause stripping of formerly intact epidermis surrounding the skin or of newly formed epidermis in the wound. Those who dress wounds should observe package insert instructions for proper dressing use and use the dressings as indicated. In many cases, dressing manufacturers also provide training in the use of their products to help wound professionals optimize clinical, humanistic, and economic outcomes.

4.3.5 LACK OF KNOWLEDGE ABOUT CLINICAL OUTCOMES

It is a challenge for busy clinicians to stay current with clinical literature. Wound care is not high on the list of priorities for physicians inundated with patients with cardiovascular disease, diabetes, or cancer. Yet for patients with these diseases, wounds are often a primary concern, because wounds can deprive patients of independence, mobility, and closeness to loved ones.[31] Examples of how healing outcomes improve with more moisture-retentive dressings on full- and partial-thickness acute and chronic clinical wounds are provided in Table 4.1. Based on these results, little doubt remains that healing is improved in the environments provided by more moisture-retentive dressings.

4.4   CONCLUSION

Science has enlightened the clinical practice of wound dressing, but only a few clinicians are using the new knowledge. The history recounted here will be incomplete until practitioners embrace the evidence on moist wound healing to provide its benefits to their patients. Change can be slow in medical practice. Practitioners were slow to accept germ theory, and even when it was accepted, counterproductive opinions stubbornly persisted. More than 100 years after Semmelweiss's discovery that physicians were transmitting infecting organisms, some prominent surgeons of the 1950s still refused to wear face masks.[5] With germ theory, the evidence gradually overpowered medical "expert opinion." Perhaps the same will happen with wound care. Will this be the generation that decides to close the gap between the ancient art of dressing wounds with gauze and the burgeoning scientific evidence that moist wound healing improves clinical, humanistic, and economic wound care outcomes?

REFERENCES

1. Wood, R.A., Disintegration of cellulose dressings in open granulating wounds, *BMJ*, 3, 1444–1445, 1976.
2. Majno, G., *The Healing Hand,* Harvard University Press, Boston, 1975.
3. Witkowski, J. and Parish, L.C., Cutaneous ulcer therapy, *Int. J. Dermatol.,* 25, 420–426, 1986.
4. Baxter. H., How a discipline came of age: a history of wound care, *J. Wound Care,* 11, 183–192, 2002.
5. Lyons, A.S. and Petrucelli, R.J., *Medicine: An Illustrated History*, Abradale Press, New York, 1987.

6. Gilje, O., On taping (adhesive tape treatment) of leg ulcers, *Acta Dermatol. Venereol.*, 28, 454–467, 1948.

7. Winter, G.D., Formation of the scab and the rate of epithelization of superficial wounds in the skin of the young domestic pig, *Nature (London)*, 193, 293–294, 1962.

8. Hinman, C.D. and Maibach, H., Effect of air exposure and occlusion on experimental human skin wounds, *Nature (London)*, 200, 377–379, 1963.

9. Pirone, L., Monte, K., Shannon, R., and Bolton, L., Wound healing under occlusion and non-occlusion in partial-thickness and full-thickness wounds in swine, *Wounds*, 2, 74–81, 1990.

10. Madden, M., Nolan, E., Finkelstein, J.L., Yurt, R.W., Smeland, J., Goodwin, C.W., Hefton, J., and Staiano-Coico, L., Comparison of an occlusive and a semi-occlusive dressing and the effect of the wound exudate upon keratinocyte proliferation, *J. Trauma*, 29, 924–930, 1989.

11. Kerstein, M.D., Gemmen, E., van Rijswijk, L., Lyder, C.H., Phillips, T., Xakellis, G., Golden, K., and Harrington, C., Cost and cost effectiveness of venous and pressure ulcer protocols of care, *Dis. Manage. Health Outcomes*, 9, 651–636, 2001.

12. Rovee, D.T., Kurowsky, C.A., Labun, J., and Downes, A.M., Effect of local wound environment on epidermal healing, in *Epidermal Wound Healing*, Maibach, H. and Rovee, D., Eds., Yearbook Medical Publishers, Chicago, 1972, Chap. 8, pp. 159–181.

13. Hien, N.T., Prawer, S.E., and Katz, H.I., Facilitated wound healing using transparent film dressing following Mohs micrographic surgery, *Arch. Dermatol.*, 124, 903–906, 1988.

14. Michie, D.D. and Hugill, J.V., Influence of occlusive and impregnated gauze dressings on incisional healing: a prospective, randomized, controlled study, *Ann. Plast. Surg.*, 32, 57–64, 1994.

15. Hutchinson, J.J. and McGuckin, M., Occlusive dressings: a microbiologic and clinical review, *Am. J. Infect. Control*, 18, 257–268, 1990.

16. Cherry, G. and Ryan, T.J., Enhanced wound angiogenesis with a new hydrocolloid dressing, in *An Environment for Healing. The Role of Occlusion*, Ryan, T.J., Ed. Royal Society of Medicine International Congress and Symposium Series No. 88, Royal Society of Medicine, London, 1985, pp. 61–68.

17. Silver, I., Oxygen tension and epithelization, in *Epidermal Wound Healing*, Maibach, H. and Rovee, D., Eds., Yearbook Medical Publishers, Chicago, 1972, Chap. 17, pp. 291–305.

18. Lawrence, J.C. and Lilly, H.A., Are hydrocolloid dressings bacteria proof? *Pharm. J.*, 239, 184, 1987.

19. Bowler, P.G., Delargy, H., Prince, D., and Fondberg, L., The viral barrier properties of some occlusive dressings and their role in infection control, *Wounds*, 5, 1–8, 1993.

20. Jonkman, M.F., *Epidermal Wound Healing between Moist and Dry*, Rijksuniversiteit Groningen, Groningen, Netherlands, 1989.

21. Bolton, L. and van Rijswijk, L., Wound dressings: meeting clinical and biological needs, *J. Dermatol. Nurs.*, 3, 146–161, 1991.

22. Bolton, L.L., Monte, K., and Pirone, L.A., Moisture and healing: beyond the jargon, *Ostomy/Wound Manage.*, 46 (1A Suppl.), 51S–64S, 2000.

23. Varghese, M., Balin, A.K., Carter, D.M., and Caldwell, D., Local environment of chronic wounds under synthetic dressings, *Arch. Dermotol.*, 122, 52–57, 1986.

24. Thomson, P.D. and Smith, D.J., Jr., What is infection? *Am. J. Surg.*, 167 (1A Suppl.), 7S–11S, 1994.

25. Hutchinson, J.J., A prospective trial of wound dressings to investigate the rate of infection under occlusion. Proceedings Advances in Wound Management Conference, Harrogate, U.K., 1994, MacMillan Magazines, Ltd., London, U.K., pp. 93–96.

26. Lawrence, J.C., Lilly, H.A., and Kidson, A., Wound dressings and the airborne dispersal of bacteria, *Lancet,* 339, 807, 1992.

27. Mertz, P., Marshall, D.A., and Eaglstein, W.H. Occlusive wound dressings to prevent bacterial invasion and wound infection, *J. Am. Acad. Dermatol.,* 12, 662–668, 1985.

28. Hudak, J., A comparative evaluation of four wound dressings for highly exuding wounds, *Proceedings 55th American Academy of Dermatology,* San Francisco, March 1997.

29. Alvarez, O.M., Mertz, P.M., and Eaglstein, W.H., The effect of occlusive dressings on collagen synthesis and re-epithelialization in superficial wounds, *J. Surg. Res.,* 35, 142–148, 1983.

30. Seaman, S., Herbster, S., Muglia, J., Murray, M., and Rick, C., Simplifying modern wound management for nonprofessional caregivers, *Ostomy/Wound Manage.,* 46, 18–27, 2000.

31. Phillips, T., Stanton, B., Provan, A., and Lew, R., A study of the impact of leg ulcers on quality of life: financial, social and psychologic implications, *J. Am. Acad. Dermatol.,* 31, 49–53, 1994.

32. Lyon, R.T., Veith, F.J., Bolton, L., Machado, F., and the Venous Ulcer Study collaborators, Clinical benchmark for healing of chronic venous ulcers, *Am. J. Surg.,* 176, 172–175, 1998.

33. Thomas, S., Banks, V., Bale, S., Fear-Price, M., Hagelstein, S., Harding, K.G., Orpin, J., and Thomas, N., A comparison of two dressings in the management of chronic wounds, *J. Wound Care,* 6, 383–386, 1997.

34. Ohlsson, P., Larsson, K., Lindholm, C., and Moller, M., A cost-effectiveness study of leg ulcer treatment in primary care, *Scand. J. Prim. Health Care,* 12, 295–299, 1994.

35. van Rijswijk, L., Multi-center leg ulcer study group. Full-thickness leg ulcers: patient demographics and predictors of healing, *J. Fam. Pract.,* 36, 625–632, 1993.

36. Sabolinski, M.L., Alvarez, O., Auletta, M., Mulder, G., and Parenteau, N.L., Cultured skin as a "smart material" for healing wounds: experience in venous ulcers, *Biomaterials,* 17, 311–320, 1996.

37. Romanelli, M., Objective measurement of venous ulcer debridement and granulation with a skin color reflectance analyzer, *Wounds,* 9, 122–126, 1997.

38. van Rijswijk, L. and Polansky, M., Predictors of time to healing deep pressure ulcers, *Wounds,* 6, 159–165, 1994.

39. Xakellis, G. and Chrischilles, E.A., Hydrocolloid versus saline-gauze dressings in treating pressure ulcers: a cost effective analysis, *Arch. Phys, Med. Rehab.,* 73, 463-469, 1992.

40. Jensen, J., Seeley, J., and Vigil, S., A 40-patient randomized clinical trial to compare the performance of ALLEVYN adhesive hydrocellular dressing and a hydrocolloid dressing in the management of pressure ulcers, *WOCN Proceedings,* June 1997.

41. Kraft, M.R., Lawson, L., Pohlmann, B., Reid-Lokos, C., and Barder, L., A comparison of Epi-Lock and saline dressings in the treatment of pressure ulcers, *Decubitus,* 6, 42–4, 46, 48, 1993.

42. Rees, R., Robson, M., Smiell, J., Perry, B., and the Pressure Ulcer Study Group, Wound repair and regeneration, *Wound Rep. Regen.,* 7, 141–147, 1999.

43. Laing, P.W., Cogley, D.I., and Klenerman, L., Neuropathic foot ulceration treated by total contact casts, *J. Bone Joint Surg.,* 74, 133–136, 1991.

44. Boulton, A.J., Meneses, P., and Ennis, W.J., Diabetic foot ulcers: a framework for prevention and care, *Wound Rep. Reg.,* 7, 7–16, 1999.

45. Gentzkow, G.D., Jensen, J.L., Pollak, R.A., Kroeker, R.O., Lerner, J.M., Lerner, M., Iwasaki, S.D. and the Dermagraft® Study Group, Improved healing of diabetic foot ulcers after grafting with a living human dermal replacement, *Wounds,* 11, 77–84, 1999.

46. Steed, D.L., Diabetic ulcer study group. Clinical evaluation of recombinant human platelet-derived growth factor for the treatment of lower extremity diabetic ulcers, *J. Vasc. Surg.,* 21, 71–81, 1995.

47. Bentkover, J.D. and Champpion, A.H., Economic evaluation of alternative methods of treatment for diabetic foot ulcer patients: cost-effectiveness of platelet releasate and wound care clinics, *Wounds,* 5, 207–215, 1993.

48. Kiecolt-Glaser, J.K., Marucha, P.T., Malarkey, W.B., Mercado, A.M., and Glaser, R., Slowing of wound healing by psychological stress, *Lancet,* 346, 1194–1196, 1995.

49. Nemeth, A., Eaglstein, W.H., Taylor, J.R., Peerson, L.J., and Falanga, V., Faster healing and less pain in skin biopsy sites treated with an occlusive dressing, *Arch. Dermatol.,* 127, 1679–1683, 1991.

50. Reig, A., Tejerina, C., Codina, J., Hidalgo, J., and Mirabet, V., Application of a new cicatrization dressing in treating second-degree burns and donor sites, *Ann. Mediterr. Burns Club,* 4, 174–176, 1991.

51. Wyatt, D., McGowan, D.N., and Najarian, M.P., Comparison of a hydrocolloid dressing and silver sulfadiazine cream in the outpatient management of second-degree burns, *J. Trauma,* 30, 857–865, 1990.

52. Doanh, N.D., Ham, N.N., Tam, N.T., Son, P.T., Dau, N.V., Grabe, M., Johansson, R., Lindgren, G., Stjernstrom, N.E., and Soderberg, T.A., The use of water extract from the bark of *Choerospondias axillaris* in the treatment of second degree burns, *Scand. J. Plast. Reconstr. Hand Surg.,* 30, 139–144, 1996.

53. Rakel, B.A., Bermel, M.A., Abbott, L.I., Baumler, S.K., Burger, M.R., Dawson, C.J., Heinle, J.A., and Ocheltree, I.M., Split-thickness skin graft donor site care: a quantitative synthesis of the research, *Appl. Nurs. Res.,* 11, 174–182, 1998.

5 Occlusive and Semipermeable Membranes

Hongbo Zhai and Howard I. Maibach

CONTENTS

5.1 INTRODUCTION

Skin occlusion is a complex issue that includes altering epidermal lipids, deoxyribonucleic acid (DNA) synthesis, epidermal turnover, pH, epidermal morphology, sweat glands, Langerhans cell stresses, and other factors.[1-17] Occlusion usually means that the skin is covered directly or indirectly by impermeable films or substances such as diapers, tape, chambers, gloves, textile garments, wound dressings, or transdermal devices,[1] but certain topical vehicles that contain fats and/or polymer oils (petrolatum, paraffin, etc.) may also generate occlusive effects.[2]

A broad selection of occlusive or semiocclusive dressings has long been employed to speed the healing processes in acute and chronic wounds.[18] These dressings keep healing tissues moist and increase superficial wound epithelialization.[2,18-22] However, occlusive or semiocclusive dressings can increase the population of microorganisms and hence induce wound infections.[2,23-25] A significant increase in the density of *Staphylococcus aureus* and lipophilic diphtheroids was observed after 24 h occlusion in eczematous and psoriatic skin.[14]

This chapter focuses on the effects of occlusive and semipermeable membranes on wound healing and summarizes related data.

5.2 EFFECTS OF OCCLUSIVE AND SEMIPERMEABLE
MEMBRANES ON WOUND HEALING

Alvarez et al.[21] compared the effects on superficial wounds in domestic pigs of:

1. Two different occlusive dressings
2. Nonocclusive wet-to-dry gauze dressings
3. Air exposure

Collagen synthesis and reepithelialization were increased in the wounds treated with occlusive dressings. Reepithelialization was increased beneath both the oxygen-impermeable and the oxygen-permeable dressings. When removed, the wet-to-dry gauze dressing and one of the occlusive dressings often damaged the new epidermis.

Surinchak et al.[26] monitored the healing process by measuring water evaporation (skin barrier function). In the first study, two wounds were created with a 2-mm biopsy punch on the backs of each of 15 rabbits and covered with occlusive and semiocclusive dressings. Water loss increased from a preoperative value of 6 g/m²/h to 55 g/m²/h after biopsy. Water loss from the occluded site returned to baseline values in 9 d as opposed to 17 d for the semioccluded sites ($P < 0.05$).

The second study followed the healing of full-thickness 4 × 4-cm wounds in five rabbits treated with fine-mesh gauze and five treated with a human amnion dressing.[26] Wound area and water loss were observed during the repair process. By visual measurement of the wound area, the injuries appeared 100% healed on day 30. The evaporimeter detected significantly increased water loss up until day 45, when original baseline values were reached. No differences were observed between the gauze and amnion groups. The evaporimeter is a simple yet accurate, noninvasive tool for measuring the wound healing endpoint based on regeneration of the epidermal water barrier.

Pinski[27] compared a series of wound dressings utilizing a human dermabrasion wound healing model. Occlusive dressings hastened healing time by as much as 50% over air-exposed sites.

Grubauer et al.[28] treated hairless mice with acetone, which removed stainable neutral lipids from the stratum corneum (SC), and compared the rate of repletion of stainable lipids, barrier recovery, and epidermal lipogenesis in animals covered with occlusive membranes or vapor-permeable membranes versus uncovered animals. Acetone treatment perturbed epidermal barrier function, which returned to normal in uncovered animals in parallel with the reappearance of SC lipid; when animals were covered with an occlusive membrane, barrier function did not recover normally. In contrast, occlusion with vapor-permeable membranes allowed barrier function to recover normally. These authors concluded that occlusive membranes prevented the increase in epidermal lipid synthesis, while a vapor-permeable membrane increased epidermal lipid synthesis in animals.

Silverman et al.[29] examined the effects of occlusive dressings on the reestablishment of the cutaneous barrier to transepidermal water loss (TEWL) after standardized skin wounds produced in human subjects. Wound repair occurred more quickly under occlusive or semiocclusive dressings than when it was allowed to proceed exposed to the environment. However, no significant improvement in the rate of reestablishment of the barrier to TEWL was observed when the covered test site was compared to uncovered control sites in each subject.

Levy et al.[30] utilized a suction blister wound model to assess drug effects on epidermal regeneration with 20 healthy volunteers. After four suction blisters were produced on the volar aspect of the forearm, the epidermis was removed to create a standardized subepidermal wound. Thereafter, the wounds were treated topically for 6 h daily for 14 days. The following treatments were compared: a topical clobetasol 17-propionate preparation under occlusion, a corticoid-free cream under occlusion, no treatment and occlusion (aluminum chamber), no treatment and no occlusion. Daily measurement of TEWL above the wounds was performed. The 0.05% clobetasol 17-propionate preparation caused a dramatic delay in TEWL decrease, while the untreated unoccluded field showed a continuous decrease over 14 days. Occlusion and corticoid-free treatment led to weak but significant delays of TEWL decrease when compared to the untreated unoccluded test field.

Visscher et al.[31] evaluated the effects of semipermeable films on human skin by following a standardized tape stripping wound by measuring of TEWL, skin hydration, rate of moisture accumulation, and erythema. Wounds treated with semipermeable films underwent more rapid barrier recovery than either unoccluded wounds or wounds under complete occlusion. Barrier films that produced intermediate levels of skin hydration during recovery produced the highest barrier repair rates.

The effects of occlusive and semipermeable membranes on wound healing and related data are summarized in Table 5.1.

5.3 CONCLUSIONS

Occlusive dressings may hasten healing time,[2,18–22,27,29] but completely occlusive dressings have some disadvantages,[21,26,28,30] particularly when compared to semiocclusive dressings. Therefore, an ideal wound dressing would require a compromise between occlusion and nonocclusion. It should absorb exudate, thus decreasing bacteria; permit fluid evaporation; and either should not be incorporated into the eschar or be sufficiently fragile to allow its removal without compromising the healing wound.

Advanced dressings attempt to specifically maintain a moist wound environment. Natural, pure, and nonwoven dressings from calcium alginate fibers can rapidly absorb and retain wound fluid to form an integral gelled structure, thereby maintaining an ideal moist wound-healing environment.[32] These dressings can also trap and immobilize pathogenic bacteria in the network of gelled fibers, stimulate macrophage activity, and activate platelets, resulting in hemostasis and accelerated wound healing.

The biologic effects of dressings remain a complex science; at a minimum, clinical relevance for humans requires a multifaceted interpretation based on our current knowledge of "validation for humans." When can we extrapolate from rodents to humans, what is the overlying "Rosetta Stone" that might relate the more "superficial" wound healing (stripping and/or solvent extraction) knowledge to split and full-thickness wounds? What can be learned from other factors (O_2, CO_2, and

TABLE 5.1
Summary Data on the Effects of Occlusive and Semipermeable Membranes on Wound Healing

Wound Models	Occlusion	Results	Ref.
Superficial wounds in domestic pigs	Wounds treated with two different occlusive dressings, nonocclusive wet-to-dry gauze dressings, and air exposure	Collagen synthesis and reepithelialization were increased in the wounds treated with occlusive dressings; reepithelialization was increased beneath both the oxygen-impermeable and oxygen-permeable dressings	21
Biopsy punch in rabbits	Wounds covered with occlusive and semiocclusive dressings	Water loss from the occluded site returned to baseline values in 9 d as opposed to 17 d for semioccluded sites	26
Full-thickness 4 × 4-cm wounds in rabbits	Wounds treated with fine-mesh gauze and a human amnion dressing	No differences observed between the gauze and amnion groups	26
Human dermabrasion wound	Wound dressings compared	Occlusive dressings hastened healing time as much as 50% over air-exposed sites	27
Acetone-induced wounds in hairless mice	Wounds covered with an occlusive membrane and a vapor-permeable membrane.	Occlusive membranes prevented the increase in epidermal lipid synthesis, while a vapor-permeable membrane increased epidermal lipid synthesis	28
Wounds produced in human subjects	Examined the effects of occlusive dressings on the reestablishment of the cutaneous barrier to transepidermal water loss	Wound repair occurred more quickly under occlusive or semiocclusive dressings than when it was allowed to proceed exposed to the environment; however, no significant improvement in the rate of reestablishment of the barrier to TEWL was observed when the covered test sites were compared to uncovered control sites in each subject	29

TABLE 5.1 (CONTINUED)
Summary Data on the Effects of Occlusive and Semipermeable Membranes on Wound Healing

Wound Models	Occlusion	Results	Ref.
Suction blister wound model in humans	Wounds treated: topical clobetasol 17-propionate preparation under occlusion, a corticoid-free cream under occlusion, no treatment and occlusion (aluminum chamber), no treatment and no occlusion	Occlusion and corticoid-free treatment led to a weak but significant delay of TEWL decrease when compared to the untreated unoccluded test field	30
Tape stripping wound in humans	Wounds treated with semipermeable films, complete occlusion, and unoccluded	Wounds treated with semipermeable films underwent more rapid barrier recovery than either unoccluded wounds or wounds under complete occlusion	31

electrolyte transport)? These represent but a few of the challenges for wound dressing developers.

Today, with the rapid development of new technologies in bioscience, we can expect greater efficacy and optimal dressings or materials that can absorb excess fluid, thus accelerating the healing of wounds without the unfavorable effects of occlusion.

REFERENCES

1. Kligman, A.M., Hydration injury to human skin, in *The Irritant Contact Dermatitis Syndrome,* Van der Valk, P.G.M. and Maibach, H.I., Eds., CRC Press, Boca Raton, FL, 1996, p. 187.
2. Berardesca, E. and Maibach, H.I., Skin occlusion: treatment or drug-like device? *Skin Pharmacol.,* 1, 207, 1988.
3. Bucks, D., Guy, R., and Maibach, H.I., Effects of occlusion, in *In Vitro Percutaneous Absorption: Principles, Fundamentals, and Applications,* Bronaugh, R.L. and Maibach, H.I., Eds., CRC Press, Boca Raton, FL, 1991, p. 85.
4. Bucks, D. and Maibach, H.I., Occlusion does not uniformly enhance penetration *in vivo,* in *Percutaneous Absorption: Drug–Cosmetics–Mechanisms–Methodology,* 3rd ed., Bronaugh, R.L. and Maibach, H.I., Eds., Marcel Dekker, New York, 1999, p. 81.
5. Faergemann, J., Aly, R., Wilson, D.R., and Maibach, H.I., Skin occlusion: effect on *Pityrosporum orbiculare,* skin P CO_2, pH, transepidermal water loss, and water content, *Arch. Dermatol. Res.,* 275, 383, 1983.

6. Matsumura, H., Oka, K., Umekage, K., Akita, H., Kawai, J., Kitazawa, Y., Suda, S., Tsubota, K., Ninomiya, Y., Hirai, H., Miyata, K., Morikubo, K., Nakagawa, M., Okada, T., and Kawai, K., Effect of occlusion on human skin, *Contact Dermatitis,* 33, 231, 1995.
7. Berardesca, E. and Maibach, H.I., The plastic occlusion stress test (POST) as a model to investigate skin barrier function, in *Dermatologic Research Techniques,* Maibach, H.I., Ed., CRC Press, Boca Raton, FL, 1996, p. 179.
8. Leow, Y.H. and Maibach, H.I., Effect of occlusion on skin, *J. Dermatol. Treat.,* 8, 139, 1997.
9. Denda, M., Sato, J., Tsuchiya, T., Elias, P.M., and Feingold K.R., Low humidity stimulates epidermal DNA synthesis and amplifies the hyperproliferative response to barrier disruption: implication for seasonal exacerbations of inflammatory dermatoses, *J. Invest. Dermatol.,* 111, 873, 1998.
10. Kömüves, L.G., Hanley, K., Jiang, Y., Katagiri, C., Elias, P.M., Williams, M.L., and Feingold, K.R., Induction of selected lipid metabolic enzymes and differentiation-linked structural proteins by air exposure in fetal rat skin explants, *J. Invest. Dermatol.,* 112, 303, 1999.
11. Fluhr, J.W., Lazzerini, S., Distante, F., Gloor, M., and Berardesca, E., Effects of prolonged occlusion on stratum corneum barrier function and water holding capacity, *Skin Pharmacol. Appl. Skin Physiol.,* 12, 193, 1999.
12. Warner, R.R., Boissy, Y.L., Lilly, N.A., Spears, M.J., McKillop, K., Marshall, J.L., and Stone, K.J., Water disrupts stratum corneum lipid lamellae: damage is similar to surfactants, *J. Invest. Dermatol.,* 113, 960, 1999.
13. Kligman, A.M., Hydration injury to human skin: a view from the horny layer, in *Handbook of Occupational Dermatology,* Kanerva, L., Elsner, P., Wahlberg, J.E., and Maibach, H.I., Eds., Springer, Berlin, 2000, p. 76.
14. Zhai, H. and Maibach, H.I., Effects of skin occlusion on percutaneous absorption: an overview, *Skin Pharmacol. Appl. Skin Physiol.,* 14, 1, 2001.
15. Zhai, H. and Maibach, H.I., Skin occlusion and irritant and allergic contact dermatitis: an overview, *Contact Dermatitis,* 44, 201, 2001.
16. Zhai, H. and Maibach, H.I., Occlusion vs. skin barrier function, *Skin Res. Technol.,* 8, 1, 2002.
17. Zhai, H., Ebel, J.P., Chatterjee, R., Stone, K.J., Gartstein, V., Juhlin, K.D., Pelosi, A., and Maibach, H.I., Hydration vs. skin permeability to nicotinates in man, *Skin Res. Technol.,* 8, 13, 2002.
18. Eaglstein, W.H,, Mertz, P.M., and Falanga, V., Wound dressings: current and future, *Prog. Clin. Biol. Res.,* 365, 257, 1991.
19. Winter, G.D., Formation of the scab and the rate of epithelization of superficial wounds in the skin of the young domestic pig, *Nature,* 193, 293, 1962.
20. Hinman, C.D. and Maibach, H.I., Effect of air exposure and occlusion on experimental human skin wounds, *Nature,* 200, 377, 1963.
21. Alvarez, O.M., Mertz, P.M., and Eaglstein, W.H., The effect of occlusive dressings on collagen synthesis and re-epithelialization in superficial wounds, *J. Surg. Res.,* 35, 142, 1983.
22. Fisher, L.B. and Maibach, H.I., Effect of occlusive and semipermeable dressings on the mitotic activity of normal and wounded human epidermis, *Br. J. Dermatol.,* 86, 593, 1972.
23. Aly, R., Shirley, C., Cunico, B., and Maibach, H.I., Effect of prolonged occlusion on the microbial flora, pH, carbon dioxide and transepidermal water loss on human skin, *J. Invest. Dermatol.,* 71, 378, 1978.

24. Rajka, G., Aly, R., Bayles, C., Tang, Y., and Maibach, H.I., The effect of short-term occlusion on the cutaneous flora in atopic dermatitis and psoriasis, *Acta Dermatol. Venereol.,* 61, 150, 1981.

25. Mertz, P.M. and Eaglstein, W.H., The effect of a semiocclusive dressing on the microbial population in superficial wounds, *Arch. Surg.,* 119, 287, 1984.

26. Surinchak, J.S., Malinowski, J.A., Wilson, D.R., and Maibach, H.I., Skin wound healing determined by water loss, *J. Surg. Res.,* 38, 258, 1985.

27. Pinski, J.B., Human dermabrasion as a wound healing model, in *Models in Dermatology,* Maibach, H.I. and Lowe, N., Eds., Karger, Basel, 1987, p. 196.

28. Grubauer, G., Elias, P.M., and Feingold, K.R., Transepidermal water loss: the signal for recovery of barrier structure and function, *J. Lipid. Res.,* 30, 323, 1989.

29. Silverman, R.A., Lender, J., and Elmets, C.A., Effects of occlusive and semiocclusive dressings on the return of barrier function to transepidermal water loss in standardized human wounds, *J. Am. Acad. Dermatol.,* 20, 755, 1989.

30. Levy, J.J., von Rosen, J., Gassmuller, J., Kleine Kuhlmann, R., and Lange, L., Validation of an *in vivo* wound healing model for the quantification of pharmacological effects on epidermal regeneration, *Dermatology,* 190, 136, 1995.

31. Visscher, M., Hoath, S.B., Conroy, E., and Wickett, R.R., Effect of semipermeable membranes on skin barrier repair following tape stripping, *Arch. Dermatol. Res.,* 293, 491, 2001.

32. Williams, C., Algosteril calcium alginate dressing for moderate/high exudate, *Br. J. Nurs.,* 8, 313, 1999.

Part III

Quantifying Repair in the Epidermis

6 Human and Swine Models of Epidermal Wound Healing

Jill Bigelman and Patricia M. Mertz

CONTENTS

6.1 INTRODUCTION

This chapter will review and discuss research studies from both human and swine models of epidermal wound healing. The research data gathered from animal and human models has heightened our understanding of the wound healing process. In 1963, Hinman and Maibach reported the use of a human model to evaluate the effect of occlusion on wound healing.[1] They made partial thickness wounds on the inner arms of healthy adult male volunteers, with each volunteer serving as his own control. The inner arm was used because relatively few hair follicles exist in this area. Their theory was that by doing this, examination of the point of origin of epithelization would be simplified, as the epithelium spreads mainly from the periphery of the wound rather than the transected hair follicle. They left the control wound exposed to air and used a polyethylene film to occlude the experimental wound. Cutaneous punch biopsies (8 mm) were taken at 3-, 5-, 7- and 9-d intervals to histologically determine the rate of reepithelization. This study demonstrated that occlusion speeds reepithelization. While this model provides an effective way of evaluating wound healing, human studies are often impractical. Volunteers may be unwilling to undergo multiple biopsies, and ethical issues concerning the use of controls must be considered.

Hartwell[2] determined that porcine skin is anatomically and physiologically more similar to human skin than is the skin of small laboratory animals. However, differences exist between porcine and human skin as well. These differences are mostly attributed to the lesser importance of skin in regulating body temperature in swine, as compared to humans.[3] The epidermis in both swine and in human skin is thick. The ratio of dermal to epidermal thickness is thought to best demonstrate their similarity, as epidermal thickness is heavily dependent on body size. This ratio has been reported to be about 10:1 to 13:1 in both swine and humans.[4] The epidermis of swine is composed of stratified squamous epithelium, thrown into many folds, resulting in the formation of both dermal papillae and interpapillary pegs; this is very similar to the situation in humans.

Both human and swine dermis are divided into the papillary and reticular dermis. Swine have a dense, less cellular, and less vascular reticular dermis than do humans. The less complex vasculature of the porcine dermis is due to the less developed adnexal structures and absence of eccrine glands in swine. Also, both pigs and humans have abundant subdermal adipose tissue, and sebaceous glands are attached to the hair follicles in a 1:1 ratio (Color Figure 6.1).*

Both swine and humans have sparse body hair relative to other animals. Their hair progresses through hair cycles independently of neighboring follicles.[5] Also, immunohistochemical staining has shown keratins 16 and 10, filaggrin, collagen IV, fibronectin, and vimentin in both swine and human skin.[6] Finally, both swine and humans are so-called tight skinned animals and have a limited capacity for early wound contraction.

Epidermis

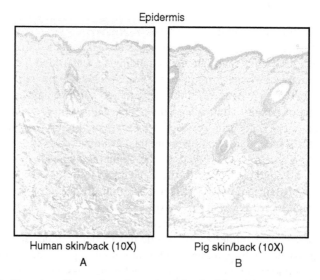

Human skin/back (10X)
A

Pig skin/back (10X)
B

FIGURE 6.1 Hematoxylin- and eosin-stained back skin of human and swine. (See color figures following page 110.)

---

* Color figures follow page 110.

Epidermal Migration Assessment

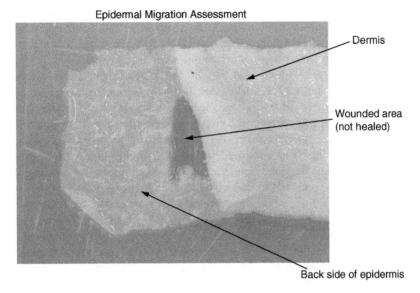

Dermis

Wounded area
(not healed)

Back side of epidermis

FIGURE 6.2 Wound healing specimen from the salt-split technique of Eaglstein and Mertz. (See color figures following page 110.)

In the mid-1970s, Eaglstein and Mertz developed a wound healing model in young domestic swine to study epidermal wound healing.[7] This model was based on models developed by Rovee and Miller[8] and by Winter.[9] Rovee and Miller used the foot pad of a guinea pig to study incisional wounds. The footpad was chosen as it is the only area of the guinea pig that has thick epidermis like the epidermis in humans. Winter's model was of partial thickness wounds in young white pigs. He examined serial histological sections of superficial wounds. The concept of working with a separated epidermis and using the establishment of a mature epidermis as an endpoint of healing, which can be examined macroscopically, resulted in the porcine model for evaluating epidermal wound healing (Color Figure 6.2).

6.2 OCCLUSIVE DRESSINGS

The ability of occlusive dressings to accelerate wound healing has been well described in the medical literature. The pioneers of this concept were Winter and Maibach, who studied wounds in swine and humans, respectively. Winter studied shallow wounds covered by polyethylene film and found that the wounds remained moist and had an increased speed of epithelization.[9] One mechanism proposed for the increased rate of resurfacing is the easier migration of epithelial cells across the moist wound bed provided by these dressings. This is important, as epidermal resurfacing is dependent on epidermal cell movement. It has been demonstrated that while occlusive dressings can reduce the magnitude and duration of mitotic activity occurring in a wound,[10] these dressings can still increase the reepithelization rate.[9] Therefore, although both cell division and migration are important in wound healing, resurfacing is dependent on cell migration.

Another hypothesized mechanism for occlusive dressings' ability to stimulate wound healing is their ability to maintain an electrical potential between wounded skin and the surrounding normal tissue. It has been demonstrated that a naturally occurring electric potential is present in moist wounds after injury and is shut off when a wound dries out.[11] Cheng et al. measured the electrical potentials in occluded wounds.[12] They created a system where small silver-chloride electrodes were connected to a voltmeter (Keithley™). One electrode was then placed in the center of a porcine wound that was covered with an occlusive dressing and the other contacted normal skin on the edge of the dressing. The electrical potential of an occluded partial-thickness wound was compared to that of a similar untreated air-exposed wound. The potentials were the same the day of wounding prior to dressing application. However, the potential of the occluded wound remained high for the 4 days needed for epithelization, while the potential of the air-exposed wound fell to a lower level. After the fourth day, the occluded wound's potential fell back to a level similar to that of the nonoccluded wound, and reepithelization was completed. This study demonstrates that occlusive dressings' ability to stimulate wound healing may be at least partially dependent on an electrical potential between wounded skin and normal tissue. In addition to speeding reepithelization, some occlusive dressings have also been shown to increase the partial pressure of oxygen beneath films, to increase local concentration of growth factors, and to have favorable effects of increasing microbial flora.[13]

Occlusive dressings have the ability to reduce tenderness at the wound site, to serve as a substitute for the role of skin as the first line of defense, and to produce a more cosmetically acceptable wound closure.[14] Linsky et al. compared half of a surgical wound covered with an occlusive dressing to the uncovered half. They concluded that in 70% of cases the half of the wound treated with an occlusive dressing was cosmetically superior.[15]

Occlusive dressings have been designed to keep wounds moist. It was feared that their use would promote wound infection because of the increased proliferation of microorganisms beneath occlusive films. Also, tissue desiccation has an antimicrobial effect, which is specifically avoided by occlusive dressing. And lastly, infection was feared because of the suppurative exudates that frequently occur in occlusively dressed wounds.[14] Yet, wound infection beneath occlusive dressings has infrequently been reported. Moreover, Buchan et al.'s study of chronic ulcers treated with occlusive dressings demonstrated that healing occurs with only rare infection despite "massive bacterial over-growth."[16]

Eaglstein et al. discovered that the time at which an occlusive dressing is applied or removed from a superficial wound is of great importance.[17] They conducted a porcine study in which polyurethane dressings were applied and removed at varied times. When dressings were applied within 2 h of wounding and were kept in place for at least 24 h, epidermal resurfacing was optimal.

Many types of occlusive dressings are available to physicians. These include film dressings, which are made of polyurethane. Film dressings are transparent and adhesive but not absorbent. Because of this, fluids tend to accumulate beneath the dressings, and bacteria tend to proliferate.[18] The bacteria found beneath these dressings tend to be normal flora rather than pathogens and have been shown to phagocytize pathogenic bacteria for the first 24 h that the film is in place.[19] The effect of these dressings on wound healing is very similar in human and animal models. Film dressings increase the rate of reepithelization in acute partial-thickness wounds in humans.[20,21] Levine et al. showed that the rate of proliferation of porcine keratinocytes increased by more than 20% beneath film occlusion.[22] Similar results were obtained in a study by Woodley and Kim, who used a human model of suction blisters to study wound healing. Suction blisters were induced in five volunteers, and the effects of a nonocclusive dressing were compared to those of a film dressing. The rate of reepithelization was greater when the film dressing was used.[23]

A hydrocolloid dressing material has also been used to promote wound healing. This type of dressing is nontransparent, adhesive, and absorbent. Therefore, it is able to absorb much of the wound fluid that is produced. Our group has shown that these dressings are able to resist bacterial penetration even when challenged with high concentrations of bacterial suspensions.[24] These dressings have also shown great concordance when studied in humans and in swine. In a study by Alvarez et al. conducted in a swine model, hydrocolloid dressings produced a greater number of resurfaced wounds on earlier days than did nonocclusive dressings or air exposure.[20] Similarly, hydrocolloid dressings were shown to accelerate the healing of wounds induced in humans.[25]

Calcium alginate dressings are made with the calcium salt of alginic acid. A hydrophilic gel is formed at the wound surface when the calcium of the alginate filaments and sodium in the blood and exudate exchange ions to produce soluble calcium–sodium alginate.[26] Hydrogels are nonadhesive, absorbent dressings. Vigilon®, a hydrogel dressing, is able to absorb twice its weight in fluid. However, this type of dressing does not exclude bacteria and may promote the growth of Gram-negative bacteria.[24] Foam dressings are absorbent but not adhesive or transparent. Therefore, they are often used for wounds that have surrounding friable skin. Calcium alginate, foam dressings, and hydrogels have been shown to increase reepithelization in acute wounds in humans, but only calcium alginate and hydrogels have shown similar results in swine.[6]

6.3 GROWTH FACTORS

The inflammatory phase of wound healing begins with the influx of neutrophils from the periphery. They are induced to migrate toward the wound by chemotactic factors produced by products of the coagulation cascade.[27] The neutrophils begin a process of phagocytizing bacteria and matrix proteins, which usually lasts a few days. However, it is not the presence of neutrophils in the wound that is critical to wound healing. Interestingly, Simpson and Ross demonstrated that neutropenia does not interfere with wound healing.[28]

Instead, macrophages are the cells of critical value. Macrophages help to fight bacterial contamination and to produce growth factors, which promote wound healing. The role of the macrophage has been substantiated by studies in which cortisone and antimacrophage serum were used to treat wounds.[29] In these studies, the rate of wound healing was markedly delayed.

Interleukin 1 (IL-1), which is produced by both macrophages and keratinocytes, possesses a wide spectrum of inflammatory, metabolic, physiologic, and immunologic properties. It was found in 1990 that the addition of exogenous IL-1α enhanced wound epithelization in a partial-thickness wound model, similar to an occlusive film dressing.[14] Although human keratinocytes express IL-1α and IL-1β, only IL-1α is active upon release.[30] Furthermore, in a second-degree burn model in swine, IL-1β did not demonstrate a stimulatory effect upon epithelization.[14]

An ultraviolet radiation (UVR) source that contains mostly UVB is known to stimulate IL-1α production by keratinocytes.[31] In a study of electrokeratome-induced partial-thickness wounds in swine, it was found that UVR exposure both prior to and after wounding stimulated epidermal repair.[14] Experiments were then conducted to elucidate whether occlusive dressings stimulate IL-1α and by that effect stimulate wound healing. Suramin, a polyanionic drug that blocks receptors for growth factors considered to be important in epithelization, was placed into wounds that were then covered with an occlusive dressing.[32] The relative rate of healing in suramin-treated wounds was 19% lower than that in non-suramin-treated wounds with the same occlusive dressing. This study suggests the role of growth factors in wound healing. Furthermore, in a study where an IL-1α receptor antagonist was applied topically under occlusion, wounds healed at same rate as wounds left open to air.[14]

Human and swine studies have shown great concordance with respect to the effects of IL-1α, while similar studies in other animals have shown different results. A study conducted by Maish et al. suggested that IL-1α may impair wound healing in rats.[33] However, IL-1α has been shown to significantly enhance healing in studies in both pigs and humans. Mertz et al. verified this hypothesis with their study involving the addition of exogenous IL-1α to partial- and full-thickness wounds in swine,[34] and Barbul reported similar results in a human study of split-thickness skin graft donor sites.[35]

6.4 WOUND INFECTION, BIOFILMS, AND ANTIMICROBIALS

Wound infection is defined as the adherence and penetration of bacteria into viable tissue and is often described using this equation: infection = dose × virulence/host resistance. Chronic wounds, which contain copious wound fluid, necrotic tissue, and deep cracks, offer an ideal environment for the proliferation of microflora. Furthermore, individuals with chronic wounds often have underlying pathology and compromised immune defense mechanisms.

There has been debate among physicians regarding treatment of clinically infected chronic wounds that contain a bacterial load of more than 1 million per g of tissue. Krizek and Robson developed this criterion during their work with skin grafts in burn patients.[36] They noticed that if the quantity of microorganisms exceeded this number, skin graft survival was unlikely. A Food and Drug Administration advisory meeting in 1997 was held in an attempt to reach a consensus regarding wound infection. It was concluded that most chronic wounds are colonized with a large number of microorganisms, and that the application of a specific number to define wound infection has no basis.

Sullivan et al. conducted a retrospective study in which they analyzed chronic leg ulcers that were cultured as part of prescreening for a clinical trial.[37] They observed that numerous bacteria are present in clinically noninfected chronic wounds and that this number does not always diminish after treatment with topical antimicrobials. It was then suspected that bacteria might live in biofilms — accumulations of microorganisms in an extracellular polysaccharide matrix (EPS). The EPS is believed to protect the bacteria from antimicrobial therapy. Biofilms have been associated with chronic infections.[38] The chronic nature of these infections may be related to a biofilm's resistance to topical and systemic antimicrobials and to the increased potential for gene transfer within a biofilm, which may convert a less virulent microorganism into a highly virulent pathogen.[39]

In a study conducted by Ceri et al., *Staphylococcus aureus* was grown in biofilms on small plastic projections. The biofilms were then exposed to antibiotics.[40] It was concluded that *S. aureus* in biofilms requires nearly a 500- to 1000-fold increase in the minimal inhibitory concentration (MIC) compared to *S. aureus* not within biofilms. This finding of greater resistance of *S. aureus* living in biofilms correlates with the lack of response of chronic wound infections to antibiotic therapy and prompted investigations by our group on biofilms found in chronic wounds. Bello and Ricotti of the University of Miami School of Medicine have used two staining methods to demonstrate that biofilms are present in chronic wounds. A modified Congo Red/Ziehl Carbol fuchsin was first used and demonstrated the presence of extracellular polysaccharide (EPS) surrounding bacteria (Color Figure 6.3).[41] Bacterial biofilm formation has recently been induced in partial-thickness wounds in swine and detected using Calcofluor White and an epifluorescent microscopy technique for visualization (Color Figure 6.4).[42] This same staining technique has demonstrated EPS in wound tissue curetted from chronic human wounds. The role of biofilm formation in reepithelization has not been studied and is an area for future investigation in both swine and human models.

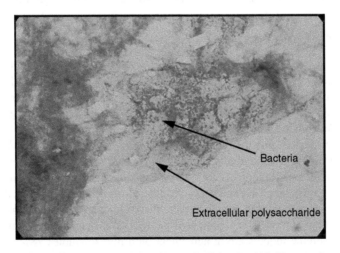

FIGURE 6.3 Modified Congo Red stain of bacteria living in a biofilm matrix made up of EPS taken from a chronic wound scraping. (See color figure following page 110.)

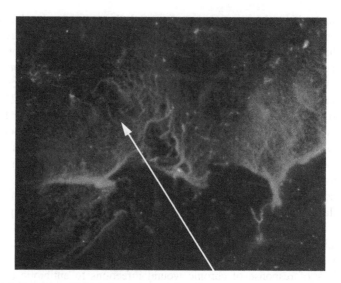

FIGURE 6.4 Calcofluor White fluorescent stain of EPS from a bacterial-induced wound biofilm from swine. (See color figure following page 110.)

The efficacy of antimicrobial use in wound healing has varied greatly in different wound models. For example, *in vitro* studies of povidone–iodine have demonstrated great toxicity to keratinocytes and fibroblasts at low concentrations.[43] However, Geronemus et al. did not observe a similar effect when testing the use of povidone–iodine in swine.[44] Overall, however, the effects of topical antimicrobials in swine correlate well with those in humans. Gruber et al. treated partial-thickness wounds in humans with 10% povidone–iodine every 6 h until wound healing was complete.[45] They found that treated wounds healed faster than air-exposed controls and concluded that povidone–iodine did not have negative effects on wound healing.

6.5 SUMMARY

Human studies remain the most accurate way to evaluate medical therapies. However, their impractical nature leads scientists to search for other methods for determining the efficacy of new treatments. Studies involving topical antimicrobials have demonstrated the relative strength of animal models as compared to *in vitro* testing. This is easily understood because *in vivo* cells are supported by an organism's homeostatic mechanisms that cells in culture lack. Yet, all animal models are not equally efficacious in their ability to predict outcomes in humans. Guinea pigs, rats, mice, and other small mammals are often selected for use in wound healing studies because they are inexpensive and easy to handle. However, there are great differences in the structure of their skin as compared to that of humans. Sullivan et al. evaluated 25 wound therapy models and compared the results in humans and animals.[6] They found that porcine models are in agreement with human studies 78% of the time. Studies in small mammals and *in vitro* agree with human studies only 53 and 57%

of the time, respectively. By using appropriate animal models it is possible to predict the results of wound healing therapies in humans with a great degree of accuracy.

ACKNOWLEDGMENT

Special thanks to Alejandro L. Cassaniga, Ysabel Bello, M.D., and Carlos Ricotti, M.D., for obtaining the images used as the figures for this chapter and to Stephen C. Davis for editorial assistance.

REFERENCES

1. Hinman, C.D. and Maibach, H., Effect of air exposure and occlusion on experimental human skin wounds, *Nature,* 200, 377–378, 1963.
2. Hartwell, S.W., *The Mechanism of Healing in Human Wounds,* Charles C. Thomas, Springfield, IL, 1955.
3. Montagna, W. and Yun, J. The skin of the domestic pig. *J. Invest. Dermatol.,* 43, 1964.
4. Vardaxis, N.J., Brans, T.A., Boon, M.E., Kreis, R.W., and Marres, L.M., Confocal laser scanning microscopy of porcine skin: implications for human wound studies, *J. Anat.,* 190, 601–611, 1997.
5. Winter, G.D., A Study of Wound Healing in the Domestic Pig, Ph.D. dissertation, Birbeck College, University of London, 1966.
6. Sullivan, T.P., Eaglstein, W.H., Davis, A.C., and Mertz, P.M., The pig as a model for human wound healing, *Wound Repair Regen.,* 9, 66–76, 2001.
7. Eaglstein, W.H., Mertz, P.M., New method for assessing epidermal wound healing: the effect of triamcinolone acetonide and polyethylene film occlusion. *J. Invest. Dermatol.,* 71(6), 382–384, 1978.
8. Rovee, D.T. and Miller, C.A., Epidermal role in the breaking strength of wounds, *Arch. Surg.,* 96, 43–52, 1968.
9. Winter, G.D., Formation of the scab and the rate of epitheliazation of superficial wounds in the skin of the young domestic pig, *Nature,* 193, 293–294, 1962.
10. Rovee, D.T., Effect of local wound environment on epidermal healing, in Maibach, H.L. and Rovee, D.T., *Epidermal Wound Healing,* Year Book Medical Publishers, Inc., Chicago, 1972, pp. 159–181.
11. Jaffe, L.F. and Vanable, J.W., Electrical fields and wound healing, *Clin. Dermatol.,* 2, 34–44, 1984.
12. Cheng, K., Tarjan, P.P., Oliveira-Gandia, M.F., Davis, S.C., Mertz, P.M., and Eaglstein, W.H., An occlusive dressing can sustain natural electrical potential of wounds, *J. Invest. Dermatol.,* 104, 662, 1995.
13. Hinman, C.C., Maibach, H., and Winter, G.D., Effect of air exposure and occlusion on experimental human skin wounds, *Nature,* 200, 377–378, 1963.
14. Alvarez, O.M., Mertz, P.M., and Eaglstein, W.H., The effect of occlusive dressings on collagen synthesis and reepithelization in superficial wounds, *J. Surg. Res.,* 35, 142–148, 1983.
15. Linsky, C.B., Rovee, D.T., and Dow, T., Effect of dressing on wound inflammation and scar tissue, in Dineen, P. and Hildick-Smith, G., Eds., *The Surgical Wound,* Lea & Febiger, Philadelphia, 1981, pp. 191–206.

16. Buchan, I.A., Andrews, J.K., and Lang, S.M., Clinical and laboratory investigation of the composition and properties of human skin wound exudates under semi-permeable dressings, *Burns,* 7, 326–334, 1981.

17. Eaglstein, W.H., Davis, S.C., Mehle, A.L., and Mertz, P.M., Optimal use of an occlusive dressing to enhance healing: effect of delayed application and early removal on wound healing, *Arch. Dermatol.,* 124, 392–395, 1988.

18. Mertz, P.M. and Eaglstein, W.H., The effect of a semi-occlusive dressing on the microbial population in superficial wounds, *Arch. Surg.,* 119, 287–289, 1984.

19. Buchan, I.A., Andrews, J.K., and Lang, S.M., Laboratory investigation of the composition and properties of pig skin wound exudate under op-site, *Burns,* 8, 39–46, 1981.

20. Alvarez, O.M., Mertz, P.M., and Eaglstein, W.H., The effect of occlusive dressings on collagen synthesis and reepithelization in superficial wounds, *J. Surg. Res.,* 35, 142–148, 1983.

21. Robbins, P., Day, C.L., and Lew, R.A., A mulitvariate analysis of factors affecting wound healing time, *J. Dermatol. Surg. Oncol.,* 10, 219–221, 1984.

22. Levine, R., Agren, M.S., and Mertz, P.M., Effect of occlusion on cell proliferation during epidermal healing, *J. Cutan. Surg. Med.,* 2, 193–198, 1998.

23. Woodley, D.T. and Kim, Y.H., A double-blind comparison of adhesive bandages with the use of uniform suction blister wounds, *Arch. Dermatol.,* 128, 1354–1357, 1992.

24. Mertz, P.M., Marshall, D.A., and Eaglstein, W.H., Occlusive wound dressings to prevent bacterial invasion and wound infection, *J. Am. Acad. Dermatol.,* 12, 662–668, 1985.

25. Nemeth, A.J., Eaglstein, W.H., Taylor, J.R., Peerson, L.J., and Falanga, V., Faster healing and less pain in skin biopsy sites treated with an occlusive dressing, *Arch. Dermatol.,* 127, 1679–1683, 1991.

26. Jarvis, P.M., Galvin, D.A.J., Blair, S.D., and McCollum, C.N., How Does Calcium Alginate Achieve Haemostasis in Surgery? 10th International Congress of Thrombosis and Haemostasis, Brussels, 8–10 July 1987.

27. Clark, R.A.F., Cutaneous tissue repair: basic biological considerations, *J. Am. Acad. Dermatol.,* 13, 701–725, 1985.

28. Simpson, D.M. and Ross, R., The neutrophilic leukocyte in wound repair. A study with antineutrophil serum, *J. Clin. Invest.,* 51, 2009–2023, 1972.

29. Leibovich, S.J. and Ross, R., The role of the macrophage in wound repair: a study with hydrocortisone and antimacrophage serum, *Am. J. Pathol.,* 71–91, 1978.

30. Mizutani, H., Black, R., and Kupper, T.S., Human keratinocytes produce but do not process pro-interleukin-1 (IL-1) beta. Different strategies of IL-1 production and processing in monocytes and keratinocytes, *J. Clin. Invest.,* 87, 1066–1071, 1991.

31. Kaiser, M.E., Davis, S.C., and Mertz, P.M., The effect of ultraviolet irradiation-induced inflammation on epidermal wound healing, *Wound Repair Regen.,* 3, 311–315, 1995.

32. Rotman, D.A., Cazzaniga, A., Helfman, R., Falanga, V., and Mertz, P.M., Sumarin application to porcine partial thickness wounds delays epithelization, *J. Invest. Dermatol.,* 98, 610, 1992.

33. Maish, G.O., Shumate, M.L., Ehrlich, H.P., Vary, T.C., and Cooney, R.N., Interleukin-1 receptor antagonist attenuates tumor necrosis factor-induced alterations in wound breaking strength, *J. Trauma,* 47, 533–537, 1999.

34. Mertz, P.M., Sauder, D.N., Davis, S.C., Kilian, P.L., Herron, A.J., and Eaglstein, W.H., IL-1 as a potent inducer of wound re-epithelization, *Prog. Clin. Biol. Res.,* 365, 473–480, 1991.

35. Barbul, A., The Effects of Interleukin 1 on the Healing of Split Thickness Donor Sites. Reported at the 47th annual session of the Forum on Fundamental Surgical Problems at the Clinical Congress of the American College of Surgeons, Chicago, Oct. 20–25, 1991.
36. Krizek, T.J. and Robson, M.C., Bacterial growth and skin graft survival, *Surg. Forum,* 18, 518, 1967.
37. Sullivan, T., Falabella, A., Valencia, I., and Mertz, P.M., Continued high-level bacterial colonization of venous stasis ulcers after topical antibiotic therapy, abstract, Wound Healing Society, 2000.
38. Pitera, C., Forging a link between biofilms and disease, *Science,* 283, 1837–1839, 1999.
39. Davis, S.C., Mertz, P.M., and Eaglstein, W.H., The wound environment: implications from research studies for healing and infection, in *Chronic Wound Care,* 3rd ed., Krasner, D., Rodeheaver, G., and Sibbald, G., Eds., HMP Communications, Wayne, PA, 2001, pp. 253–263.
40. Ceri, H., Olson, M.E., Strenik, C., Read, R.R., Morck, D., and Buret, A., The Calgary biofilm device: new technology for rapid detection of antibiotic susceptibilites of bacterial biofilms, *J. Clin. Microbiol.,* 1771–1776, 1999.
41. Bello, Y.M., Falabella, A.F., Cazzaniga, A.L., Harrison-Balestra, C., and Mertz, P.M., Are Biofilms Present in Chronic Wounds? Abstract 283, Vol. 117, No. 2, August 2001, p. 437, Society of Investigative Dermatology, Miami, FL, May 9, 2001.
42. Ricotti, C.A., Cazzaniga, A., Feiner, A.M., Davis, S.C., and Mertz, P.M., Epifluorescent microscopic visualization on an *in vitro* biofilm formed by a *Pseudomonas aeruginosa* wound isolate and of an *in vivo* polymicrobial biofilm obtained from an infected wound, Abstract 1019, *J. Inv. Dermatol.,* 12(1), July 2003, Symposium of Advanced Wound Care, April 2003.
43. Cooper, M.L., Laxer, J.A., and Hansbrough, J.F., The cytotoxic effects of commonly used topical antimicrobial agents on human fibroblasts and keratinocytes. *J. Trauma,* 31, 775–784, 1991.
44. Geronemus, R.G., Mertz, P.M., and Eaglstein, W.H. Wound healing: the effects of topical antimicrobial agents, *Arch. Dermatol.,* 115, 1311–1314, 1979.
45. Gruber, R.P., Vistness, L., and Pardoe, R., The effect of commonly used antiseptics on wound healing, *Plast. Reconstr. Surg.,* 55, 472–476, 1975.

7 Noninvasive Physical Measurements of Wound Healing

Marco Romanelli, Diego Mastronicola, and Giovanni Gaggio

CONTENTS

7.1 INTRODUCTION

Chronic ulcerative skin lesions affect around 1.5% of the population and represent a considerable medical and social problem. The population affected by this pathology is generally geriatric and often suffers from concomitant illnesses. Chronic ulcers have different causes and can be divided into the following main categories: vascular ulcers (venous, arterial, mixed), diabetic foot ulcers, pressure ulcers, and ulcers of other etiologies. The above pathologies refer to chronic and disabling conditions that profoundly affect the patients' quality of life and often lead to psychological disturbances, such as depression.

New treatments for these pathologies have led to improvements in lesion management and in the quality of the assistance provided by medical and paramedical staff, but lesion-monitoring methodologies have not kept pace with this progress. The techniques used to obtain a valid wound assessment are currently based on the use of transparent acetate sheets, which are positioned on the lesion so as to trace its perimeter manually, measuring the depth of the lesion by placing a cotton swab inside it, or filling the lesion cavity with hypoallergenic material to produce a cast, which is then measured to obtain the volume of the lesion. However, most clinical diagnoses depend on visual observation of the lesion. This is obviously an inaccurate, nonstandardized, slow, and above all subjective method, which depends on the experience of the physician.

The effective and accurate monitoring of skin lesions should be performed by measuring in an objective, precise, and reproducible way the complete status and evolution of the skin lesion.[1] The main goal of current research projects is to design a system that can monitor the qualitative and quantitative evolution of a skin lesion with an easy-to-use technological system.

The shape characteristics of a small skin section can be calculated using three-dimensional (3D) scanners,[2,3] in particular, systems based on active optical approaches. Some of these systems also support the integrated acquisition of the color of the scanned region, and color plays a very important role in the analysis of the status of a skin lesion. The quality of current 3D scanning devices allows accurate geometric and chromatic characterizations of the skin lesion to be achieved. This objective characterization allows numerical measures to be assessed according to a flexible set of parameters; the data may then be stored in a database, and the skin damage may be easily monitored over time. Such devices have two different categories of potential applications: medical treatment, to improve the efficacy of therapeutic regimens, and pharmacological scientific research, to assess the quality and effectiveness of new chemicals or clinical procedures.

Once a 3D model of the lesion has been produced, the assessment of significant parameters must be performed either in an automatic manner or through the contribution of a dermatologist. Two related actions can be performed:

First, the required shape-based measurements are calculated.
Second, the associated color information is segmented to produce an image,
    in which color segmentation is integrated with the shape characterization.

7.2   VIDEO IMAGE ANALYSIS

Previous attempts at monitoring the evolution of lesions in a more objective manner include systems based on the acquisition of two-dimensional (2D) images or video streams.[4,5] In these studies, a characterization of the tissue status is reconstructed from the segmentation of the RGB image, and some 2D measurements are inferred from this segmentation (e.g., the wound area computed in the 2D image projection space). Calibration specimens are generally placed in proximity to the lesion, to allow color calibration and reconstruction of linear measurements.

Laser scanning systems were introduced some years ago and have been adopted to produce very accurate 3D digital models in many different applications, including the film and advertising industries, industrial quality control, rapid prototyping, and cultural heritage. The accuracy of the scanning systems has improved in the last few years and prices have also decreased, making these devices affordable for a wider community of potential users. The integration into a single system of capabilities that can capture the shape and surface reflection characteristics (i.e., color) makes 3D scanning an invaluable resource in all those applications where it is necessary to sample both of these surface attributes. The acquisition speed of some of these scanning devices (generally less than 1 sec to take a range map) is suitable for scanning human beings, who can easily stay still for such a short time.

From a purely technical point of view, an integrated system for wound assessment must support the following functionalities:

- Three-dimensional geometrical acquisition of skin lesions with accuracy on the order of 0.2 mm.
- Acquisition of the color attribute of the skin section considered.
- Mapping of the color information on the 3D geometry of the lesion.
- Characterization of significant measures for the objective monitoring of various types of skin lesions. This includes both automatic measurements, such as the surface extent of the lesion, its perimeter, the depth of the lesion in selected locations, the volume delimited by the lesion surface, and the hypothetical skin surface, as well as any point-to-point distance requested by the medical user.
- Segmentation of the color attribute and integration of the segmented interpretation with the numeric measures taken by the 3D lesion geometry. Color characterization is important, since areas with different colors correspond to different states of the tissue.
- Storage of all the acquired/computed data in a database, organized on *per patient* and *per examination* bases.

Obviously, all of the above functionalities have to be provided to the prospective clinical user with an easy-to-use guide, which should allow an intuitive use of the system as much as possible. The final system chosen must be extremely reliable, since diagnosis and medical treatment will depend on the system characterization of the lesion status.

7.3 SHAPE CHARACTERIZATION

The main clinical parameters involve the measurement of lengths, surface extension, and volume. Point-to-point distances can be obtained very easily. Point pairs are selected on the 3D model through a point-and-click technique; the segment connecting the points is displayed immediately, together with the associated length. The perimeter of the wound is first specified by the user with an interactive approach and then refined by the system. Selection of the border of the lesion is performed in a semiautomatic manner: first, the user draws a closed poly-line covering the border of the lesion; then the system improves the fit of this border with the 3D data by considering the shape and the color gradient of the selected areas. The initial poly-line is refined, with the creation of new points whose coordinates are located in 3D space according to surface curvature and color gradient estimation. The method used is based on the snake approach.[6,7] The user has complete control over the shape defined by this refinement phase and can modify the location of any point that delimits the lesion boundary. Once the perimeter of the lesion has been selected, the assessment of its length is straightforward.

Once the wound perimeter is known, the corresponding wound bed is isolated and measured to obtain the wound surface. Perimeter, surface, and volume measurements are obviously performed on the 3D mesh and therefore take into account any possible roughness.

7.4 CHROMATIC ASSESSMENT

Characterization of the chromatic data is another analysis of particular importance in wound assessment. The color of different tissues can be linked to different conditions of the lesion. A segmentation step is therefore needed in order to reduce the different color shades in the lesion region to a few, user-defined color clusters, which are directly linked to different clinical conditions of the tissue. Standard image segmentation techniques are therefore applied to the lesion image.

In general, three main classes are used by clinicians: black necrotic eschar, yellow slough, and red granulation tissue. Once the lesion region has been segmented into a few classes, the system produces numerical data computed on the corresponding 3D mesh, such as the perimeter, the surface area, and the percentage of each class with respect to the wound size. The segmented chromatic characterization and the computed data can be saved in the database and can be used for comparison of the status of the lesion at different intervals.[8]

Recently, we monitored the efficacy of debridement through the use of tristimulus colorimetric assessment in chronic wounds.[9] In this study, we were comparing a hydrogel and an enzymatic preparation, which were applied once a day for 2 weeks. The colorimetric evaluation was more accurate than clinical scoring in assessing granulation tissue, and it has been shown to possess high reproducibility, with the advantage of avoiding the bias involved in clinical scoring.

7.5 HIGH-FREQUENCY ULTRASOUND

A noninvasive assessment of the skin structure can be obtained by high-frequency ultrasound (Figure 7.1). This technology has shown consistent results in dermatology in the acquisition of data on different dermatological diseases, such as skin cancer, psoriasis, and scleroderma, as well as in wound healing.[10,11] Noninvasive assessment of skin structure using this technique allows accurate measurement and quantification of edema in venous insufficiency, providing greater information for the understanding of this fundamental pathogenic factor.[12] The technique has been shown to be an objective, valid, and reproducible instrument for the evaluation of the healing process up to the point of scar formation.[13]

Using 20-MHz B-mode high resolution ultrasonography, it is possible to obtain a specific image of the skin and an identification of physiological and pathological skin structures (Color Figure 7.2).* Major changes observed in the skin involve epidermal atrophy and dermal modifications, but high-frequency ultrasound is used to identify

---

* Color figures follow page 110.

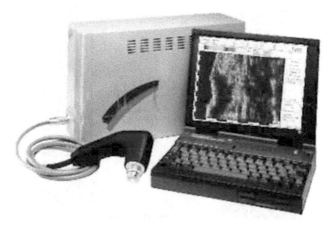

FIGURE 7.1 A portable 20-MHz ultrasound device.

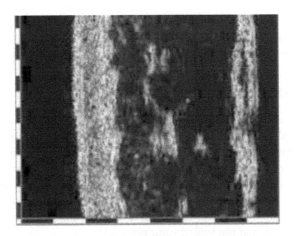

FIGURE 7.2 A 20-MHz ultrasound scan of normal skin. (See color figure following page 110.)

the ultrastructure in chronic wounds, hypertrophic scars (Color Figure 7.3), keloids, and normal surrounding skin.[14] The use of an aqueous transmission gel over the wound bed allows for optimal recording without any direct contact with the lesion.

The parameters analyzed are the depth between skin surface, the inner limit of the dermis, and the tissue density. The depth measurement, expressed in millimeters, gives an estimate of wound and scar thickness. The values of echogenicity are an expression of tissue density and are characterized by a high echogenicity of the dermis, compared to a relative hypoechogenicity of the subcutaneous fat. Moreover, a significant correlation has been found between echogenicity and the duration of scars.

This technique also makes possible an accurate evaluation and quantification of the amount of granulation and sloughy and necrotic tissue, together with measurements of the length and width of the wound.[15] The technique has enormous advantages over other methods such as callipers, xeroradiography, and punch biopsies.[16]

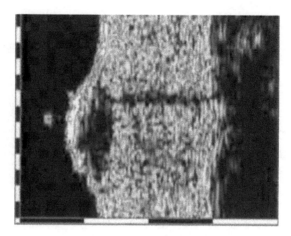

FIGURE 7.3 A 20-MHz ultrasound scan of a hypertrophic scar. (See color figure following page 110.)

High-frequency ultrasound is a safe, objective, noninvasive and painless method for the evaluation of the wound healing process, allowing an accurate evaluation of epithelialization, formation of granulation tissue, and contraction of ulcers.

7.6 LASER DOPPLER SYSTEMS

Adequate perfusion is fundamental to the maintenance of the normal structure and function of the skin and in the healing process. There are several problems in microcirculation in epidermal diseases that have been difficult to clarify due to the absence of appropriate instrumentation. Different techniques are available for measuring skin blood flow, such as skin temperature measurement, dynamic capillaroscopy, isotope techniques, percutaneous measurement of partial oxygen pressure, assessment of capillary pressure, fluorescence videomicroscopy, videodensitometry, and photoplethysmography.[17]

The different layers of local skin microcirculation can be directly detected by laser Doppler flowmetry and laser Doppler perfusion imaging. Laser Doppler devices are noninvasive; they are based on the Doppler effect and a laser light source such as a low-power helium–neon laser (2 to 5 mW, $\lambda = 632.8$ nm) or semiconductor laser diodes with near-infrared light of 780 nm. The main differences between these two laser sources is that laser diodes are multichannel instruments, and the light generated can penetrate more deeply into cutaneous tissue.[18]

The photons of monochromatic light emitted by lasers penetrate into tissue and are reflected by stationary and moving tissue components. Stationary tissue scatters and reflects the incident photons at the same frequency, while red blood cells moving with a certain speed reflect the waves, which go through Doppler shifts in their frequency. The radiation returning to the instrument is composed of two components: the nonshifted waves reflected from nonmoving tissue elements and the frequency-modulated light. A proportion of shifted light is backscattered to the system where the signal is detected by an optoelectronic device and processed. The voltage output is proportional to the velocity and concentration of the moving red cells and gives a measurement of tissue perfusion.

The development of laser Doppler flowmetry dates back to 1972. Since 1975, this technique has been used for the assessment of skin blood flow in humans.[19]

Laser Doppler flowmetry is widely used because it is a noninvasive, simple, objective, and fast instrumental measurement that quantifies cutaneous blood flow 1 to 2 mm under the skin surface (including the upper papillary plexus) and provides a continuous or near-continuous record. The monochromatic, coherent laser light is conducted by glass fibers to a probe, attached to the skin by means of adhesive discs. The movement of blood cells leads to a scattering of the laser light, generated by a low-powered helium-neon source, inducing a Doppler shift.

The backscattered signal containing data on flux, cell concentration, and cell velocity is displayed on screens, and the data may be recorded by a computer.[20]

Capillaries and dermal vessels are usually present at a depth of 1 mm and can be easily evaluated with this technique. This measurement is able to monitor perfusion in the wound bed, adjacent normal skin, and scars. Two parameters are monitored with the patient supine and relaxed: resting flow and healing potential index (HPI) (ml of blood/100 g of tissue/min). HPI represents the ratio of resting flow values for the ulcer and the adjacent normal skin.

It has been shown that blood flow in all types of chronic ulcers is 170% higher than in normal skin and that a potential healing index of less than 100% is not a good prognosis. Blood flow in hypertrophic scars and keloids is 180% higher than in normal skin.[21] However there are some limitations with this technique, such as the necessity for contact with the organs evaluated, the potential for pain or sepsis when applying the probe to skin surface, and poor accuracy in the determination of tissue volume.

Since 1993, a development of the laser Doppler flowmetry called laser Doppler imaging has been available; it combines laser Doppler and scanning techniques and overcomes the above limitations.[22] This instrument is equipped with a moving mirror and light collection system instead of optical fibers.

This technique displays on the screen of a computer a two-dimensional color-coded image of the local flux, in which each color corresponds to a different level of perfusion. It can therefore be used for evaluating tissue viability and ischemic areas.[23]

With regard to colors, blue-violet is an expression of poor flux, whereas green, yellow, and red correspond to areas with higher flux. Grey areas represent regions where no flux can be detected.

Although some authors do not recommend these exams for routine use in wound healing studies,[24] laser Doppler flowmetry and laser Doppler perfusion imaging (LDPI) have been used in the evaluation of wound healing and for definition of ischemia, inflammation, and reperfusion. They could be useful in delimiting areas that need debridement.

Laser Doppler flowmetry has been used to assess patch test reaction, providing quantitative and more comparable data, as well as accurate statistical analysis (although expensive and time-consuming.)[25] The advantage of this method is that it can visualize subclinical reactions through blood flow changes at a time when clinical assessment cannot detect any erythema.[26]

The use of laser Doppler flowmetry or LDPI has been reported in the evaluation of immediate wheal-and-flare reactions,[27] tuberculin reactions,[28] and ultraviolet-induced erythema.[25] Vasodilating effects of various systemic and topical drugs or blood flow changes in response to the effect of chemical mediators can also be measured by laser Doppler flowmetry.[29]

Laser Doppler flowmetry is useful in the evaluation of wound healing, microangiopathy in diabetic patients, and burn depth; it has also been used to monitor flaps and replants.[30]

The laser Doppler flowmeter–measured resting flux has been shown to be elevated (and reversible with treatment) in venous disorders,[31] while remaining approximately at a normal value in peripheral arterial obliterative disease.[32]

Laser Doppler flowmetry has been used in stage 2 and 3 pressure ulcers for the continuous evaluation of local skin microcirculation, and it has been shown that the local blood flow increased at the ulcer edge at rest and after heat stress at 44°C, when compared to surrounding skin.[33]

Concomitant evaluation using laser LDPI and capillary microscopy within venous ulcers and ischemic ulcers is capable of differentiating the distribution of microcirculation in granulation tissue, nongranulation tissue, adjacent normal skin, and distant skin.[34,35] In fact, up to 85% of the laser Doppler signal is generated by deeper layers of skin microcirculation characterized by a thermoregulatory function, while the superficial nutritive layers are well detected by capillary microscopy, which detects the density and morphology of visible capillaries.[36]

Laser Doppler imaging is also an accurate technique for the early and objective assessment of burn depth, as well as a useful instrument in assessing the timing of surgical treatment. High flux indicates a favorable prognosis for wound healing, whereas low flux is an expression of difficult or impossible spontaneous wound closure. With this instrument, it is also possible to assess the whole burn without direct contact with the burn surface.[37]

Laser Doppler flowmetry has been used to assess local blood flow changes in scleroderma, in which the blood flow of sclerotic plaques is higher than normal, and in rosacea,[38] which is characterized by a lesional blood flow three to four times higher than normal (control patients). Scanning laser Doppler flowmetry allows the measurement of increased cutaneous blood flow in psoriatic plaques and the assessment of its decrease with various treatment modalities, thanks to the rapidity of evaluation and the ability to cover a large area of skin surface. This method also seems very useful as an adjunct instrument in the differentiation between benign and malignant pigmented skin lesions.[39] Currently, this noninvasive instrument is not directly applicable to clinical practice but is reliable in several fields of dermatologic research, providing excellent monitoring of cutaneous microcirculation.

7.7 TRANSCUTANEOUS OXIMETRY

The observation of the existence of an exchange of O_2 and CO_2 between skin and ambient air was first made by Gerlach in 1851.[40]

Transcutaneous oximetry is an effective technique widely used in the evaluation of local skin microcirculation, nutrition, and tissue ischemia. Several methods for noninvasive measurements of tissue O_2 are available.[41] One of these is the transcutaneous partial oxygen ($tcpO_2$) technique, based on the electrochemical reduction of oxygen, which is measured on the skin surface with a calibrated Clark electrode. The $tcpO_2$ measurement provides information about the content of tissue oxygenation in superficial skin layers. The post-heating reactive hyperemia responses of $tcpO_2$ can be used as relative measures of the vasodilatory capacity of skin microvessels. The $tcpO_2$ values depend on cutaneous circulation, arterial oxygen tension (pO_2), oxygen consumption in skin tissue, and oxygen diffusibility through the skin itself. The values measured represent the partial pressure of oxygen diffusing from the capillaries and provide data on the oxygenation of superficial skin layers. The $tcpO_2$ values from undamaged skin can vary depending on the body region, and it has been noticed that low values are associated with failure in wound healing.[42] In tissue with inflammatory reaction, the dramatic increase in local metabolism and the infiltration of a large number of cells requiring oxygen may increase the consumption of oxygen in the skin, leading to low $tcpO_2$ values. The $tcpO_2$ and transcutaneous partial carbon dioxide ($tcpCO_2$) values have been measured in a large number of skin conditions and clinical situations, such as evaluation and management of leg ulcers,[43] the assessment of skin involvement in patients with morphea and scleroderma,[44] investigation into hypertrophic scars,[45] and the understanding of the action and efficacy of vasoactive drugs.[46] These values can be influenced by many local factors such as blood flow, thickness of the epidermis, metabolism of the epidermis and glands, conductivity of the gases, and the production and consumption of such gases *in situ*. The epidermal barrier must also be considered in the measurement of $tcpO_2$, since the stratum corneum represents an important resistance to oxygen diffusion; its removal (using a stripping technique or other methods) is recommended when studying the skin, for a better reproducibility of the assessment.[47]

Other perfusion analyses, such as arteriography, capillaroscopy, plethysmography, and videomicroscopy, are considered difficult to perform and too invasive.

7.8 pH MEASUREMENT

pH is defined as the negative logarithm of the activity of hydrogen ions in an aqueous solution and is used to express acidity and alkalinity on a scale of 0 to 14. There are few reports on the noninvasive measurement of skin surface pH.

In 1892, Hesus first determined the acid nature of the skin surface,[48] and since then a large number of studies have confirmed his observation and defined the representative range of pH for the population as a whole. The first study on the scientific assessment of skin surface pH was performed by Schade and Marchionni using an electrometric technique.[49] More recently, the normal range of values of skin surface pH[50] has been established. Normal values of pH in intact skin range from 4.8 to 6.0 due to the presence of the acid mantle, while the interstitial fluid is characterized by neutral values. The values are more alkaline for subjects over age 80 years.

In recent years, a central role for the acid mantle as a regulating factor in stratum corneum homeostasis has been emerging, and this has been shown to be very relevant to the integrity of barrier function. Until now, no diseases have been associated with an increase or decrease in skin surface pH. However, alteration in the skin pH (and the organic factors influencing it) seems to play a role in the pathogenesis, prevention, and healing of several cutaneous diseases, such as irritant contact dermatitis, atopic dermatitis, and ichthyosis; it also plays a role in wound healing.

Measurements of cutaneous pH are used in assessing sudden changes in pH following exposure to external factors, such as acid or alkaline products, and in assessing the state of acute or chronic cutaneous diseases.

Significant improvements in the methodology and instrumentation of skin surface pH measurement took place during the last century. Two major methods are currently used for measuring cutaneous pH: the colorimetric technique and the glass electrode potentiometric (GEP) measurement.

The most common pH instrument, in use since 1972, is a flat glass electrode connected to a meter and applied to the skin, with one or two drops of bi-distilled water interposed between the electrode and the skin.[51] The use of a flat electrode is necessary to provide good contact with the skin surface, providing high accuracy and sensitivity for the assessment. The measurement is noninvasive and the electric current is low and constant and causes no skin damage. In contrast, the colorimetric procedure with dye pH indicators is less accurate, owing to the interference of many factors.

The recommended regions for GEP measurement of pH are the forehead in the midline, 3 cm above the nasion, and the cheek below the zygomatic bone, but if necessary, measurements can be performed on any area of the skin.

The electrode is attached to the skin for an interval of 10 sec until stabilization of the reading. Measurements are performed at a room temperature that is below 23°C and a relative humidity of less than 65%, because sweat can influence the results. Readings should be taken 12 h after the application of detergents or creams to the skin.

One new instrument for pH reading is based on pH transistor technology, in which the sensor is an ion-sensitive field effect transistor.[52] This noninvasive technique for the measurement of skin surface pH has been used in the past to assess the barrier properties of the stratum corneum and also to evaluate the relationship between changes in superficial skin microflora and the development of skin irritation. In fact, researchers have already noted that a relationship exists between the acidity of the skin surface and its antimicrobial activity.

Many reports have been published on the relationship between skin pH and the incidence of cutaneous diseases. In acute eczema (with erosions), the pH is alkaline due to extracellular components. Some authors have found an increase in skin surface pH in xeroderma, atopic dermatitis, and seborrheic dermatitis.[53]

Glibbery and Mani[54] used glass electrodes for the measurement of skin surface pH on ulcers and control sites and showed a link between acid medium and healing. Wound bed pH has been proven to be fundamental in the healing of chronic wounds, since prolonged acidification of the wound bed enhances the healing rate of chronic leg ulcers; the pH of nonhealing chronic venous leg ulcers and pressure ulcers was shown to be alkaline or neutral when compared to that of normal perilesional skin.

Sayeg et al.[55] used reproducible wound pH measurements in experimental and clinical studies to predict skin graft survival and found this assessment useful in the determination of the percentage success or failure of the surgical treatment of burns and chronic ulcers.

The use of occlusive dressings in wound healing provides the optimum environment for normal repair and regeneration, and the acidic wound fluid collected during moist wound healing has been shown to inhibit bacterial growth and to promote fibroblast proliferation.[56] Using a foam dressing on venous leg ulcers, we were able to change the wound bed pH from an alkaline to an acidic environment and to maintain this acidic state until dressing removal, 72 h later.[57]

Currently, the use of skin pH measurements is limited to the assessment of the effects of various materials and environmental factors on the skin surface, but we believe that wound bed pH measurement can provide highly useful information about the changes in bacterial burden in chronic wounds.

7.9 INFRARED THERMAL IMAGING SYSTEMS

The skin represents a thermal interface between the body and the environmental temperature; it is influenced by both internal and external factors, and the link between temperature and diseases has been observed for millennia.

The study of body temperature is based on the three fundamental methods of heat transmission: conduction (fluid thermometers, thermistors, and thermocouples), convection, and radiation (radiation thermometers, infrared imaging system). Many of these instruments alter the heat exchange between the skin and the environment, but an ideal temperature measurement technique should in no way interfere with this exchange.

Another essential parameter in the measurement of skin temperature is reproducibility, and the thermal radiation system is thoroughly reliable in this sense. It provides a high-speed, two-dimensional temperature recording, does not need direct contact, and does not interfere with the skin.

Thermal imaging is a highly efficient instrument for the assessment of skin temperature, providing both thermal and spatial resolution. Thermography is a noninvasive method and represents one of the most technically developed methods of thermal imaging, which, when correctly used under controlled conditions, supersedes the effectiveness of other thermometers. Through the use of thermography, temperatures can be evaluated and recorded, allowing visualization of heat flow.

Three types of thermography are currently in use: liquid crystal thermography, infrared thermography, and microwave thermography[58] (Color Figure 7.4).

Infrared thermography has been found to be a fast and stable method, which is relatively impervious to user technique. The technology used is based on electro-optical systems for the detection of infrared radiation emitted by the skin. Cadmium–mercury–telluride or indium–antimonide are the detectors most commonly used to generate an electrical signal; at this point, a scanning optical arrangement allows the creation of a two-dimensional image.[59] This real-time imaging, in association with efficient online processing, allows greater ease of use and higher quality

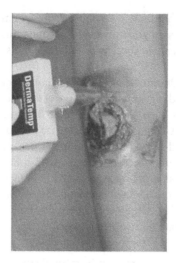

FIGURE 7.4 Skin temperature measurement on the surrounding skin of an infected ulcer. (See color figure following page 110.)

of information, while the use of digital infrared cameras has improved spatial and thermal resolutions enormously.

Even though it is nonspecific, thermal imaging can be used to monitor many clinical conditions. Increased skin temperature has long been associated with infection; therefore, thermography could provide a useful means to evaluate and monitor the healing process in complicated chronic wounds. Inflammation with increased local perfusion may be detected clearly and early, thanks to the precise relationship between skin perfusion and temperature.

This technique is therefore reliable in monitoring local heat and quantifying the degree, extent, and response to therapy.[60] Reduction of body temperature assessed by thermal index has been used to evaluate the efficacy of analgesic and anti-inflammatory agents.[61] Increases in skin temperature have been measured during erythema and urticarial eruptions.[62] Equally, a reduction in skin temperature can be found in a large number of conditions where there is a decrease in tissue perfusion, such as venous ulceration.

Low wound bed temperatures have been shown to delay healing rate, mainly because there is a decrease in oxygen release.[63]

Moreover, a region with poor vascularization, generating a cold area on the thermography, will probably result in delayed or impaired healing, while a hot, well-perfused region can be expected to heal correctly.

Even though the cost for these techniques is currently high, new possibilities are emerging through the use of low-cost portable thermal imaging cameras, and high-resolution thermal imaging will improve our knowledge of skin temperature physiology and measurement. The elevated resolution and noninvasiveness of thermographic systems make them valuable options for the detection and diagnosis of several skin diseases or abnormalities, such as infections, inflammation, or malignancies characterized by increased skin temperature.

7.10 CONCLUSION

Over the past few years, a number of highly developed objective and noninvasive techniques for wound assessment have been brought into use. These techniques are important research tools in investigating the different phases of wound healing and in determining therapeutic effects. Since noninvasive measurements can be performed repeatedly on the same wound site, changes during wound healing may be monitored. Our knowledge about the physical properties of acute and chronic wounds is likely to increase in the near future, thanks to this greater interaction with the engineering field. Because of its importance in wound healing, the use of noninvasive measurements can be expected to progress with new techniques and methods to be applied in research and in clinical practice.

REFERENCES

1. Romanelli, M. et al., Technological advances in wound bed measurements, *WOUNDS,* 14, 58, 2002.
2. Chen, F., Brown G.M., and Song, M., Overview of three-dimensional shape measurement using optical methods, *Opt. Eng.,* 39, 10, 2000.
3. Bernardini, F. and Rushmeier, H.E., The 3D model acquisition pipeline, *Computer Graphics Forum,* 21, 149, 2002.
4. Mekkes, J.R. and Westerhof, W., Image processing in the study of wound healing, *Clin. Dermatol.,* 13, 401, 1995.
5. Solomon, C. et al., The use of video image analysis for the measurements of venous ulcers, *Br. J. Dermatol.,* 133, 565, 1995.
6. Gonzales, R.C. and Woods, R.E. *Digital Image Processing,* Addison-Wesley Publishing Company, Philadelphia, 1993, p. 85.
7. Kass, M., Witkin, A.P., and Terzopoulos, D., Snakes: active contour model, *ICCV87 Proc.,* 259, 1987.
8. Herbin, M. et al., Assessment of healing kinetics through true color image processing, *IEEE Trans. Med. Imaging,* 12, 39, 1993.
9. Romanelli, M., Objective measurements of venous ulcer debridement and granulation with a skin colour reflectance analyser, *WOUNDS,* 9, 122, 1997.
10. Altermyer, P. et al., General phenomenon of ultrasound in dermatology, in *Ultrasound in Dermatology,* Altermyer, P., El-Gammal, S., and Hoffmann, K., Eds., Springer-Verlag, Berlin, 1991, p. 55.
11. Whiston, R.J., Melhuish, J., and Harding, K.G., High resolution ultrasound imaging in wound healing, *WOUNDS,* 5, 116, 1993.
12. Gniadecka, M., Localization of dermal edema in lipodermatosclerosis, lymphedema and cardiac insufficiency, *J. Am. Acad. Dermatol.,* 35, 37, 1996.
13. Katz, S.M. et al., Objective measurement of hypertrophic burn scar. A preliminary study on tonometry and ultrasonography, *Ann. Plast. Surg.,* 14, 121, 1985.
14. Van Den Kerckhove, E., et al., Reproducibility of repeated measurements on postburn scars with Dermascan C, *Skin Res. Technol.,* 9, 81, 2003.
15. Dyson, M. et al., Wound healing assessment using 20 MHz ultrasound and photography, *Skin Res. Technol.,* 9, 116, 2003.
16. Rippon, M.G. et al., Ultrasound assessment of skin and wound tissue; comparison with histology, *Skin Res. Technol.,* 4, 147, 1998.

17. Bongard, O. and Bounameaux, H., Clinical investigation of skin microcirculation, *Dermatology,* 186, 6, 1993.
18. Vongsavan, N. and Mattews, B., Some aspects of the use of laser Doppler flow meters for recording tissue blood flow, *Exp. Physiol.,* 78, 1, 1993.
19. Stern, M.D., *In vivo* evaluation of microcirculation by coherent light scattering, *Nature,* 254, 56, 1975.
20. Nilsson, G.E., Tenland, T., and Oberg, P.A., Evaluation of a laser Doppler flowmeter for measurement of tissue blood flow, *IEEE Trans. Biomed. Eng.,* 27, 597, 1980.
21. Timar-Banu, O. et al. Development of noninvasive and quantitative methodologies for the assessment of chronic ulcers and scars in humans, *Wound Repair Regen.,* 9, 123, 2001.
22. Wardell, K., Jakobsson, A., and Nilsson, G.E., Laser Doppler perfusion imaging by dynamic light scattering, *IEEE Trans. Biomed. Eng.,* 40, 309, 1993.
23. Gschwandtner, M.E. et al., Laser Doppler imaging and capillary microscopy in ischemic ulcers, *Atherosclerosis,* 142, 225, 1999.
24. Graham, J.S. et al. Bioengineering methods employed in the study of wound healing of sulfur mustard burns, *Skin Res. Technol.,* 8, 57, 2002.
25. Bircher, A.J., Guy, R.H., and Maibach, H.I., Skin pharmacology and dermatology, in *Laser-Doppler Blood Flowmetry,* Shepard, A.P. and Oberg, P.A., Eds., Kluwer Academic, Boston, 1990, p. 141.
26. Wahlberg, J.E., Skin irritancy evaluated by laser Doppler flowmetry, *Acta. Pharm. Nord.,* 4, 113, 1992.
27. Van Neste, D. et al., Agonist–antagonist interactions in the skin: comparison of effects of loratadine and cetirizine on skin vascular responses to prick tests with histamine and substance P, *J. Dermatol. Sci.,* 4, 172, 1992.
28. Harrison, D.K. et al., A preliminary assessment of laser Doppler perfusion imaging in human skin using the tuberculin reaction as a model, *Clin. Phys. Physiol. Meas.,* 14, 241, 1993.
29. Heden, P., Plastic and reconstructive surgery, in *Laser-Doppler Blood Flowmetry,* Shepard, A.P., and Oberg, P.A., Eds., Kluwer Academic, Boston, 1990, p. 175.
30. Olavi, A., Kolari, P.J., and Esa, A., Edema and lower leg perfusion in patients with post-traumatic dysfunction, *Acupunt. Electrother. Res.,* 16, 11, 1991.
31. Fagrell, B., Peripheral vascular diseases, in *Laser-Doppler Blood Flowmetry,* Shepard, A.P. and Oberg, P.A., Eds., Kluwer Academic, Boston, 1990, p. 214.
32. Schubert, V., The influence of local heating on skin microcirculation in pressure ulcers, monitored by a combined laser Doppler and transcutaneous oxygen tension probe, *Clin. Physiol.,* 6, 413, 2000.
33. Gschwandtner, M.E. et al., Microcirculation in venous ulcer and the surrounding skin: findings with capillary microscopy and a laser Doppler imager, *Eur. J. Clin. Invest.,* 29, 708, 1999.
34. Gschwandtner, M.E., Laser Doppler imaging and capillary microscopy in ischemic ulcers, *Atherosclerosis,* 142, 225, 1999.
35. Bollinger, A. and Fagrell, B., *Clinical Capillaroscopy. A Guide to Its Use in Clinical Research and Practice,* Hofgrefe and Hubert, Toronto, 1990, p. 7.
36. Fagrell, B., Vital microscopy and the pathophysiology of deep venous insufficiency, *Int. Angiol.,* 14, 18, 1995.
37. Essex, T.J.H. and Byrne, P.O., A laser Doppler scanner for imaging blood flow in skin, *J Biomed. Eng.,* 13, 189, 1991.
38. Sibenge, S. and Gawkrodger, D.J., Rosacea: a study of clinical patterns, blood flow and the role of *Demodex folliculorum, J. Am. Acad. Dermatol.,* 26, 590, 1992.

39. Tur, E. and Brenner, S., Cutaneous blood flow measurements for the detection of malignancy in pigmented skin lesion, *Dermatology*, 184, 8, 1992.
40. Gerlach, J.V., Über das hautatmen, *Arch. Anat. Physiol.*, 431, 1851.
41. Sheffield, P.J., Measuring tissue oxygen tension: a review. *Undersea Hyper. Med.*, 25, 179, 1998.
42. Rooke, T.W., The use of transcutaneous oximetry in the noninvasive vascular laboratory, *Int. Angiol.*, 11, 36, 1992.
43. Nemeth, A.J., Eaglstein, W.H., and Falanga, V., Clinical parameters and transcutaneous oxygen measurements for the prognosis of venous ulcer, *J. Am. Acad. Dermatol.*, 20, 186, 1989.
44. Silverstein, J.L. et al., Cutaneous ipoxia in patients with systemic sclerosis (scleroderma), *Arch. Dermatol.*, 124, 1379, 1988.
45. Berry, R.B. et al., Transcutaneous oxygen tension as index of maturity in hypertrophic scars treated by compression, *Br. J. Plast. Surg.*, 38, 163, 1985.
46. Romanelli, M. et al., The effect of topical nitroglycerin on transcutaneous oxygen, *Br. J. Dermatol.*, 124, 354, 1991.
47. Takiwaki, H. et al., The influence of cutaneous factors on the transcutaneous pO_2 and pCO_2 at various body sites, *Br. J. Dermatol.*, 125, 243, 1991.
48. Hesus, E., Die Reaktion des Schweissen beim gesunden Menschen, *Monatsschr. Prakt. Dermatol.*, 14, 343, 1892.
49. Schade, H. and Marchionni, A., Der Sauremantel der Haut nach Gaskettenmessungen. *Klin. Wochenschr.*, 7, 12, 1928.
50. Dikstein, S. and Zlotogorski, A., Skin surface hydrogen ion concentration (pH), in Levegue, J.L., Ed., *Cutaneous Investigation in Health and Disease: Noninvasive Methods and Instrumentation,* Marcel Dekker, New York, 1988, p. 59.
51. Peker, J. and Wahlbas, W.. Zur Methodic der pH-Messung der Hautoberflache, *Dermatol. Wochenschr.*, 158, 572, 1972.
52. von Kaden, H., Oelssner, W., Kaden, A., and Schirmer, E., Die Bestimmung des pH-Wertes *in vivo* mit Ionensensitiven Feldeffekttransistoren, *Z. Med. Lab. Diagn.*, 32, 114, 1991.
53. Anderson, D.S., The acid-base balance of the skin, *Br. J. Dermatol.*, 63, 283, 1951.
54. Glibbery, A.B. and Mani, R., pH in leg ulcers, *Int. J. Microcirc. Clin. Exp.*, 2, 109, 1992.
55. Sayeg, N., Dawson, J., Bloom, N., and Sthal, W., Wound pH as a predictor of skin graft survival, *Curr. Surg.*, 45, 23, 1988.
56. Varghes, M.C. et al., Local environment of chronic wounds under synthetic dressings, *Arch. Dermatol.*, 122, 52, 1986.
57. Romanelli, M. et al., Evaluation of surface pH on venous leg ulcers under Allevyn dressings, in *International Congress and Symposium Series, No. 227,* Suggett, A., Cherry, G., Mani, R., and Eaglstein, W., Eds., Royal Society of Medicine Press, London, 1998, p. 57.
58. Yang, W.J. and Yang, P.P., Literature survey on biomedical applications of thermography, *Biomed. Mater. Eng.*, 2, 7, 1992.
59. Putley, E.H., The development of thermal imaging systems, in *Recent Advances in Medical Thermology,* Ring, E.F.J. and Phillips, B., Eds., Plenum Press, New York, 1984, p. 151.
60. Collins, A.J. and Ring, E.F.J., Measurement of inflammation in man and animals by radiometry, *Br. J. Pharmacol.*, 44, 145, 1972.
61. Ring, E.F.J., Thermal imaging and therapeutic drugs, in *Biomedical Thermology,* Gautherie, M., Ed., Alan R. Liss, New York, 1982, p. 463.

62. Stuttgen, G., Dermatology and thermography, in *Thermological Methods,* Engel, J.M., Flesch, U., and Stuttgen, G., Eds., Verlag Chemie, Weinheim, 1984, p. 257.
63. Ring, E.F.J., Skin temperature measurement, *Bioeng. Skin,* 2, 15, 1986.

8 Micro Wound Healing Models

Hongbo Zhai and Howard I. Maibach

CONTENTS

8.1 INTRODUCTION

Theoretically, it would be ideal to evaluate topical wound agents in the actual clinical situation. However, since the wound healing process is complex, and aspects of the natural wound, such as wound induction (physical or chemical), depth (superficial or deep), size (regular or irregular), site-to-site variability, and environmental factors (infection or not), may vary,[1-4] it is difficult to evaluate the effects of therapy upon the repair process. To objectively measure treatment effects, quantitative wound models are important.

This chapter presents micro wound healing models and summaries of related data.

8.2 MODELS

8.2.1 TAPE STRIPPING

Yang et al.[5] utilized three hairless mice wound models (lipid solvent–acetone-induced disruption of barrier function, cellophane tape stripping-induced mechanical wound, and detergent-induced irritant dermatitis) to determine the healing effect of a lipid mixture (cholesterol, ceramide, palmitate, and linoleate 4.3:2.3:1:1.08). The lipid mixture accelerated barrier repair after disruption of the barrier by solvent treatment or tape stripping (mechanical), and by certain detergents such as Sarkosyl and dodecylbenzensulfuric acid. However, following barrier disruption with other detergents, sodium dodecyl sulfate and ammonium lauryl sulfosuccinate, the lipid mixture did not improve recovery.

Reed et al.[6] compared skin barrier recovery rates in humans of different races and both genders with a tape stripping model. Neither the number of tape strippings required to perturb the barrier nor the rates of barrier recovery were significantly different in white versus Asian subjects or in female versus male subjects. However, patients with skin types II/III required only 30 ± 2 tape strippings to perturb the barrier, while those with skin types V/VI required 67 ± 7 tape strippings. Furthermore, while barrier function in skin type II/III recovered by approximately 20% by 6 h and 55% by 48 h, barrier function in skin type V/VI, independent of race, recovered more quickly, 43% and 72% at 6 and 48 h, respectively. The authors concluded that darkly pigmented skin displays both a more resistant barrier and one that recovers more quickly after perturbation by tape stripping than does the skin of individuals with lighter pigmentation.

Tanaka et al.[7] evaluated the recovery of barrier function following complete stratum corneum (SC) removal by tape stripping in patients with atopic dermatitis (AD) and age-matched healthy control subjects. They reported no difference between the groups in the recovery process of the water barrier function of the SC.

Zettersten et al.[8] compared the ability of equimolar and cholesterol- and free fatty acids (FFA)-dominant molar lipid mixtures (2% in propylene glycol/n-propanol, 7:3) versus vehicle alone on barrier recovery rates at 0, 3, 6, 24, and 48 h and 1 week after tape stripping of aged hairless mice (>18 months) and chronologically aged human skin (80 $\pm$ 5 years). A single topical application of the equimolar mixture allowed normal recovery in young mice but improved barrier recovery in chronologically aged mice ($P < 0.06$). Moreover, a 3:1:1:1 mixture with cholesterol as the dominant lipid further accelerated barrier recovery at 3 and 6 h ($P < 0.01$ and $P < 0.03$, respectively, versus 1:1:1:1). Likewise, the cholesterol-dominant, optimal molar ratio mixture significantly accelerated barrier recovery in chronologically aged human skin at 6 h ($P < 0.005$; n = 6). In contrast, in aged mice, a FFA-dominant mixture significantly delayed barrier recovery at 3, 6, and 24 h ($P < 0.005, 0.05$, and 0.001, respectively). The optimized ratios of physiologic lipids accelerated barrier recovery in both chronologically aged murine epidermis and aged human skin.

Denda and Tsuchiya[9] measured the recovery of skin barrier functions following tape stripping on volar forearm skin in human volunteers over 24 h. Barrier recovery rate was significantly lower between 20:00 h and 23:00 h than that at other time points. The skin surface temperature and the basal transepidermal water loss reached their highest values at about 03:00 h, while the cortisol level in the saliva was highest at 09:00 h. These researchers suggested significant time-dependent variation in skin barrier repair independent of changes in skin temperature and cortisol level.

Loden and Barany[10] compared the ability of "skin-identical lipids" in a petrolatum-rich cream base and pure petrolatum to facilitate barrier repair in detergent- and tape-stripped–perturbed human skin. Barrier recovery and inflammation were instrumentally monitored for 14 d. Treatment with the two products gave no indication that "skin-identical lipids" in a cream base are more efficient than pure petrolatum at promoting normalization in either of the two experimental insults.

8.2.2 Lipid Solvent

This model was partially described in Section 8.2.1.[5]

Grubauer et al.[11] treated hairless mice with acetone, which removed stainable neutral lipids from the SC, and compared the rate of repletion of stainable lipids, barrier recovery, and epidermal lipogenesis in animals covered with occlusive membranes or vapor-permeable membranes versus uncovered animals. Acetone treatment perturbed epidermal barrier function, which normalized in uncovered animals in parallel with the reappearance of SC lipid. When animals were covered with an occlusive membrane, barrier function did not recover normally. In contrast, occlusion with vapor-permeable membranes allowed barrier function to recover normally. Occlusive membranes prevented the increase in epidermal lipid synthesis, while a vapor-permeable membrane increased epidermal lipid synthesis. The authors suggested that transepidermal water flux was an indicative signal for recovery of barrier structure and function.

Man et al.[12] determined the effects of lipids alone or in various mixtures on acetone-treated hairless mouse skin and assessed barrier recovery. Ceramide and fatty acid alone, and their complex derivatives (cholesterol esters and cerebrosides), and two-component mixtures of fatty acid plus ceramide, cholesterol plus fatty acid, or cholesterol plus ceramide delayed barrier recovery. In contrast, complete mixtures of ceramide, fatty acid, and cholesterol allowed normal barrier recovery. Moreover, fluorescent-labeled cholesterol, fatty acid, and ceramide rapidly traversed the stratum corneum with uptake into the epidermal nucleated layers. Finally, incomplete, but not complete, mixtures produced abnormal lamellar bodies, leading to abnormal stratum corneum intercellular membrane bilayers. These authors concluded that:

1. Topical applications of individual lipids or incomplete mixtures of lipids interfere with barrier recovery, while complete mixtures of cholesterol, fatty acid, and ceramide allow normal barrier repair.
2. Incomplete mixtures of topical lipids inhibit barrier recovery at the level of the lamellar body, resulting in abnormal intercellular membrane structures in the stratum corneum, abnormalities that do not occur when a complete lipid mixture is provided.

Zhai et al.[13] assessed the efficacy of a topical agent in barrier recovery after acetone-induced acute water loss barrier disruption *in vivo* in humans. The upper back of volunteers was rubbed with acetone-soaked cotton balls until elevated rates of transepidermal water loss (TEWL) occurred (>20 g/m^2/h). The topical agent was then applied to the acetone-treated skin sites once daily for 5 d. Resolution evaluation used TEWL measurements, and the data were expressed as the percentage recovery in water barrier function. In comparison with placebo control, the topical agent significantly enhanced barrier recovery, especially within the first 72 h ($P < 0.05$).

8.2.3 SURFACTANT IRRITANT DERMATITIS

This model was also partially described in Section 8.2.1.[5,10]

Wilhelm et al.[14] investigated the repair phase in surfactant-induced irritant dermatitis from short-term exposure to three structurally different surfactants in humans. Sodium lauryl sulfate (SLS), dodecyl trimethyl ammonium bromide (DTAB), and potassium soap were the model irritants. Surfactant solutions (0.5%) were applied for 24 h to the volar aspect of the forearm of 11 volunteers. Visual scoring and biometrics were used to assess irritant reactions and the healing process. SLS and DTAB induced similar degrees of erythema, whereas SLS induced significantly higher TEWL increase. Although both erythema and TEWL were highest 1 h after surfactant exposure, skin dryness appearance showed delayed onset. Minimum hydration values were measured as late as 7 d following surfactant exposure. Dryness was significantly more pronounced in areas exposed to SLS than in areas exposed to DTAB. Complete repair of the irritant reaction induced by either SLS or DTAB was achieved 17 d post surfactant exposure. Stratum corneum hydration was the last feature to return to baseline values. Potassium soap did not significantly influence skin function.

Zhai et al.[15] conducted *in vivo* human studies to evaluate the efficacy of a topical agent after SLS-induced water barrier disruption. Occlusive chambers with 1% SLS were applied to the upper backs of volunteers for 24 h. The chambers were removed, and the topical agent applied on the SLS-treated skin sites daily for 5 d. Water barrier restoration was monitored by measuring TEWL. Results showed that a topical agent produced more rapid improvement in barrier function than its placebo vehicle, markedly accelerating repair at 48 h ($P < 0.01$), and persisting throughout the experiment ($P < 0.05$), in comparison with SLS-control sites. They concluded that topical agents might accelerate the repair rates of water barrier function in SLS-treated human skin.

Levin et al.[16] assessed the efficacy of low- and medium-potency corticosteroids on SLS-induced irritant dermatitis in humans. The dorsal side of hands was irritated with 10% SLS five times in 1 d. Once on day 1 and twice daily on days 2 through 5, 1% hydrocortisone, 0.1% betamethasone-17-valerate, and vehicle cream (petrolatum) were applied subsequently. Visual grading, bioengineering techniques, and squamometry were used to quantify skin response. Corticosteroids were ineffective in treating the surfactant-induced irritant dermatitis when compared with the vehicle and with the untreated control.

8.2.4 ALLERGIC CONTACT DERMATITIS

Zhai et al.[17] developed an *in vivo* human model system for the bioengineering and visual quantification of the effect of topical agents on nickel allergic contact dermatitis (ACD). Fourteen nickel patch test-positive subjects were included in a placebo-controlled, double-blind study after a prescreening procedure with a standard diagnostic patch test with nickel sulfate in 54 healthy human volunteers. Five percent nickel sulfate in petrolatum in a Finn Chamber was applied to forearm skin for 48 h to create a standardized dermatitis. Thereafter, the dermatitis was treated with a model topical agent and a placebo control while endpoint parameters were recorded daily for 10 d. Resolution was quantified by four parameters: visual scoring (VS), TEWL, skin blood flow volume (BFV), and skin color (a* value). The model agent reduced cutaneous allergic reactions, especially on days 8 to 10, in comparison with the placebo control.

8.2.5 BLISTERS

Frosch and Kligman[18] developed a blister wound model induced by topical administration of 1:1 aqueous solution of ammonium hydroxide (AH) to human skin. Using a 0.5-ml fresh solution of AH placed in a well held on the skin, an intraepidermal blister formed in an average time of 13 min. The blister roof can be used for physicochemical analyses of the horny layer, while the wound base is suitable for studies of wound healing or bacterial infections. Healing of this wound model is rapid without scarring. Grove et al.[19] utilized this model with a modification to observe the effect of aging. They measured two groups, young adults (aged 18 to 30 years) and older adults (aged 65 to 75 years). The time required for blister formation was greatly prolonged in the aged.

Leyden and Bartelt[20] compared the effects of topical antibiotics, a wound protectant, and antiseptics on the rate of wound healing and bacterial growth using a modification of a method employing ammonium hydroxide-induced intradermal blisters inoculated with *Staphylococcus aureus*. Each volunteer had six blister wounds induced (three per forearm). Two wounds were treated with antibiotic ointments (neomycin–polymyxin B–bacitracin or polymyxin B–bacitracin); the other wounds were treated with a wound protectant and antiseptics. All wounds were treated twice daily. A control wound remained untreated. All wounds were covered with an occlusive dressing during the study. The time to healing (100% epithelialization) was evaluated for each wound. Wounds were cultured for bacterial growth after two treatments. Contaminated blister wounds treated with either the neomycin–polymyxin B–bacitracin ointment or polymyxin B–bacitracin healed significantly faster (mean 9 d) than control wounds or those receiving the wound protectant or antiseptics. Only the neomycin–polymyxin B–bacitracin combination effectively eliminated bacterial contamination of the wounds after two applications (within 16 to 24 h after contamination with *S. aureus*). The overall clinical appearance and healing rates of antibiotic ointment-treated wounds were superior to the control and the other treatments.

Levy et al.[21] utilized a suction blister wound model to assess drug effects on epidermal regeneration in 20 healthy volunteers. After four suction blisters were created on the volar aspect of the forearm, the epidermis was removed to create a standardized subepidermal wound. Thereafter, the wounds were treated topically for 6 h daily during 14 days. The following were compared: clobetasol 17-propionate preparation under occlusion, corticoid-free cream under occlusion, no treatment and occlusion (aluminum chamber), no treatment and no occlusion. Daily measurements of TEWL were performed. The 0.05% clobetasol 17-propionate preparation caused a dramatic delay in TEWL decrease, whereby the untreated unoccluded field showed a continuous decrease over the observation period of 14 days. Occlusion and corticoid-free treatment led to weak but significant delays of TEWL decrease when compared to the untreated unoccluded test field. The authors concluded that this model seems to describe reepithelialization in a reliable manner and can be used for *in vivo* assessment of drug effects on migrating and proliferating epithelial cells.

8.2.6 OTHERS

Bolton and Constantine[22] described a partial-thickness incision wound model in guinea pigs. They used a movable and adjustable blade device to make uniform-depth wounds. They also studied a cantharidin blister bed wound model in small animals.

Pinski[23] compared wound dressings by using a human dermabrasion wound healing model and reported that occlusive dressings hastened healing time by as much as 50% over air-exposed sites.

Surinchak et al.[24] monitored the healing process by water evaporation. In the first study, two wounds were created with a 2-mm biopsy punch on the backs of each of 15 rabbits and covered with occlusive or semiocclusive dressings. Water loss increased from a preoperative value of 6 $g/m^2/h$ to 55 $g/m^2/h$ after surgery. Water loss from the occluded site returned to baseline values in 9 d, as opposed to 17 d for the semioccluded sites ($P < 0.05$).

The second study followed the healing of full-thickness 4 × 4-cm wounds in five rabbits treated with fine-mesh gauze and five treated with a human amnion dressing.[24] Wound area and water loss were observed during the repair process. Visual measurement of the wound area indicated that the injuries were 100% healed on day 30. The evaporimeter detected significantly increased water loss up to day 45, when the original baseline values were reached. No differences were observed between the gauze and amnion groups. The evaporimeter presents a simple yet accurate, noninvasive tool measuring the wound healing endpoint based on regeneration of the epidermal water barrier.

Experimental micro wound models are summarized in Table 8.1.

8.3 CONCLUSIONS

Since wound healing is complex, defining the sequence of biological events leading to skin healing is aided by animal and human wound models that determine species-specific responses and discriminate the effects of imposed variables on specific aspects of healing.[1-4] In the evaluation of topical agents, such an experimental procedure is essential.

However, to date, no one standardized wound model to evaluate topical agents has been established. Each model described here has advantages and limitations. One good human model may offer substantial advantages over uncontrolled patient-use situations. However, some human models are accompanied by discomfort and may leave scars. Hence, animal wound models may provide an alternative, but no one animal, with its complex anatomy and biology, will simulate wound healing in humans for all compounds. Therefore, a realistic estimate of human wound healing for topical agents is determined by *in vivo* studies in humans. Furthermore, application of noninvasive bioengineering techniques in evaluating effects of topical

TABLE 8.1
Experimental Micro Wound Models

Wound Models			
Animals	**Humans**	**Clinical Relevance**	**Ref.**
Three wound models on hairless mice: lipid solvent–acetone-induced disruption of barrier function, cellophane tape stripping-induced mechanical wound, detergent-induced irritant dermatitis		The lipid mixture accelerated barrier repair following disruption of the barrier by solvent treatment or tape stripping (mechanical), and by certain detergents such as Sarkosyl and dodecylbenzensulfuric acid but failed to do so after treatment with other detergents, sodium dodecyl sulfate and ammonium lauryl sulfosuccinate	5
	Tape stripping model on different races and both genders in humans	Darkly pigmented skin displayed both a more resistant barrier and one that recovered more quickly after perturbation by tape stripping than did the skin of individuals with lighter pigmentation	6
	Tape stripping in patients with atopic dermatitis (AD) and age-matched healthy control subjects	No difference in the recovery process of the water barrier function of the SC between the two groups	7
Tape stripping on aged hairless mouse	Tape stripping on chronologically aged human skin	Ratios of physiologic lipids accelerated barrier recovery in both chronologically aged murine epidermis and aged human skin	8
	Tape stripping on volar forearm skin in human volunteers	Barrier repair was time-dependent	9
	Detergent- and tape-stripped–perturbed human skin	There was no different of two products at promoting normalization in either of the two experimentally perturbed areas	10
Acetone-induced disruption of barrier function on hairless mice		Occlusive membranes prevented the increase in epidermal lipid synthesis; but a vapor-permeable membrane increased epidermal lipid synthesis in animals; the transepidermal water flux is the signal for recovery of barrier structure and function	11

TABLE 8.1 (CONTINUED)
Experimental Micro Wound Models

Wound Models		Clinical Relevance	Ref.
Animals	**Humans**		
Acetone-treated hairless mouse skin		Topical applications of individual lipids or incomplete mixtures of lipids interfere with barrier recovery, while complete mixtures of cholesterol, fatty acid, and ceramide allow normal barrier repair; incomplete mixtures of topical lipids appear to inhibit barrier recovery at the level of the lamellar body resulting in abnormal intercellular membrane structures in the stratum corneum, abnormalities that do not occur when a complete lipid mixture is provided	12
	Acetone-induced acute water loss barrier disruption in humans	Topical agent accelerated barrier repair within the first 72 h post acetone damage	13
	Surfactant-induced irritant dermatitis in humans	Emphasized the importance of extended periods needed before a patient with irritant contact dermatitis can be reexposed to irritant substances; the evaluation of the irritation potential of diverse surfactants depended significantly on the feature (erythema vs. hydration and TEWL) measured	14
	Sodium lauryl sulfate (SLS)-induced water barrier disruption in humans	Topical agents accelerated the repair rates of water barrier function in SLS-treated human skin	15
	SLS-induced irritant dermatitis on humans	Corticosteroids were ineffective in treating the surfactant-induced irritant dermatitis	16
	Nickel allergic contact dermatitis (ACD) in humans	Model agent reduced cutaneous allergic reactions, especially on days 8 to 10, in comparison with the placebo control	17
	Blister wound model by aqueous solution of ammonium hydroxide to human skin	The blister base is suitable for studies of wound healing, bacterial infections, etc.; healing of this wound model is rapid without scarring	18

TABLE 8.1 (CONTINUED)
Experimental Micro Wound Models

Wound Models			
Animals	**Humans**	**Clinical Relevance**	**Ref.**
	Blister wound model by aqueous solution of ammonium hydroxide to both of young and aged human skin	Time required for blister formation was greatly prolonged in the aged	19
	Ammonium hydroxide-induced intradermal blisters with modification *in vivo* in human	Overall clinical appearance and healing rates of wounds treated with the triple antibiotic were ranked superior to all treatments (and no treatment) except the other antibiotic ointment	20
	Suction blister wound model *in vivo* human skin	A 0.05% clobetasol 17-propionate preparation caused a dramatic delay in TEWL decrease, whereby the untreated unoccluded field showed a continuous decrease over the observed period of 14 days; occlusion and corticoid-free treatment led to a weak but significant delay of TEWL decrease when compared to the untreated unoccluded test field	21
Partial-thickness incision wound model and cantharidin blister bed wound model in small animals		This device made uniform-depth wounds that reduced the variation in depth; these authors also created the cantharidin blister bed wound model in small animals	22
	Human dermabrasion wound healing model	Occlusive dressings hastened healing time as much as 50% over air-exposed sites	23
Biopsy punch full-thickness wound in rabbits		Occluded sites showed markedly increased wound healing compared to nonoccluded sites (9 d versus 17 d, respectively)	24

agents may provide accurate, highly reproducible, and objective observations in quantifying the healing process.

Although a well-designed, double-blind, placebo-controlled clinical trial is the "gold standard," an ideal experimental model should be convenient, simple, reproducible, economic, and clinically relevant. Skin healing data appear to correlate better between the human and the domestic pig than between the human and the mouse, guinea pig, or rat.

REFERENCES

1. Rovee, D.T., Kurowsky, C.A., Labun, J., and Downes, A.M., Effect of local wound environment on epidermal healing, in *Epidermal Wound Healing*, Maibach, H.I., and Rovee, D.T., Eds., Year Book Medical Publishers, Chicago, 1972, p. 159.
2. Pollack, S.V., The wound healing process, *Clin. Dermatol.*, 2, 8, 1984.
3. Rovee, D.T., Linsky, C.B., and Bothwell, J.W., Experimental models for the evaluation of wound repair, in *Animal Models in Dermatology*, Maibach, H.I., Ed., Churchill Livingstone, Edinburgh, 1975, p. 253.
4. Bolton, L., Vasko, A-J., and Monte, K., Quantification of wound healing, in *Cutaneous Biometrics*, Schwindt, D.A. and Maibach, H.I., Eds., Kluwer Academic/Plenum Publishers, New York, 2000, p. 205.
5. Yang, L., Mao-Qiang, M., Taljebini, M., Elias, P.M., and Feingold, K.R., Topical stratum corneum lipids accelerate barrier repair after tape stripping, solvent treatment and some but not all types of detergent treatment, *Br. J. Dermatol.*, 133, 679, 1995.
6. Reed, J.T., Ghadially, R., and Elias, P.M., Skin type, but neither race nor gender, influence epidermal permeability barrier function, *Arch. Dermatol.*, 131, 1134, 1995.
7. Tanaka, M., Zhen, Y.X., and Tagami, H., Normal recovery of the stratum corneum barrier function following damage induced by tape stripping in patients with atopic dermatitis, *Br. J. Dermatol.*, 136, 966, 1997.
8. Zettersten, E.M., Ghadially, R., Feingold, K.R., Crumrine, D., and Elias, P.M., Optimal ratios of topical stratum corneum lipids improve barrier recovery in chronologically aged skin, *J. Am. Acad. Dermatol.*, 37, 403, 1997.
9. Denda, M. and Tsuchiya, T., Barrier recovery rate varies time-dependently in human skin, *Br. J. Dermatol.*, 142, 881, 2000.
10. Loden, M. and Barany, E., Skin-identical lipids versus petrolatum in the treatment of tape-stripped and detergent-perturbed human skin, *Acta. Dermatol. Venereol.*, 80, 412, 2000.
11. Grubauer, G., Elias, P.M., and Feingold, K.R., Transepidermal water loss: the signal for recovery of barrier structure and function, *J. Lipid. Res.*, 30, 323, 1989.
12. Man, M.Q., Feingold, K.R., and Elias, P.M., Exogenous lipids influence permeability barrier recovery in acetone-treated murine skin, *Arch. Dermatol.*, 129, 728, 1993.
13. Zhai, H., Leow, Y.H., and Maibach, H.I., Human barrier recovery after acute acetone perturbation: an irritant dermatitis model, *Clin. Exp. Dermatol.*, 23, 11, 1998.
14. Wilhelm, K.P., Freitag, G., and Wolff, H.H., Surfactant-induced skin irritation and skin repair. Evaluation of the acute human irritation model by noninvasive techniques, *J. Am. Acad. Dermatol.*, 30, 944, 1994.
15. Zhai, H., Poblete, N., and Maibach, H. I., Sodium lauryl sulphate damaged skin *in vivo* in man: a water barrier repair model, *Skin Res. Technol.*, 4, 24, 1998.
16. Levin, C., Zhai, H., Bashir, S., Chew, A.L., Anigbogu, A., Stern, R., and Maibach, H.I., Efficacy of corticosteroids in acute experimental irritant contact dermatitis? *Skin Res. Technol.*, 7, 214, 2001.
17. Zhai, H., Chang, Y.C., Singh, M., and Maibach, H.I., *In vivo* nickel allergic contact dermatitis: human model for topical therapeutics, *Contact Dermatitis*, 40, 205, 1999.
18. Frosch, P.J. and Kligman, A.M., Rapid blister formation in human skin with ammonium hydroxide, *Br. J. Dermatol.*, 96, 461, 1977.

19. Grove, G.L., Duncan, S., and Kligman, A.M., Effect of ageing on the blistering of human skin with ammonium hydroxide, *Br. J. Dermatol.*, 107, 393, 1982.

20. Leyden, J.J. and Bartelt, N.M., Comparison of topical antibiotic ointments, a wound protectant, and antiseptics for the treatment of human blister wounds contaminated with *Staphylococcus aureus*, *J. Fam. Pract.*, 24, 601, 1987.

21. Levy, J.J., von Rosen, J., Gassmuller, J., Kleine Kuhlmann, R., and Lange, L., Validation of an *in vivo* wound healing model for the quantification of pharmacological effects on epidermal regeneration, *Dermatology*, 190, 136, 1995.

22. Bolton, L.L. and Constantine, B.E., Partial-thickness wound models in small animals, in *Models in Dermatology*, Maibach, H.I. and Lowe, N., Eds., Karger, Basel, 1987, p. 190.

23. Pinski, J.B., Human dermabrasion as a wound healing model, in *Models in Dermatology*, Maibach, H.I. and Lowe, N., Eds., Karger, Basel, 1987, p. 196.

24. Surinchak, J.S., Malinowski, J.A., Wilson, D.R., and Maibach, H.I., Skin wound healing determined by water loss, *J. Surg. Res.*, 38, 258, 1985.

Part IV

Physical and Chemical Factors Affecting Repair

9 Wound Microbiology and the Use of Antibacterial Agents

Robert S. Kirsner, Lucy K. Martin, and Anna Drosou

CONTENTS

9.1 INTRODUCTION

Epidermal wound healing is a well-orchestrated cascade of events that lead to repair when the underlying dermis is also compromised, but lead to regeneration when only the epidermis is injured. This process, should it occur in a timely fashion, is termed acute wound healing, typically with restoration of skin integrity occurring within a period of days to weeks. Classically, acute wound healing is considered to occur in three overlapping phases termed the inflammatory, proliferative, and remodeling phases, respectively.[1] Conversely, when this process is disrupted and healing is prolonged, delayed, or does not occur, the wound is termed a chronic wound.[2] An exact time when acute wound healing becomes chronic does not exist; instead, the time depends upon patient-related variables such as age and comorbid conditions, and wound-related variables such as the location of the wound, its size, depth, and shape, and the method by which it was created.

The most common types of chronic wounds include venous leg ulcers, diabetic foot ulcers secondary to neuropathy, pressure ulcers, and ulcers secondary to vascular disease. A chronic wound may take months to heal or may not show a tendency to heal at all. This unfortunately is not rare, as less than 25% of diabetic foot ulcers enrolled in the standard care arms in recent clinical trials healed during the study period and less than half of diabetic foot ulcers heal in clinical practice.[3,4] Significant attention has focused on chronic wounds, especially those that have failed to heal, as they are associated with substantial costs in both human and financial terms. Among the many factors suggested as being causal in retarding healing is an abnormal microbiologic environment of the wound. Therefore, knowledge of wound microbiology is essential.

Wound microbiology affects healing in a number of ways. Bacteria may be present in abundant numbers; the criteria for and the definition of "abundant" may depend upon the type and virulence of the bacteria and on host characteristics as well. For example, the abnormal presence of bacteria in wounds prolongs the inflammatory phase of wound healing, which may delay the process by which wounds start to heal. Bacteria present in wounds consume glucose and oxygen and therefore may lead to tissue anoxia. Cell lysis is promoted by a low pH and tissue anoxia.[5]

Although it is possible for acute wounds to lack bacteria, most if not all chronic wounds contain bacteria; this bacterial presence has been termed "bioburden." Bioburden refers to the metabolic load imposed by bacteria.[6] Often, the balance between the bioburden and the host defenses determines whether infection or detrimental effects on healing will occur.[6,7] Some authors believe that the density of microorganisms is the critical factor in determining whether a wound is likely to heal,[8–12] and others believe specific pathogens are of primary importance in delayed healing.[13–18] However, not all are convinced of the importance of bacteria in delayed healing.[19–25] This chapter will focus on bacteria in wounds and on attempts to eradicate those bacteria to eliminate any detrimental influence that they may have on the healing process.

9.2 BIOFILMS AND PLANKTONIC BACTERIA

Bacteria grow in various forms. Best known are free-floating or planktonic bacteria. An alternative way in which bacteria may grow is in *biofilms* — complex communities of bacteria (as well as other microorganisms) that adhere to solid surfaces.[26] The microorganisms in biofilms are embedded in an extracellular polysaccharide matrix or glycocalyx.[27] Bacterial biofilms are known to be in a sessile or adherent form, which differs from the planktonic or free-living form of bacteria. These biofilms have been implicated in chronic infections and are known to be resistant to antimicrobial agents.[26] The ways in which biofilms are resistant to different antimicrobial agents include an inability of the antimicrobial agent to penetrate the depth of the biofilm, a slower rate of growth of the biofilm bacteria due to nutrient limitation,[28] or the adoption of a distinct bacterial phenotype as a response to growth on a surface.[29]

Reports of evidence supporting the presence of biofilms on the surface of chronic human wounds as well as in animal models involving partial-thickness wounds are relatively new.[30,31] As tight attachment is among the hallmark features of biofilms, attempts to treat biofilms with agents that prevent attachment or promote the detachment of biofilms would theoretically be advantageous.[27] Biofilms have the ability to survive in hostile environments and contain different structures including channels in which circulation of nutrients can occur. Cells in different areas of the biofilm exhibit diverse patterns of gene expression.[32,33] It is believed that an acylated homoserine lactone (acyl-HSL) is responsible for the maturation of the biofilm.[34] One special characteristic of biofilms is known as quorum sensing. Quorum sensing is a way in which bacteria communicate; this process allows bacteria to survive without consuming all of their nutrients and allows biofilms to dispose of their waste products.[28]

Biofilms can be caused by a single organism or a combination of a variety of different species of bacteria (or other microorganisms, including fungi).[27] The same species of bacteria that cause biofilms can also occur as planktonic bacteria. Due to factors mentioned above related to resistance, antibiotic therapy destroys planktonic cells without harming biofilms.[35] It should be mentioned that much of the information learned about bacteria and wounds is from studies of planktonic bacteria. Much more needs to be and will be learned about the role of biofilm bacteria in healing and wounds.

9.3 THE IMPORTANCE OF BACTERIA WITHIN WOUNDS

It is important to distinguish between colonization and infection. Some acute wounds and virtually all chronic wounds contain bacteria, and many heal. Occlusive dressings speed healing and reduce pain and scarring, but they also encourage microbial proliferation in wounds.[22,36] Yet the infection rate is lower under occlusive dressings than under conventional dry dressings.[37,38] Therefore, the mere presence of bacteria is not necessarily detrimental. Whether faster healing using occlusive dressings is related to the increased number of bacteria is under investigation.

When clinical signs of infection are present, such as pain and tenderness, redness, warmth, and swelling in the surrounding and adjacent tissue, as seen in patients experiencing cellulitis or lymphangitis, the clinical importance of microbiologic findings of bacteria is obvious.[38] These features and perhaps wound histology may be used to distinguish infection from colonization. Histology may also be useful, as by definition, infection involves invasion of viable tissue by pathogens.[39] On the other hand, colonization refers to the presence of multiplying bacteria without immunological reaction or clinical symptoms.[40]

However, another situation may exist when clinical signs of infection are not present or are blunted by patient characteristics (diabetes, age, concomitant medications, etc.), yet a wound has increased exudate or odor or simply fails to heal. This is an intermediate state on the spectrum from colonization to infection and may represent situations where normal healing is compromised with or without tissue invasion. It is this situation that is the focus of many involved with chronic wound care.

9.4 MICROBIOLOGY OF WOUNDS

Extensive information has been published on the effects of specific types of microorganisms on wound healing. The majority of wounds are polymicrobial, with both aerobes and anaerobes present. Aerobic pathogens such as *Staphylococcus aureus, Pseudomonas aeruginosa*, and beta-hemolytic streptococci have been most frequently cited as the causes of delayed wound healing and infection.[15,17,18,41–46] At a consensus meeting of the European Tissue Repair Society and the European Wound Management Association in 1998, the general opinion was that the presence of beta-hemolytic (group A) streptococci or *P. aeruginosa* in a chronic wound was an indicator of the need for antimicrobial therapy.

However, it may be that polymicrobial bacteriology could play a role in healing. In a study of the bacteriology of chronic leg ulcers in 52 patients, Trengove et al.[25] reported that no single microorganism or group of microorganisms was more detrimental to wound healing than any other (inclusive of *S. aureus, P. aeruginosa*, beta-hemolytic streptococci, anaerobes, and coliform bacteria). However, a significantly lower probability of healing was observed if four or more bacterial groups were present in any ulcer,[25] and this indicates that microbial interactions may have induced an enhanced pathogenic effect. Similarly, Bowler and Davies[47] reported a greater diversity of microorganisms in infected leg ulcers than in noninfected leg ulcers (means of 5.1 and 3.6 isolates per wound, respectively). These observations support an earlier view of Kingston and Seal,[48] who argued that all species associated with a microbial disease should be considered potentially synergistic, rather than a single species being causative, as is commonly perceived. Additionally, certain organisms make the identification of other bacteria difficult. For example, *Proteus* sp., which has a high incidence in venous ulcers, has a swarming characteristic hiding the presence of other organisms. Alternative culture conditions or methods may help obviate this.[49]

In a paper published in 1964, in addition to describing the type of bacteria, Bendy et al. described the effect of bacterial number on the healing of decubitus ulcers and found that healing progressed only when the bacterial load was $<10^6$ colony-forming units (CFU)/ml of wound fluid. In that study, quantification was determined by using superficial wound swab samples.[50] Similar observations have been made using counts from tissue biopsy specimens, with skin graft survival in experimental wounds,[51] in pressure ulcer healing,[52] and in delayed closure of surgical wounds.[53] Work from Robson and Heggers, among others, suggests that acute or chronic wound infection exists when the microbial load is $>10^5$ CFU/g of tissue.[53]

However, Pruitt et al.[54] reported that quantitative cultures were incapable of differentiating between burn wound colonization and infection, and they described histological analysis as being the most effective and rapid method for determining invasive burn wound infection.

Keep in mind that immunocompromised patients can have infection at less than 10^5 colonies.[5] While classically one thinks of "immunocompromised" as referring to someone who has human immunodeficiency virus (HIV) infection, has or is being treated for cancer, or is a transplant recipient, a broader definition including diabetics, the elderly, and the infirm may be worthwhile. It is also important to consider that certain organisms, such as group A beta-hemolytic streptococcus, are known to cause infection at lower concentrations (less than 10^5 organisms/g tissue) even in the immunocompetent.[6,52,55]

9.5 SAMPLING TECHNIQUES

Identifying wound bacteria is essential in the treatment of wounds. In addition to delaying healing, bacteria present in wounds can lead to cellulitis, osteomyelitis, bacteremia, or sepsis; therefore, proper identification and management should be addressed.[5] The two major methods of identifying wound bacteria are tissue biopsy and swab culture. Both have the common goal of identifying bacteria in both a qualitative and a quantitative fashion. The gold standard used to determine bacterial bioburden is tissue biopsy;[35] using this technique, one may be able to identify both the type and quantity of bacteria reliably.

The acquisition of deep tissue during biopsy following initial debridement and cleansing of superficial debris is recognized as the most useful method for determining the microbial load and the presence of invasive pathogens.[56–58] Tissue is obtained aseptically and is then weighed, homogenized, serially diluted, and cultured on selective and nonselective agar media under aerobic and anaerobic conditions to provide quantitative and qualitative information. It is rationalized that determining the bacteria in tissue as opposed to on the surface of a wound may have greater clinical significance. Tissue biopsies, however, are not always performed for various reasons,[59] such as high cost, pain, damage to healing tissue, unavailability of materials used to process tissue biopsies, and the need for expertise in obtaining a sample.

Additionally, the relative delay in obtaining results from this technique has suggested other possibilities including a rapid Gram stain technique, which may reliably predict a microbial load of $>10^5$ CFU/g of tissue if a single microorganism was seen on the slide preparation.[9,12] However, in diabetic foot infections and burn wounds, both of which involve complex microbial ecosystems, a poor correlation between Gram stain and culture results from deep tissue biopsy specimens has been reported.[60] Regarding the speed of obtaining results, it appears that culture results serve different needs depending upon the situation. For acute infections, culture results serve to confirm the choice of empiric therapy prescribed. In this case, the clinician does not have the luxury of waiting for culture results prior to prescribing therapy. For chronic wounds, where antimicrobial treatment is being considered to reverse the inhibitory effect of bacteria within the wound, the clinician can await the results prior to instituting therapy.

The swab culture is a relatively simple procedure and does not have the above-mentioned disadvantages.[61] Wound swabbing most frequently involves the use of a cotton-tipped swab to sample superficial wound fluid and tissue debris, enabling a semiquantitative and qualitative analysis of the wound microflora. An alginate-tipped swab can also be used to perform a fully quantitative analysis, since the swab will dissolve and release all associated microorganisms when transferred to an appropriate diluent.

Swab sampling has been challenged on the bases that the superficial microbiology does not reflect that of deeper tissue[62,63] and that subsequent cultures do not correlate with the presence of pathogenic bacteria.[64] Also, if a swab sample is taken inappropriately (i.e., prior to wound cleansing and removal of devitalized superficial debris), the resulting culture has been considered to reflect only surface contamination[65] and may provide misleading or useless information.[56] However, since the majority of wounds are contaminated with endogenous microorganisms from the external environment, any microorganisms present in deeper tissue are also likely to be present in the superficial debris. Consequently, it is most likely that superficial wound fluid and tissue debris display a full spectrum of the wound aerobic and anaerobic microflora, some of which may be involved in pathogenesis and some of which may not be.

Anaerobes are not regarded as detrimental to normal wound healing.[18,20, 21,66] Compared with aerobic and facultative microorganisms, the culture, isolation, and identification of anaerobic bacteria is more time consuming, labor intensive, and expensive and is often deemed to be too demanding for many diagnostic microbiology laboratories. This concept has recently been challenged.[67]

Several studies have demonstrated a correlation between surface cultures and tissue biopsy cultures. Levine et al.[68] demonstrated a close correlation between quantitative swab and tissue biopsy specimen counts in open burn wounds, and Armstrong et al.[69] observed no difference in the isolation rate of microorganisms from deep tissue and superficial curettage in 112 diabetic foot ulcer infections. Using an experimental rat model, Bornside and Bornside[70] demonstrated that tissue counts of 10^5 CFU/g were equivalent to a 10^3 CFU/ml count obtained from a moist swab. Similarly, Thomson[58] demonstrated a correlation between a semiquantitative surface swab count (1+ to 4+) and a fully quantitative biopsy specimen count in burn wounds; 1+ growth from a swab correlated with a tissue count of 10^2 to 10^3 CFU/g, and 4+ correlated with a tissue count of approximately 10^7 CFU/g. Other studies[24,47] also demonstrated a close correlation between the isolation of microorganisms in superficial and deep tissue.

Rudensky et al. compared wound swab cultures, tissue aspiration, and tissue biopsies and found that tissue biopsies were the most effective method.[65] However, it is possible the results are altered due to surface colonization in devitalized tissue. Proper swab culture technique is required, with prior cleansing of the surface tissue before obtaining swab cultures in addition to pressure application to exude fluid from the wound tissue.[35,68] Once again it should be highlighted that proponents of the equivalency of wound swabs point out that wound contamination most often occurs from sources external to the wound. Thus, superficial tissue is likely to harbor a diversity of microorganisms, one or more of which may invade deeper tissue, and it is highly unlikely that superficial tissue will be "sterile" while deeper tissue is "infected." Most wounds are colonized with microorganisms, and failure to isolate them is likely a consequence of poor microbiological technique.

As technology expands, new techniques in bacteriologic identification emerge. Examples include certain fluorescent-stained microbes visualized under ultraviolet light. Deoxyribonucleic acid (DNA) analysis using gene probes, DNA fingerprinting, and DNA amplification are other examples.[71,72] Serologic analysis can also be used to identify microbes, providing information on antigenic determinants in bacterial cell walls, capsules, and flagella.

9.6 WHEN TO CULTURE A WOUND

Routine culturing of wounds is not indicated; instead, culturing should be reserved for wounds that are either clinically infected or those that have no clinical signs of infection but are deteriorating or failing to heal. In the former situation, a surface swab sample can provide useful data regarding the presence of potential pathogens, the diversity of microorganisms involved, and direct antimicrobial therapy. In the latter situation, optimally a tissue biopsy culture for qualitative and quantitative analysis should be obtained or, if not available, a swab culture may suffice. A swab sample can also provide a semiquantitative estimation of the microbial load (i.e., light growth to heavy growth, or $>10^5$ CFU/ml), which is considerably easier to perform than a fully quantitative analysis. A correlation between semiquantitative swab data and quantitative biopsy data has previously been demonstrated.[58,68–70,73,74] Although wound cleansing is considered necessary to avoid the pointless exercise of sampling superficial devitalized tissue,[62–65] Hansson et al. observed no difference in the qualitative and quantitative microbiology of leg ulcers, whether or not they were cleansed prior to sampling with absorbent disks.[23]

9.7 MANAGEMENT OF BACTERIA IN WOUNDS

Although systemic antibiotic therapy is essential for advancing cutaneous infections and those that involve deeper tissues, wounds that exhibit only localized signs of infection or are failing to heal but do not have clinical signs of infection (having a clinically important bioburden) may initially be treated with topical agents. Topical antimicrobial agents include both antiseptics and antibiotics.

In support of this concept are recent guidelines on the treatment of pressure ulcers issued by the European Pressure Ulcer Advisory Panel, which recommended that systemic antibiotics not be required for pressure ulcers that exhibit only clinical signs of local infection.[75] Since leg ulcers and foot ulcers often exhibit a microflora similar to that found in pressure ulcers, such advice could probably be extended to cover a wider variety of chronic wound types. In the absence of advancing cellulitis, bacteremia, fever, or pain, topical antimicrobial agents (antibiotics or antiseptics) may offer the most useful first line of treatment.

9.7.1 Antiseptics

Antiseptics are agents that destroy or inhibit the growth and development of microorganisms in or on living tissue. Unlike antibiotics, which act selectively on a specific target, antiseptics have multiple targets and a broader spectrum of activity that includes bacteria, fungi, viruses, protozoa, and even prions.[76,77] Several antiseptic categories exist including alcohols (ethanol), anilides (triclocarban), biguanides (chlorhexidine), bisphenols (triclosan), chlorine compounds, iodine compounds, silver compounds, peroxygens, and quaternary ammonium compounds. Among the most commonly used products in clinical practice today are povidone–iodine, chlorhexidine, alcohol, acetate, hydrogen peroxide, boric acid, silver nitrate, silver sulfadiazine, and sodium hypochlorite.

Several antiseptic agents are useful primarily for cleansing intact skin; they are used for preparing patients preoperatively, prior to injections or venous punctures, pre- and postoperative scrubbing in the operating room, and handwashing by medical personnel. Some contain a detergent, which renders them too harsh for use on nonintact skin.[78] The usefulness of antisepsis on intact skin is well established and broadly accepted.[19] However, the use of antiseptics as prophylactic antiinfective agents for open wounds such as lacerations, abrasions, burns, and chronic ulcers has been an area of intense controversy for several years.

Two official guidelines have been released concerning antiseptic use on wounds. Povidone–iodine (PVP-I) has been approved by the U.S. Food and Drug Administration (FDA) for short-term treatment of superficial and acute wounds.[79] The approval states that PVP-I has not been found to either promote or inhibit wound healing. On the other hand, guidelines for the treatment of pressure ulcers by the U.S. Department of Health and Human Services strongly discourage the use of antiseptics and promote the use of normal saline for cleansing pressure ulcers.[80]

The main rationale for using antiseptics on open wounds is prevention of infection and therefore increased rate of the healing process. It is well established that infections can delay healing, cause failure to heal, and even cause wound deterioration.[81] Consequently, although creation of an optimal environment for the wound healing process is currently the primary objective of wound care, prevention of infection still plays a critical role in wound management. Another argument for the use of antiseptics is that they are considered preferable to topical antibiotics with regard to the development of resistance. Antiseptics work by eliminating all pathogenic bacteria in the wound, while antibiotics are effective only for certain bacteria, which are sensitive to them. Although resistance to antiseptics has been reported, it is significantly less than that reported with antibiotic usage.[82] According to McDonnell and Russell, some acquired mechanisms of resistance (especially to heavy metals) have been shown to be clinically significant, but in most cases the results have been speculative.[76] Moreover, development of resistance against povidone–iodine, which is the most commonly used antiseptic today, in practice does not exist.[83] Payne et al. state that the sensible use of antiseptics could help decrease the usage of antibiotics, preserving their advantage for clinically critical situations.[84]

Antiseptics are also considered superior to topical antibiotics because they are less likely to cause contact sensitization. Aminoglycosides, especially neomycin, have a much higher sensitization rate than PVP-I.[85] Moreover, patients allergic to one antibiotic may acquire a cross-allergy to other antibiotics as well. The sensitization rate to povidone–iodine, the most commonly used antiseptic, has been found to be only 0.73%.[85,86]

A main concern prior to applying a topical agent on a wound is to ensure that it is safe. Agents that are cytotoxic or cause delay of wound healing are regarded with reservation. The strongest argument against the use of antiseptics on wounds is the fact that antiseptics have been found, mainly in *in vitro* models, to be cytotoxic to cells essential for the wound healing process, such as fibroblasts, keratinocytes, and leukocytes.[87–89] However, this cytotoxicity seems to be concentration dependent, since several antiseptics in low concentrations are not cytotoxic although they maintain their antibacterial activity *in vitro*.[85] Since *in vitro* results are not always predictive of what may happen *in vivo*, numerous studies have been conducted on animal and human models. The results of these studies are conflicting and will be presented below.

A second argument against the use of antiseptics on open wounds, first stated by Fleming in 1919,[90] is that antiseptics are not as effective against bacteria that reside in wounds as they are against bacteria *in vitro*. The presence of exudate, serum, or blood seems to decrease their activity. However, several bacteriological studies show that antiseptics may decrease the bacterial counts of wounds.[91,92]

9.7.2 Iodine Compounds

Since the first discovery of the natural element iodine in 1811 by the chemist Bernard Courtois, iodine and its compounds have been broadly used for prevention of infection and treatment of wounds.[93] However, molecular iodine can be very toxic for tissues, so formulations composed by combining iodine with a carrier that decreases iodine availability were developed. PVP-I results from the combination of molecular iodine and polyvinylpyrrolidone. PVP-I is available in several forms (solution, cream, ointment, scrub). The scrub form contains detergent and should be used only on intact skin. Cadexomer iodine consists of spherical hydrophilic beads of cadexomer-starch, which contain iodine, are highly absorbent, and release iodine slowly in the wound area. It is available as an ointment and as a dressing. Numerous studies have been conducted to determine the safety and efficacy of iodine compounds on healing wounds.

9.7.2.1 Effects of Iodine Compounds on the Bacterial Load of Wounds

9.7.2.1.1 PVP-I

Several animal studies have examined the effects of PVP-I on the bacterial load of wounds. These results have not proven the efficacy of PVP-I; however, the results of numerous clinical trials show that it is effective in reducing the bacterial load of wounds. Rodeheaver et al.[94] found that PVP-I solutions significantly reduce bacterial load 10 min after the application of the antiseptic. This effect did not persist, as there was no decreased rate of infection or decreased bacteria number 4 d after a single PVP-I application. Another study,[95] which evaluated contaminated 12-h-old lacerations in a guinea pig model, failed to find any decrease of wound bacterial counts after irrigation with PVP-I in comparison to normal saline. However, most of the human trials performed prove the efficacy of povidone–iodine in clinical situations. In an uncontrolled study, Georgiade and Harris[96] showed that PVP-I controlled bacterial growth in 50 patients. Gravett et al.[97] found that 1% PVP-I solution reduced the incidence of infection in sutured lacerations in 395 patients. In a recent study[98] on venous leg ulcers, the combination of PVP-I with a hydrocolloid dressing was shown to reduce the bacterial load and increase the healing rate in comparison to the hydrocolloid dressing alone.

Viljanto,[99] in surgical wounds in 294 pediatric patients, found that a 5% PVP-I aerosol increased infection, which the author related to excipients (glycerol, citrate-phosphate buffer, polyoxyethylated nonylphenol) in the aerosol. Follow-up experiments found that the 5% aerosol caused pronounced leukocyte migration, a 5% solution without excipients caused slighter inhibition, and a 1% solution was practically no different than the control (saline). Subsequently, spraying wounds with a 1% PVP-I solution had no effect on wound healing and significantly decreased infection rate. Increased bactericidal activity is found at lower concentrations.[100]

Conversely, some studies have not confirmed the previously mentioned results. PVP-I soaking was not found to significantly decrease bacterial counts in acute traumatic contaminated wounds that required debridement, while saline soaking caused increased counts. PVP-I solution was not found to be an effective substitute for wound cleaning and debridement.[101]

9.7.2.1.2 Cadexomer Iodine

The efficacy of cadexomer iodine has been shown in both animal and human models. Using a porcine model, Mertz et al.[102] found daily cadexomer iodine significantly reduced methicillin-resistant *Staphylococcus aureus* (MRSA) and total bacteria in the wounds in comparison to no-treatment control and vehicle (cadexomer) at all time points. Danielsen et al.[103] found negative culture results in an uncontrolled series treating ulcers with cadexomer iodine that were colonized with *Pseudomonas aeruginosa* in 65 and 75% of patients after 1 and 12 weeks of treatment, respectively.

9.7.2.2 Effects of Iodine Compounds on the Wound Healing Process

9.7.2.2.1 PVP-I

The literature regarding the effect of PVP-I on wound healing in animal wound models is conflicting. Briefly, in some studies PVP-I was found to cause no inhibition of wound reepithelialization,[104,105] while in others it retarded healing.[106] Similarly conflicting results regarding the effect on tensile strength have been reported, with PVP-I causing increased tensile strength[107] or reduced tensile strength[108] or having no effect.[109] It has also been found to have no effect on collagen[108] and granulation tissue production or to cause an insignificant reduction.[110] Moreover, it has been shown to increase revascularization.[111]

Clinical studies evaluating the influence of PVP-I in wound healing are numerous. Most of them showed no decrease in wound healing rate from the use of povidone–iodine. The aforementioned study by Viljanto[99] found no effect on wound healing when a 1% solution was used. Niedner[78] concluded that neither suction blister healing[112] nor healing after Moh's surgery[113] or burns[114] is negatively influenced by PVP-I.

Piérard-Franchimont et al.[98] examined the effect of PVP-I in combination with a hydrocolloid dressing on venous leg ulcers and found that healing rate was accelerated. Lee et al., in a noncontrolled study, found reduction of infection and promotion of healing in patients with longstanding (6 months to 16 years) decubitus and venous ulcerations.[115] In a review of *in vivo* studies, Mayer and Tsapogas[116] summarized the data by concluding that PVP-I was not found to negatively influence wound healing in comparison to the control group or to other treatments. Table 9.1 summarizes the effects of PVP-I on both infection and healing.

9.7.2.2.2 Cadexomer Iodine

In animal models, cadexomer iodine has been reported to increase epidermal regeneration and epithelialization in both partial-thickness and full-thickness wounds.[91,117] However, cadexomer iodine appears to have no effect on granulation tissue formation, neovascularization, or wound contraction.[78]

Cadexomer iodine has also been the subject of many clinical studies, in which it was found to be effective and beneficial to wound healing. Nine clinical trials comparing the effects on chronic venous ulcers of cadexomer iodine vs. other treatments showed enhancement of wound healing. The other treatments compared to cadexomer iodine included "standard treatment" (cleansing with diluted hydrogen peroxide or dilute potassium permanganate baths and covering with either a zinc paste dressing or nonadherent dressings, mainly paraffin-impregnated or saline dressings, or saline wet-to-dry compressive dressings, or gentian violet and polymyxin–bacitracin ointment, or support bandaging/stocking and a dry dressing),[118–123] dextranomer[124] and hydrocolloid dressing, or paraffin gauze dressings.[125] In one study, no control group was used since the main purpose of the study was to examine the safety of cadexomer iodine as far as the development of sensitivity is concerned.[126] In several of these studies, the ulcers had been recalcitrant or nonresponding to previous treatments. All these studies found that cadexomer iodine did not inhibit healing but actually accelerated it. Moreover, observations of other positive effects included reduction of pain; removal of pus, debris, and exudate; and stimulation of granulation tissue formation.[127] As an example, Moberg et al.,[128] in a randomized trial, compared cadexomer iodine with standard treatment in patients with decubitus ulcers. Cadexomer iodine significantly accelerated the healing rate and reduced pus, debris, and pain.

9.7.2.3 Iodine Compounds: Summary

In summary, from reviewing numerous *in vivo* studies of iodine compounds, we can conclude that in humans PVP-I and cadexomer iodine do not have a negative effect on healing, while cadexomer iodine possibly accelerates it in chronic human wounds.

TABLE 9.1
Povidone–Iodine

Wound Type	Species	Number of Wounds Treated	Control/Comparator	Effect on Healing	Effect on Infection	Ref.
Partial thickness wounds	Pigs	48 (8 wounds for each group)	Mafenide acetate Sodium hypochlorite Hydrogen peroxide Acetic acid No treatment	No effect (81% reepithelialization, with 1% PI, after 4 d vs. 69% for the no treatment group, nonsignificant difference)	Slightly decreased bacterial counts (yet still >10^5, statistical difference from control not calculated)	748
Leg ulcers	Humans	34 (17 patients)	No treatment Silver sulfadiazine Chlorhexidine (all groups treated with hydrocolloid dressing)	Increase (4 to 18% improvement of healing rate, 2 to 9 weeks faster vs. untreated, $P < 0.01$)	N/A	149
Lacerations contaminated with *S. aureus*	Guinea pigs	48 (12 animals)	Saline Cefazolin No treatment	N/A	No effect (4.63 log *S. aureus* recovered from wounds 2 h after irrigation vs. 5.47, 6.13, and 6.37 for no treatment, cefazolin, and saline groups respectively; nonsignificant difference)	95
Burns	Humans	50	N/A	N/A	Decrease (77% of wound cultures had no bacterial growth after QID application vs. 42 and 33% for the BID/TID and QOD/QD application groups, $P < 0.001$)	96

Partial thickness	Pigs	600 wounds (in 4 animals, 300 for each group)	No treatment	No influence (4.55 d needed for 50% of wounds to reepithelialize with pharmadine (9 to 12% PI solution) vs. 4.6 for control, relative rate of healing +1%; nonsignificant difference)	N/A	104
Sutured lacerations	Humans	395	No treatment (all wounds were initially irrigated with saline)	N/A	Decrease (1% rate of purulent wounds and 5.47% wound sepsis rate vs. 6.19 and 15.4% in the control group)	97
Partial and full thickness	Rats Humans	40 rats (20 for each group) 20 humans (10 for each group)	Saline	No effect (12.2 and 9.3 d mean healing time for Betadine vs. 12.4 and 9.5 for saline in partial thickness wounds in rats and humans; 19.2 vs. 19.5 in full thickness wounds in rats, nonsignificant difference)	N/A	105
Incisional	Mice	120 (2 animals)	Vehicle Steroids No treatment	Decreased strength/no effect on collagen	N/A	109
Full thickness wounds	Mice	23 (13 control, 10 PI)	No treatment	Decrease (11.8 d for complete reepithelialization vs. 7.2 for control, $P < 0.01$)	N/A	106

TABLE 9.1 (CONTINUED)
Povidone–Iodine

Wound Type	Species	Number of Wounds Treated	Control/Comparator	Effect on Healing	Effect on Infection	Ref.
Burns, chronic wounds	Humans	759 (90 PI solution and sugar, 515 PI solution, PI ointment and sugar, 154 standard treatment)	Standard therapy	Increase (0% need for skin graft for the triple combination group, 4.5% for the PI solution/sugar group vs. 40.3% for the control group)	Decrease	150
Pressure ulcers	Humans	40 (15 SSD,15 PVP-I, 14 saline)	Saline PVP-I	N/A	No effect (60% of patients responded to treatment after 14 d vs. 60% and 90% at the saline and SSD groups)	136
Acute, heavily contaminated wounds	Humans	33	Saline No treatment	N/A	No effect (bacterial counts similar to no treatment group after 10 min; saline soaking increased bacterial counts, P <.0001)	101
Decubitus ulcers Stasis ulcers	Humans	18	N/A	Increase (67% of ulcers cured after 6 weeks, 33% of ulcers improved)	Decrease (2 out of 14 infected lesions continued being infected after 6 weeks, P <0.001)	151

Wound type	Model	Number	Treatment	Effect	Effect	Ref.
Incisional wounds	Guinea pigs	120 (60 animals)	Saline / Shur-Clens	Decrease (Betadine surgical scrub significantly delayed epidermal and dermal healing vs. all groups, but increased significantly tensile strength after 21 d vs. all groups)	N/A	107
Partial thickness	Pigs	54 (9 animals)	Distilled water / Alcohol 70%	N/A	Decrease (5.94 log bacterial counts after 24 h vs. 7.53 and 7.28 in the water and alcohol groups, $P < 0.05$)	102
Incisional	Rats	341	Ringer's solution	No effect on strength (17.52 g/mm^2 tensile strength after 1 week vs. 17.90 in the Ringer's solution group; nonsignificant difference)	N/A	108
Full thickness	Guinea pigs	10 for each group	No treatment	No effect (nonsignificant decrease by 19% of thickness of the granulation layer in comparison to control)	N/A	78
Venous ulcers	Humans	30 (15 patients)	No treatment (both groups treated with hydrocolloid dressings)	Increase (increased healing rate with PVP-I treatment, especially during the first 4 weeks of treatment, $P < 0.05$)	Decrease (less neutrophilic vasculitis and fewer bacterial clumps in PVP-I treated group, significance not calculated)	98
Contaminated wounds	Guinea pigs		Saline	N/A	Decrease (?) (1.31 log reduction of bacteria 10 min after, $P < 0.001$; no effect 4 d after a single application; no effect on infection rate)	94

TABLE 9.1 (CONTINUED)
Povidone–Iodine

Wound Type	Species	Number of Wounds Treated	Control/Comparator	Effect on Healing	Effect on Infection	Ref.
Femoral vessels section	Rats	150 animals	Saline, Chlorhexidine	Toxicity (marked difference of 10% PI solutions on histological assessment, damage to vascular endothelium and thrombosis, vs. saline and chlorhexidine)	N/A	152
Surgical wounds	Humans	500 (242 PI, 258 control)	Saline	N/A	Decrease (2.9% wound sepsis rate vs. 15.1% in the control group, $P < 0.001$)	153
Surgical wounds	Humans	294	Saline	No effect (cell morphology similar to saline-impeded control)	Decrease (2.6% infection rate with 1% PI solution after appendectomy vs. 8.5% in the control group; however, 19% infection rate with 5% PI solution vs. 8% in the control group)	99

Both can be effective in reducing bacterial numbers and decreasing the likelihood of infection. Results of animal studies depend on many variables and should be interpreted with caution. The studies of PVP-I have had conflicting results, especially in the animal models, and have prompted concern on the part of many clinicians. Nevertheless, the results from the studies evaluating cadexomer iodine are clear and leave no doubt that this newer iodine compound is effective without having any negative influence on wound healing rate; instead, an acceleration of wound healing has been observed.

9.7.3 Silver Compounds

Silver compounds have widely been used as wound antiseptics, mainly in burns. Silver sulfadiazine (SSD) and silver nitrate ($AgNO_3$) are among the most commonly used. Silver sulfadiazine is the most broadly used treatment for the prevention of infection in patients with burn wounds.[129,130] Combinations of SSD with cerium nitrate[131] and nanocrystalline silver-releasing systems (Acticoat® dressing)[132] have been developed in order to increase its efficacy and/or reduce its toxicity. The newer silver formulations, such as Acticoat, seem to increase the rate and degree of microbial killing, decrease exudate formation, and can remain active for days.[133]

Animal studies examining the effects of SSD and $AgNO_3$ on wounds have shown no significant effect on epithelialization rate.[106] SSD was also found to increase the rate of neovascularization. In another study in rats, silver compounds were found to promote wound healing, reduce the inflammatory and granulation phases of healing, and influence metal ion binding.[134] Moreover, Geronemus et al.[104] found an increased reepithelialization rate in domestic pigs with the use of SSD. However, Leitch et al.[135] found SSD to cause inhibition of wound contraction in an acute wound rat model. Likewise, Niedner and Schopf[110] found a slight, nonsignificant reduction of granulation tissue formation with the use of $AgNO_3$.

Little controversy exists over the role of silver products in burn wounds; however, the use of silver in other wounds is less widely accepted. Kucan et al.[136] examined the effects of SSD on bacterial counts in patients with infected chronic pressure ulcers. They found SSD to be effective in decreasing the bacteria to below 10^5/g tissue in all the ulcers treated. In a randomized trial with venous ulcers, SSD 1% cream statistically reduced the ulcer size compared to the placebo,[137] while in another study it was found to be well tolerated and effective on wound cleansing and granulation tissue formation.[138] Livingstone et al.[139] studied the effect of $AgNO_3$ and an antibiotic solution (neomycin plus bacitracin) on reducing autogenous skin graft loss due to infection in patients with thermal injury. They found both medications to be effective in comparison to the control group (Ringer's lactate solution), but the antibiotic solution was associated with the rapid emergence of drug-resistant organisms, while $AgNO_3$ was not.

Summarizing, it appears that silver compounds have no negative effect on wounds, and may even accelerate wound healing clinically. Their *in vivo* antimicrobial activity is not in question. Table 9.2 summarizes the published data on silver compounds.

TABLE 9.2
Silver Compounds

Wounds	Species	Number of Wounds Treated	Control/Comparator	Effect on Healing	Effect on Infection	Ref.
Venous stasis ulcers	Humans	86 (28 SSD 1% cream, 29 copper tripeptide copper, 29 placebo)	Placebo Copper tripeptide complex	Increase (44% decrease in lesion size vs. 18.7 and 22.5% for the other groups, $P < 0.05$)	N/A	137
Leg ulcers	Humans	34	No treatment Chlorhexidine Povidone–iodine (all groups treated with hydrocolloid dressing)	No effect (mild improvement of healing rate vs. untreated, 2 to 7%, nonsignificant difference)	N/A	149
Partial thickness	Pigs	600 wounds (in 4 animals, 200 for each group)	No treatment Vehicle	Increase (3.1 d needed for 50% of wounds to reepithelialize with Silvadine (1% sulfadiazine silver) vs. 4.3 for untreated control and 3.4 for vehicle; relative rate of healing +25%)	N/A	104
Full thickness	Mice	46 (13 control, 18 silver sulfadiazine, 15 silver nitrate)	No treatment	No effect (7.1 and 8.9 d for complete reepithelialization with silver sulfadiazine and silver nitrate vs. 7.2 for control; nonsignificant difference)	N/A	106
Pressure ulcers	Humans	40 (15 SSD, 15 PVP-I, 14 saline)	Saline PVP-I	N/A	Decrease (90% of patients responded to treatment after 14 d vs. 60% in the saline and PVP-I groups, $P < 0.022$)	136

Wound	Model	n	Treatment	Wound healing	Infection/bacterial effect		Ref
Incisional wounds	Rat	50 (10 wounds for each group)	Deionized water (silver nitrate 0.01%, 0.1%, 1%; SSD 0.5 g; deionized water)	Increase (all wounds completely closed by day 8 for 1%, 0.1% silver nitrate and SSD vs. half wounds closed for the 0.01% silver nitrate and water groups; significance not calculated)	N/A	N/A	134
Grafting after burn injury	Humans	52 (19 silver nitrate, 18 neomycin + bacitracin, 15 Ringer's lactate)	Ringer's lactate Neomycin plus bacitracin	N/A	Decrease (16% graft failure, mostly due to infection, vs. 33 and 53% for topical antibiotics and Ringer's lactate groups, $P = 0.02$; 1 out of 3 infection cases of emergence of antibiotic-resistant bacteria in the silver nitrate group vs. 6 out of 6 and 4 out of 8 for the other groups, $P < 0.05$)	N/A	139
Full thickness	Guinea pigs	10 for each group	No treatment	No effect (nonsignificant decrease by 25% of thickness of the granulation layer with $AgNO_3$ solution in comparison to control)	N/A	N/A	110
Partial thickness	Pigs	72 (24 for each group: silver coated dressing moistened once, daily, and petrolatum gauze)	Petrolatum gauze	Increase (100 and 96% of wounds reepithelialized by day 7 in silver-treated groups vs. 33% for petrolatum gauze group, $P < 0.0001$)	N/A	N/A	154
Burns	Humans	30	Silver nitrate vs. Acticoat®	N/A	Decrease (5 wounds with $>10^5$ counts in Acticoat-treated group vs. 16 in silver nitrate group and 1 secondary bacteremia vs. 5)	N/A	132

9.7.4 OLD AND EMERGING ANTIMICROBIALS

Many essential oils possess antimicrobial properties, and tea tree oil in particular (derived from the Australian native plant *Melaleuca alternifolia*) has been recognized for its efficacy against MRSA and has consequently been considered as an alternative treatment for mupirocin-resistant MRSA.[139] Additional safety and clinical efficacy data need to be generated.

Honey is an ancient remedy gaining renewed popularity as an alternative treatment for infections caused by antibiotic-resistant bacteria. Both honey and sugar (in a paste form) are considered useful as topical antimicrobial agents, primarily as a consequence of their high osmolarity and ability to minimize water availability to bacteria.[140] Although the dilution of honey in the presence of wound fluid is likely to reduce the efficacy of its osmotic effect, the slow and sustained production of hydrogen peroxide by some types of honey (e.g., manuka honey) is capable of maintaining an antimicrobial effect at a concentration approximately 1000-fold lower (and less toxic) than that commonly used in antiseptics (i.e., 3%).[141] Also, components of manuka honey, such as flavonoids and aromatic acids, demonstrate antimicrobial properties.[142] Honey may also serve as a wound deodorizing agent; this effect is attributed to the glucose that is metabolized by bacteria as opposed to proteinaceous necrotic tissue, resulting in the production of lactic acid and not the malodorous compounds generated by protein degradation. Honey's usefulness in infected wounds has been attributed to its high glucose content and low pH, both of which stimulate macrophages.[143]

Prior to antibiotics, the use of larvae (maggots) as a wound debridement treatment was routine.[144,145] This biosurgical debridement has played a minor role in wound management during the last 50 years. Its popularity gradually increased again during the 1990s, as alternative treatments have been sought in an attempt to combat the surge in infections caused by antibiotic-resistant bacteria. Larval therapy is currently being used in the treatment of a variety of infected acute and chronic wounds, including those colonized by resistant bacteria such as methicillin-resistant *S. aureus*.[146,147] The fly maggots of *Lucilia sericata* are capable of physically and enzymatically degrading devitalized tissue in a safe, effective manner. During this process, potentially pathogenic bacteria may be destroyed as part of the natural feeding process, but endogenous antimicrobial secretions are also considered to play an important role in microbial elimination.[146,147] Additional data suggest that fly larvae may stimulate fibroblast proliferation *in vitro*.

9.8 CONCLUSION

Appreciation of the role of bacteria in healing is critical. Bacteria may be a detriment to patients by causing infection or prolonging or preventing healing. To fully recognize the effect of bacteria upon healing for any given patient, the way in which bacteria live, the number and type of bacteria, and characteristics of the host are all important. In addition to planktonic forms, bacteria may live in tightly adherent and resistant colonies as biofilms. For planktonic bacteria, studies suggest that greater than 10^5 CFU of bacteria per gram of tissue is detrimental to healing, but for certain bacteria and in certain patients, lower levels may be important as well. Both qualitative and quantitative cultures will assist in evaluating problematic wounds, but random cultures of patients with wounds are not recommended. To appropriately treat an abnormal bacterial burden and to decrease the development of host resistance, a variety of topical treatment options may be utilized, including the use of novel agents.

REFERENCES

1. Kirsner, R.S. and Bogensberger, G., The wound healing process, in *Wound Healing: Alternatives in Management,* 3rd ed., McColluch, J.M., Kloth, L.C., and Feedar, J.A., Eds., F.A. Davis Company, Philadelphia, 2001.
2. Schultz, G.S., Sibbald, R.G., Falanga, V., Ayello, E.A., Dowsett, C., Harding, K., Romanelli, M., Stacey, M.C., Teot, L., and Vanscheidt, W., Wound bed preparation: a systematic approach to wound management, *Wound Repair Regen.,* 11 Suppl 1, S1–S28, 2003.
3. Margolis, D.J., Kantor, J., and Berlin, J.A., Healing of diabetic neuropathic foot ulcers receiving standard treatment. A meta-analysis, *Diabetes Care,* 22, 692–695, 1999.
4. Margolis, D.J., Kantor, J., Santanna, J., Strom, B.L., and Berlin, J.A., Effectiveness of platelet releasate for the treatment of diabetic neuropathic foot ulcers, *Diabetes Care,* 24, 483–488, 2001.
5. Corum, G.M., Characteristics and prevention of wound infection, *J. ET Nurs.,* 20, 21–25, 1993.
6. Stotts, N.A. and Whotney, J.D., Identifying and evaluating wound infection, *Home Healthcare Nurse,* 17(3), 159–164, 1999.
7. Robson, M.C., Wound infection: a failure of wound healing caused by an imbalance of bacteria, *Surg. Clin. North Am.,* 77, 637–650, 1977.
8. Heggers, J.P., Defining infection in chronic wounds: does it matter? *J. Wound Care,* 7, 389–392, 1998.
9. Heggers, J.P., Robson, M.C., and Doran, E.T., Quantitative assessment of bacterial contamination of open wounds by a slide technique, *Trans. Roy. Soc. Trop. Med. Hyg.,* 63, 532–534, 1969.
10. Mangram, A.J., Horan, T.C., Pearson, M.L., Silver, L.C., and Jarvis, W.R., Guideline for prevention of surgical site infection, *Am. J. Infect. Control,* 27, 97–134, 1999.
11. Raahave, D., Friis-Moller, A., Bjerre-Jespen, K., Thiis-Knudsen, J., and Rasmussen, L.B., The infective dose of aerobic and anaerobic bacteria in postoperative wound sepsis, *Arch. Surg.,* 121, 924–929, 1986.
12. Robson, M.C., Lessons gleaned from the sport of wound watching, *Wound Rep. Regen.,* 7, 2–6, 1999.
13. Danielsen, L.E., Balslev, G., Döring, N., Høiby, S.M., Madsen, M., Ågren, M., Thomsen, H.K., Fos, H.H.S., and Westh, H., Ulcer bed infection. Report of a case of enlarging venous leg ulcer colonised by *Pseudomonas aeruginosa, APMIS,* 106, 721–726, 1998.
14. Lavery, L.A., Harkless, L.B., Felder-Johnson, K., and Mundine, S., Bacterial pathogens in infected puncture wounds in adults with diabetes, *J. Foot Ankle Surg.,* 33, 91–97, 1994.
15. Madsen, S.M., Westh, H., Danielsen, L., and Rosdahl, V.T., Bacterial colonisation and healing of venous leg ulcers, *APMIS,* 104, 895–899, 1996.

16. Pallua, N., Fuchs, P.C., Hafemann, B., Völpel, U., Noah, M., and Lütticken, R., A new technique for quantitative bacterial assessment on burn wounds by modified dermabrasion, *J. Hosp. Infect.,* 42, 329–337, 1999.

17. Schraibman, I.G., The significance of beta-haemolytic streptococci in chronic leg ulcers, *Ann. Roy. Coll. Surg. Med.,* 7292, 123–124, 1990.

18. Sehgal, S.C., and Arunkumar, B.K., Microbial flora and its significance in pathology of sickle cell disease leg ulcers, *Infection,* 20, 86–88, 1992.

19. Annoni, F., Rosina, M., Chiurazzi, D., and Ceva, M., The effects of a hydrocolloid dressing on bacterial growth and the healing process of leg ulcers, *Int. Angiol.,* 8, 224–228, 1989.

20. Eriksson, G., Eklund, A.E., and Kallings, L.O., The clinical significance of bacterial growth in venous leg ulcers, *Scand. J. Infect. Dis.,* 16, 175–180, 1984.

21. Gilchrist, B. and Reed, C., The bacteriology of chronic venous ulcers treated with occlusive hydrocolloid dressings, *Br. J. Dermatol.,* 121, 337–344, 1989.

22. Handfield-Jones, S.E., Grattan, C.E.H., Simpson, R.A., and Kennedy, C.T.C., Comparison of a hydrocolloid dressing and paraffin gauze in the treatment of venous ulcers, *Br. J. Dermatol.,* 118, 425–427, 1988.

23. Hansson, C., Hoborn, J., Moller, A., and Swanbeck, G., The microbial flora in venous leg ulcers without clinical signs of infection, *Acta Dermatol. Venereol. (Stockh.),* 75, 24–30, 1995.

24. Sapico, F.L., Witte, J.L., Canawati, H.N., Montgomerie, J.Z., and Bessman, A.N., The infected foot of the diabetic patient: quantitative microbiology and analysis of clinical features, *Rev. Infect. Dis.,* 6, 171–176, 1984.

25. Trengove, N.J., Stacey, M.C., McGechie, D.F., and Mata, S., Qualitative bacteriology and leg ulcer healing, *J. Wound Care,* 5, 277–280, 1996.

26. Bello, Y.M., Falabella, A.F., DeCaralho, H., Nayyar, G., and Kirsner, R.S., Infection and wound healing, *Wounds,* 13(4), 127–131, 2001.

27. Costerton, J.W., Lewandowski, Z., Caldwell, D.E., Korber, D.R., and Lappin-Scott, H.M., Microbial biofilms, *Annu. Rev. Microbiol.,* 49, 711–745, 1995.

28. Bowler, P.G. and Davies, B.J., The microbiology of infected and noninfected leg ulcers, *Int. J. Dermatol.,* 38, 101–106, 1999.

29. Costerton, J.W., Stewart, P.S., and Greenberg, E.P., Bacterial biofilms: a common cause of persistent infections, *Science,* 284, 1318–1322, 1999

30. Serralta, V.W., Harrison-Balestra, C., Cazzaniga, A.L., Davis, S.C., and Mertz, P.M., Lifestyles of bacteria in wounds: presence of biofilms? *WOUNDS,* 13, 29–34, 2001.

31. Bello, Y.M., Falabella, A.F., Cazzaniga, A.L., Harrison-Balestra, C., and Mertz, P.M., Are biofilms present in human chronic wounds? Presented at the Symposium on Advanced Wound Care and Medical Research Forum on Wound Repair in Las Vegas, NV, April 30–May 3, 2001.

32. DeBeer, D., Stoodley, P., Roe, F., and Lewandowski, Z., Effects of biofilm structures on oxygen distribution and mass transfer. *Biotech. Bioeng.,* 43, 1131–1135, 1994.

33. Davies, D.G., Chakrabarty, A.M., and Geesey, G.G., Exopolysaccharide production in biofilm: substration activation of alginate gene expression by *Pseudomonas aeruginosa, Appl. Environ. Microbiol.,* 59, 1181–1186, 1993.

34. Kolter, R. and Losick, R., One for all and all for one, *Science,* 280, 226–227, 1998.

35. Marrie, T.J., Nelligan, J., and Costerton, J.W., A scanning and transmission electron microscopic study of an infected endocardial pacemaker lead, *Circulation,* 66, 1339–1341, 1982.

36. Lance George, W., Other infections of skin, soft tissue, and muscle, in *Anaerobic Infections in Humans,* Finegold, S.M. and Lance George, W., Eds., Academic Press, Inc., San Diego, CA, 1989, pp. 1491–1492.

37. Boulton, A.J.M., Meneses, P., and Ennis, W.J., Diabetic foot ulcers: a framework for prevention and care, *Wound Repair Regen.,* 7, 7–16, 1999.

38. Hutchinson, J.J. and Lawrence, J.C., Wound infection under occlusive dressings, *J. Hosp. Infect.,* 17, 83–94, 1991.

39. Bucknall, T.E., Factors affecting healing, in *Wound Healing for Surgeons,* Bucknall, T.E., and Ellis, H., Eds., Bailliere-Tindall, London, 1984, pp. 42–74.

40. White, R.J., Cooper, R., and Kingsley, A., Wound colonization and infection: the role of topical antimicrobials, *Br. J. Nurs.,* 10, 563–578, 2001.

41. Brook, I., Aerobic and anaerobic microbiology of necrotising fasciitis in children, *Pediatr. Dermatol.,* 13, 281–284, 1996.

42. Daltrey, D.C., Rhodes, B., and Chattwood, J.G., Investigation into the microbial flora of healing and non-healing decubitus ulcers, *J. Clin. Pathol.,* 34, 701–705, 1981.

43. Gilliland, E.L., Nathwani, N., Dore, C.J., and Lewis, J.D., Bacterial colonisation of leg ulcers and its effect on the success rate of skin grafting, *Ann. Roy. Coll. Surg. Engl.,* 70, 105–108, 1988.

44. Halbert, A.R., Stacey, M.C., Rohr, J.B., and Jopp-McKay, A., The effect of bacterial colonisation on venous ulcer healing., *Australas. J. Dermatol.,* 33, 75–80, 1992.

45. MacFarlane, D.E., Baum, K.F., and Serjeant, G.R., Bacteriology of sickle cell leg ulcers, *Trans. Roy. Soc. Trop. Med. Hyg.,* 80, 553–556, 1986.

46. Twum-Danso, K., Grant, C., Al-Suleiman, S.A., Abdel-Khaders, S., Al-Awami, M.S., Al-Breiki, H., Taha, S., Ashoor, A.A., and Wosornu, L., Microbiology of postoperative wound infection: a prospective study of 1770 wounds, *J. Hosp. Infect.,* 21, 29–37, 1992.

47. Bowler, P.G. and Davies, B.J., The microbiology of infected and noninfected leg ulcers, *Int. J. Dermatol,* 38, 72–79, 1999.

48. Kingston, D. and Seal, D.V., Current hypotheses on synergistic microbial gangrene, *Br. J. Surg.,* 77, 260–264, 1990.

49. Cooper, R. and Lawrence, J.C., The isolation and identification of bacteria from wounds, *J. Wound Care,* 5, 335–340, 1996.

50. Bendy, R.H., Nuccio, P.A., Wolfe, E., Collins, B., Tamburro, C., Glass, W., and Martin, C.M., Relationship of quantitative wound bacterial counts to healing of decubiti. Effect of topical gentamicin, *Antimicrob. Agents Chemother.,* 4, 147–155, 1964.

51. Krizek, T.J., Robson, M.C., and Kho, E., Bacterial growth and skin graft survival, *Surg. Forum,* 18, 518–519, 1967.

52. Robson, M.C. and Heggers, J.P., Bacterial quantification of open wounds, *Mil. Med.,* 134, 19–24, 1969.

53. Robson, M.C. and Heggers, J.P., Delayed wound closures based on bacterial counts, *J. Surg. Oncol.,* 2, 379–383, 1970.

54. Pruitt, B.A., Jr., McManus, A.T., Kim, S.H., and Goodwin, C.W., Burn wound infections: current status, *World J. Surg.,* 22, 135–145, 1998.

55. Kerstein, M.D., Wound infection: assessment and management, *Wounds Compend. Clin. Res. Pract.,* 8, 141–144, 1996.

56. Fowler, E., Wound infection: a nurse's perspective, *Ostomy Wound Manage.,* 44, 44–53, 1998.

57. Neil, J.A. and Munro, C.L., A comparison of two culturing methods for chronic wounds, *Ostomy Wound Manage.,* 43, 20–30, 1997.

58. Thomson, P.D. and Smith, D.J., What is infection? *Am. J. Surg.,* 167, 7s–11s, 1994.

59. Bill, T., Ratliff, C., Donovan, A., Knox, L., Morgan, R., and Rodeheaver, G., Quantitative swab culture versus tissue biopsy: a comparison in chronic wounds, *Ostomy Wound Manage.,* 47, 34–37, 2001.

60. Taddonio, T.E., Thomson, P.D., Tait, M.J., Prasad, J.K., and Feller, I., Rapid quantification of bacterial and fungal growth in burn wounds: biopsy homogenate Gram stain versus microbial culture results, *Burns,* 14, 180–184, 1988.

61. Stotts, N.A., Determination of bacterial bioburden in wounds, *Adv. Wound Care,* 8, 46–52, 1995.

62. Gradon, J. and Adamson, C., Infections of pressure ulcers: management and controversies, *Infect. Dis. Clin. Pract.,* 1, 11–16, 1995.

63. Perry, C.R., Pearson, R.L., and Miller, G.A., Accuracy of cultures of material from swabbing of the superficial aspect of the wound and needle biopsy in the preoperative assessment of osteomyelitis, *J. Bone Joint Surg.,* 73A, 745–749, 1991.

64. Brown, D.J. and Smith, D.J., Bacterial colonization/infection and the surgical management of pressure sores, *Ostomy Wound Manage.,* 45, 119s–120s, 1999.

65. Rudensky, B., Lipschitz, M., Isaacsohn, M., and Sonnenblick, M., Infected pressure sores: comparison of methods for bacterial identification, *South. Med. J.,* 85, 901–903, 1992.

66. Majewski, W., Cybulski, Z., Napierala, M., Pukacki, F., Staniszewski, R., Pietkiewicz, K., and Zapalski, S., The value of quantitative bacteriological investigations in the monitoring of treatment of ischaemic ulcerations of lower legs, *Int. Angiol.,* 14, 381–384, 1995.

67. Bowler, P.G., Duerden, B.I., and Armstrong, D.G., Wound microbiology and associated approaches to wound management, *Clin. Microbiol. Rev.,* 14, 244–269, 2001.

68. Levine, N.S., Lindberg, R.B., Mason, A.D., and Pruitt, B.A., The quantitative swab culture and smear: a quick, simple method for determining the number of viable bacteria on open wounds, *J. Trauma,* 16, 89–94, 1976.

69. Armstrong, D.G., Liswood, P.J., and Todd, W.F., Prevalence of mixed infections in the diabetic pedal wound. A retrospective review of 112 infections, *J. Am. Podiatr. Med. Assoc.,* 85, 533–537, 1995.

70. Bornside, G.H. and Bornside, B.B., Comparison between moist swab and tissue biopsy methods for quantitation of bacteria in experimental incisional wounds, *J. Trauma,* 19, 103–105, 1979.

71. Van Belkum, A., DNA fingerprinting of medically important microorganisms by use of PCR, *Clin. Microbiol. Rev.,* 7, 174–184, 1994.

72. Hogg, S.J., Cooper, R.A., and Harding, K., Genotypic Variability in Streptococci from Venous Leg Ulcers, in Proceedings of the 5th European Conference on Advances in Wound Management, Cherry, G.W., Gottrup, F., Lawrence, J.C. et al., Eds., Macmillan, London, 1996, pp. 243–245.

73. Lawrence, J.C., The bacteriology of burns, *J. Hosp. Infect.,* 6, 3–17, 1985.

74. European Pressure Ulcer Advisory Panel, Guidelines on treatment of pressure ulcers, *EPUAP Rev.,* 1, 31–33, 1999.

75. Vindenes, H. and Bjerknes, R., Microbial colonisation of large wounds, *Burns,* 21, 575–579, 1995.

76. McDonnell, A.G. and Russell, A.D., Antiseptics and disinfectants: activity, action and resistance, *Clin. Microbiol. Rev.,* 12, 147–179, 1999.

77. Taylor, D.M., Inactivation of unconventional agents of the transmissible degenerative encephalopathies, in *Principles and Practice of Disinfection, Preservation and Sterilization*, 3rd ed., Russell, A.D., Hugo, W.B., and Ayliffe, G.A.J., Eds., Blackwell Science, Oxford, U.K., 1999.

78. Niedner, R., Cytotoxicity and sensitization of povidone iodine and other frequently used anti-infective agents, *Dermatology*, 195(suppl 2), 89–92, 1997.

79. 56 Federal Register 33644 at 33662.

80. Bergstrom, N., Bennet, M.A., Carlson, C.E. et al., Clinical Practice Guideline No 15: Treatment of Pressure Ulcers, Agency for Health Care Policy and Research, Public Health Service, U.S. Department of Health and Human Services, Rockville, MD, 1994, AHCPR Publication 95–0652.

81. Dow, G., Browne, A., and Sibbald, R.G., Infection in chronic wounds: controversies in diagnosis and treatment, *Ostomy Wound Manage.*, 45, 23–40, 1999.

82. Eriksson, G., Eklund, A., and Kallings, L., The clinical significance of bacterial growth in venous leg ulcers, *Scand. J. Infect. Dis.*, 16, 175–180, 1984.

83. Fleischer, W. and Reimer, K., Povidone–iodine in antisepsis: state of the art, *Dermatology*, 195(suppl 2), 3–9, 1997.

84. Payne, D.N., Gibson, S.A.W., and Lewis, R., Antiseptics: a forgotten weapon in the control of antibiotic resistant bacteria in hospital and community settings, *J. Roy. Soc. Health.*, 118, 18–22, 1998.

85. Drosou, A., Falabella, A.F., and Kirsner, R.S., Antiseptics on wounds: an area of controversy, *Wounds*, 15, 149–166, 2003.

86. Kirsner, R.S., Infection and intervention, *Wounds*, 15, 127–128, 2003.

87. Lineaweaver, W., Howard, R., Soucy, D. et al., Topical antimicrobial toxicity, *Arch. Surg.*, 120, 267–270, 1985.

88. Greenberg, L. and Ingalls, J.W., Bactericide/leukocide ratio: a technique for the evaluation of disinfectants, *J. Am. Pharmaceut. Assoc.*, 47, 531–533, 1958.

89. Cooper, M.L., Laxer, J.A., and Hansbrough, J.F., The cytotoxic effects of commonly used topical antimicrobial agents on human fibroblasts and keratinocytes. *J. Trauma*, 31, 775–784, 1991.

90. Fleming, A., The action of chemical and physiological antiseptics in a septic wound, *Br. J. Surg.*, 7, 99–129, 1919.

91. Mertz, P.M., Davis, S., Brewer, L., and Franzen, L., Can antimicrobials be effective without impairing wound healing? The evaluation of a cadexomer iodine ointment, *Wounds*, 6, 184–193, 1994.

92. Skog, E., Amesjo, B., Troeng, T. et al., A randomized trial comparing cadexomer iodine and standard treatment in the outpatient management of chronic venous ulcers, *BMJ*, 109, 77–83, 1983.

93. Fleischer, W. and Reimer, K., Povidone iodine in antisepsis: state of art, *Dermatology*, 195 (suppl 2), 3–9, 1997.

94. Rodeheaver, G., Bellamy, W., Kody, M. et al., Bactericidal activity and toxicity of iodine-containing solutions in wounds, *Arch. Surg.*, 117, 181–185, 1982.

95. Howell, J.M., Stair, T.O., Howell, A.W. et al., The effect of scrubbing and irrigation with normal saline, povidone iodine, and cefazolin on wound bacterial counts in a guinea pig model, *Am. J. Emerg. Med.*, 11, 134–138, 1993.

96. Georgiade, N.G. and Harris, W.A., Open and closed treatment of burns with povidone iodine, *Plast. Reconstruct. Surg.*, 52, 640–644, 1973.

97. Gravett, A., Sterner, S., Clinton, J.E. et al., A trial of povidone iodine in the prevention of infection in sutured lacerations, *Ann. Emerg. Med.*, 16, 167/47–171/51, 1987.

98. Piérard-Franchimont, C., Paquet, P., Arrese, J.E. et al., Healing rate and bacterial necrotizing vasculitis in venous leg ulcers, *Dermatology,* 194, 383–387, 1997.

99. Viljanto, J., Disinfection of surgical wounds without inhibition of wound healing, *Arch. Surg.,* 115, 253–256, 1980.

100. Berkelman, R.L., Holland, B.W., and Anderson, R.L., Increased bactericidal activity of dilute preparations of povidone iodine solutions, *J. Clin. Microbiol.,* 15, 635–639, 1982.

101. Lammers, R.L., Fourré, M., Calahan, M.L. et al., Effect of povidone iodine and saline soaking on bacterial counts in acute, traumatic, contaminated wounds, *Ann. Emerg. Med.,* 19, 709/155–714/160, 1990

102. Mertz, P.M., Oliveira-Gandia, M.F., and Davis, S.C., The evaluation of a cadexomer iodine wound dressing on methicillin resistant *Staphylococcus aureus* in acute wounds, *Dermatol. Surg.,* 25, 89–93, 1999.

103. Danielsen, L., Cherry, G.W., Harding, K., and Rollman, O., Cadexomer iodine in ulcers colonized by *Pseudomonas aeruginosa, J. Wound Care,* 6, 169–172, 1997.

104. Geronemus, R.G., Mertz, P.M., and Eaglstein, W.H., Wound healing: the effects of topical antimicrobial agents, *Arch. Dermatol.,* 15, 1311–1314, 1979.

105. Gruber, R.P., Vistnes, L., and Pardoe, R., The effect of commonly used antiseptics on wound healing, *Plast. Reconstruct. Surg.,* 55, 472–476, 1975.

106. Kjolseth, D., Frank, J.M., Barker, J.H. et al., Comparison of the effects of commonly used wound agents on epithelialization and neovascularization, *J. Am. Coll. Surg.,* 179, 305–312, 1994.

107. Menton, D.N. and Brown, M., The effects of commercial wound cleansers on cutaneous wound healing in guinea pigs, *Wounds,* 6, 21–27, 1994.

108. Mulliken, J.B., Healey, N.A., and Glowacki, J., Povidone iodine and tensile strength of wounds in rats, *J. Trauma,* 20, 323–324, 1980.

109. Kashayap, A., Beezhold, D., Wiseman, J., and Beck, W.C., Effect of povidone-iodine dermatologic ointment on wound healing, *Am. Surg.,* 61, 486–491, 1995.

110. Niedner, R. and Schopf, E., Inhibition of wound healing by antiseptics, *Br. J. Dermatol.,* 115 (suppl 31), 41–44, 1986.

111. MacRae, S.M., Brown, B., and Edelhauser, H.F., The corneal toxicity of presurgical antiseptics, *Am. J. Ophthalmol.,* 97, 221–232, 1984.

112. Hopf, K., Grandy, R., Stahl-Bayliss, C., and Fitzmartin, R., The effect of betadine cream vs. silvadene cream on reepithelialization in uninfected experimental wounds, *Proc. Burn Assoc.,* 23, 166, 1991.

113. Robins, P., Day, C.L., Jr., and Lew, R.A., A multivariate analysis of factors affecting wound healing time, *Dermatol. Surg. Oncol.,* 10, 219–222, 1984.

114. De Kock, M., van der Merwe, A.E., and Swarts, C., A Comparative Study of Povidone Iodine Cream and Silver Sulfadiazine in the Topical Treatment of Burns, in Proceedings of the First Asian/Pacific Congress of Medicine Services, Selwyn, S., Ed., Royal Society of Medicine Services, London, 1998, pp. 65–71.

115. Lee, B.Y., Trainor, F.S., and Thoden, W.R., Topical application of povidone–iodine in the management of decubitus and stasis ulcers, *J. Am. Geriatr. Soc.,* 27, 302–306, 1979.

116. Mayer, D.A. and Tsapogas, M.J., Povidone–iodine and wound healing: a critical review, *Wounds,* 5, 14–23, 1993.

117. Lamme, E.N., Gustafsson, T.O., and Middelkoop, E., Cadexomer iodine shows stimulation of epidermal regeneration in experimental full thickness wounds, *Arch. Dermatol. Res.,* 290, 18–24, 1998.

118. Laudanska, H. and Gustavson, B., Inpatient treatment of chronic varicose venous ulcers. A randomized trial of cadexomer iodine versus standard dressings, *J. Int. Med. Res.*, 16, 428–435, 1988.
119. Hillstrom, L., Iodosorb compared to standard treatment in chronic venous ulcers: a multicenter study, *Acta Chir. Scand.*, Suppl 544, 53–56, 1988.
120. Skog, E., Arnesjo, B., Troeng, T. et al., A randomized trial comparing cadexomer iodine and standard treatment in the outpatient management of chronic venous ulcers, *Br. J. Dermatol.*, 109, 77–83, 1983.
121. Holloway, G.A., Johansen, K.H., Barnes, R.W., and Pierce, G.E., Multicenter trial of cadedxomer iodine to treat venous stasis ulcers, *West. J. Med.*, 151, 35–38, 1989.
122. Ormiston, M.C., Seymour, M.T.J., Venn, G.E., Cohen, R.I., and Fox, J.A., Controlled trial of iodosorb in chronic venous ulcers, *Br. Med. J.*, 291, 308–310, 1985.
123. Harcup, J.W. and Saul, P.A., A study of the effect of cadexomer iodine in the treatment of venous leg ulcers, *Br. J. Clin. Pract.*, 40, 360–364, 1986.
124. Tarvainen, K., Cadexomer iodine (iodosorb) compared with dextranomer (debrisan) in the treatment of chronic leg ulcers, *Acta Chir. Scand.*, Suppl 544, 57–59, 1988.
125. Hansson, C. et al., The effects of cadexomer iodine paste in the treatment of venous leg ulcers compared with hydrocolloid dressing and paraffin gauze dressing, *Int. J. Dermatol.*, 37, 390–396, 1998.
126. Floyer, C. and Wilkinson, J.D., Treatment of venous leg ulcers with cadexomer iodine with particular reference to iodine sensitivity, *Acta Chir. Scand.*, Suppl 544, 60–61, 1988.
127. Apelqvist, J. and Ragnarson Tennvall, G., Cavity foot ulcers in diabetic patients: a comparative study of cadexomer iodine and standard treatment. An economic analysis alongside a clinical trial, *Acta Dermatol. Venereol.*, 76, 231–235, 1996.
128. Moberg, S., Hoffman, L., Grennert, M.L., and Holst, A., *J. Am. Geriatr. Soc.*, 31, 462–465, 1983.
129. Klasen, H.J., A historical review of the use of silver in the treatment of burns. II. Renewed interest for silver, *Burns*, 26, 131–138, 2000.
130. Monafo, W.W. and West, M.A., Current treatment recommendations for topical burn therapy, *Drugs*, 40, 364–373, 1990.
131. de Gracia, C.G., An open study comparing topical silver sulfadiazine and topical silver sulfadiazine–cerium nitrate in the treatment of moderate and severe burns, *Burns*, 27, 67–74, 2001.
132. Tredget, E.E., Shankowsky, H.A., Groeneveld, A., and Burrell, R., A matched-pair, randomized study evaluating the efficacy and safety of Acticoat silver-coated dressing for the treatment of burn wounds, *J. Burn Care Rehabil.*, 19, 531–537, 1998.
133. Demling, R.H. and DeSanti, L., Effects of silver on wound management, *Wounds*, 13, 5–15, 2001.
134. Lansdown, A.B., Sampson, B., Laupattarakasem, P., and Vuttivirojana, A., Silver aids healing in the sterile skin wound: experimental studies in the laboratory rat, *Br. J. Dermatol.*, 137, 728–735, 1997.
135. Leitch, I.O., Kucukcelebi, A., and Robson, M.C., Inhibition of wound contraction by topical antimicrobials, *Aust. N.Z. J. Surg.*, 63, 289–293, 1993.
136. Kucan, J.O., Robson, M.C., Heggers, J.P. et al., Comparison of sliver sulfadiazine, povidone iodine and physiologic saline in the treatment of pressure ulcers, *J. Am. Geriatr. Soc.*, 29, 232–235, 1981.

137. Bishop, J.B., Phillips, L.G., Mustoe, T.A., VanderZee, A.J., Wiersema, L., Roach, D.E., Heggers, J.P., Hill, D.P., Jr., Taylor, E.L., and Robson, M.C., A prospective randomized evaluator-blinded trial of two potential wound healing agents for the treatment of venous stasis ulcers, *J. Vasc. Surg.,* 16, 251–257, 1992.

138. Ouvry, P.A., A trial of silver sulfadiazine in the local treatment of venous ulcers, *Phlebologie,* 42, 673–679, 1989.

139. Livingstone, D.H., Cryer, H.G., Miller, F.B. et al., A randomized prospective study of topical antimicrobial agents on skin grafts after thermal injury, *Plast. Reconstruct. Surg.,* 86, 1059–1064, 1990.

140. Carson, C.F., Riley, T.V., and Cookson, B.D., Efficacy and safety of tea tree oil as a topical antimicrobial agent, *J. Hosp. Infect.,* 40, 175–178, 1998.

141. Molan, P.C., The role of honey in the management of wounds, *J. Wound Care,* 8, 415–418, 1999.

142. Cooper, R.S. and Molan, P.C., Honey in wound care, *J. Wound Care,* 8, 340, 1999.

143. Moch, D., Fleischmann, W., and Russ, M., The BMW (biosurgical mechanical wound treatment) in diabetic foot, *Zentralbl. Chir.,* 124 (Suppl 1), 69–72, 1999.

144. Mumcuoglu, K.Y., Ingber, A., Gilead, L., Stessman, J., Friedmann, R., Schulman, H., Bichucher, H., Ioffe-Uspensky, I., Miller, J., Galun, R., and Raz, I., Maggot therapy for the treatment of intractable wounds, *Int. J. Dermatol.,* 38, 623–627, 1999.

145. Thomas, S., Andrews, A., and Jones, M., Maggots are useful in treating infected or necrotic wounds, *BMJ,* 318, 807, 1999.

146. Thomas, S. and Jones, M., The use of larval therapy in wound management, *J. Wound Care,* 7, 521–524, 1998.

147. Prete, P.E., Growth effects of *Phaenicia sericata* larval extracts on fibroblasts: mechanism for wound healing by maggot therapy, *Life Sci.,* 60, 505–510, 1997.

148. Bennett, L.L., Rosenblum, R.S., Perlov, C. et al., An *in vivo* comparison of topical agents on wound repair, *Plast. Reconstruct. Surg.,* 108, 675–685, 2001.

149. Fumal, I., Braham, C., Paquet, P., Pierard-Franchimont, C., and Pierard, G.E., The beneficial toxicity paradox of antimicrobials in leg ulcer healing impaired by a polymicrobial flora: a proof-of-concept study, *Dermatology,* 204 (Suppl 1), 70–74, 2002.

150. Knutson, R.A., Merbitz, L.A., Creekmore, M.A., et al., Use of sugar and povidone–iodine to enhance wound healing: five years' experience, *South. Med. J.,* 74, 1329–1335, 1981.

151. Lee, B.Y., Trainor, F.S., and Thoden, W.R., Topical application of povidone–iodine in the management of decubitus and stasis ulcers, *J. Am. Geriatr. Soc.,* 27, 302–306, 1979.

152. Severyns, A.M., Lejeune, A., Rocoux, G., and Lejeune, G., Non-toxic antiseptic irrigation with chlorhexidine in experimental revascularization in the rat, *J. Hosp. Infect.,* 17, 197–206, 1991.

153. Sindelar, W.F. and Mason, G.R., Irrigation of subcutaneous tissue with povidone–iodine solution for prevention of surgical wound infections, *Surg. Gynecol. Obstet.,* 148, 227–231, 1979.

154. Olson, M.E., Wright, J.B., Lam, K., and Burrell, R.E., Healing of porcine donor sites covered with silver-coated dressings, *Eur. J. Surg.,* 166, 486–489, 2000.

10 Oxygen and Skin Wound Healing

Thomas K. Hunt

CONTENTS

SUMMARY

Despite skin's superficial position, lack of oxygen is one of the most frequent reasons why it fails to heal. Oxygen concentrations, i.e., PO_2, in wounds are low, and most of the variations in collagen deposition, angiogenesis, and epithelization in human wounds are due to variations of local PO_2. The rates are directly proportional to the PO_2. This proportionality extends from zero to well above the "normal" wound levels found in ideal wounds and patients.

Lack of blood perfusion is the root cause in most cases of wounds that fail to heal. Lack of perfusion may be due to heart failure, vasoconstriction, arterial hypoxemia, hypertension, repetitive scarring (venous disease), and arterial disease. Vasoconstriction and vascular diseases are by far the most important. While the normal oxygen demands of wounds are relatively low, they are heightened by excessive inflammation. The result is a lower PO_2 that prolongs healing and may cause excessive scarring in the long run. When more oxygen is made available to healing tissue, more is used, and some of the added consumption contributes to accelerated healing and greater resistance to infection.[1,2,3]

When blood flow, i.e., perfusion through wounds, is slow, breathing oxygen is rarely helpful. Blood perfusion can often be raised by treating vasoconstriction due to pain, cold, drugs, stress, or blood volume loss. Transfusion is rarely needed. Breathing oxygen, even to hyperbaric levels, is often helpful when diffusion barriers rather than perfusion are the main obstacles to oxygenation.

10.1 INTRODUCTION AND HISTORY

The now-obvious link between poor perfusion and healing failure was long ignored. Even to this day, relatively few practitioners consciously use even the simplest means to optimize skin tissue perfusion. Surgeons have noted for centuries that wounds in poorly perfused tissues heal poorly or not at all and, furthermore, are excessively prone to infection. What was missed was the link between poor perfusion and tissue hypoxia and the importance of oxygen itself to healing and resistance to infection. My grandmother told me long ago to use warm wet soaks for infected wounds because warmth improves circulation (and oxygenation, though she did not know it).

A Russian experimentalist measured inadequate epithelization at high altitude six decades ago. Mountaineers observed failure to clear skin infections at high altitude, but medical interest in oxygen in wound healing began only in the 1960s, when it was noted that hyperbaric oxygen therapy stimulated growth of granulation tissue in ischemic and irradiated wounds. Jacques Cousteau's divers observed that their work-wounds healed most rapidly when they lived in their undersea habitat at 30 ft. underwater. Unfortunately, the medical belief at that time was that oxygen breathing could not change tissue oxygen concentration. Instead, more hemoglobin was believed to be the *only* way. That is, dissolved oxygen was thought insignificant in oxygen transport. This conviction left little room for these observations, and the conviction has changed very slowly. It is difficult now to understand how medicine missed the significance of pain, pallor, or cyanosis with cold, all being corrected with warmth. (Think pain due to hypoxia.)

The breakthrough came when technology to measure oxygen concentration, i.e., PO_2, in tissue proved that:

1. PO_2 in skin and subcutaneous tissue is highly variable according (largely) to the rate of local skin perfusion.
2. PO_2 is considerably lower in wounds than in uninjured tissue.
3. Both normal skin and wound PO_2 can be raised by oxygen supplementation if the right conditions exist.
4. Healing significantly improves when the local concentration of oxygen is elevated.

With objective numerical measurement, a number of obstacles to maintaining and elevating PO_2 in tissue were found. Details of how oxygen travels from blood to its point of use became available. Two of the most valuable findings were quantification of how vulnerable PO_2 in skin and subcutaneous tissue is to vasoconstriction and how much vasoconstriction contributes to poor healing and infection.

10.2 OXYGEN IN NORMAL AND INJURED SKIN AND SUBCUTANEOUS TISSUE

Electrodes that are made to exclude air detect little oxygen on human skin surface (0 to 10 mmHg in most places). Oxygen flux across the keratin layer from the outside is quite slow. Warming of the skin to produce hyperemia and overcome the diffusion barrier of keratin with a transcutaneous oximeter raises surface PO_2 to about two-thirds of the arterial PO_2 if perfusion is normal. Tape-stripped skin exposes the basal layers to a relatively normal PO_2 for only a day. The exudate and its coagulum soon form a diffusion barrier, and inflammatory cells increase oxygen consumption. If, however, a friction blister is kept intact or a water vapor–impermeable/oxygen-permeable plastic sheet is used to cover the wound, the stripped surface PO_2 is almost that of air, or higher if oxygen is blown onto it. This does not apply to burn blisters, in which PO_2 is zero, as it is in the skin beneath. As the electrodes are advanced deeper into the normal dermis and then into subcutaneous tissue, the PO_2 becomes totally dependent on arterial oxygen tension and all its vagaries.[4]

To summarize a very important paper by Silver that is out of print and available only in libraries:[4] The stratum corneum is a diffusion barrier. Oxygen supply to the basal layers of (human) skin comes almost entirely from the arterial blood. Epithelium that is migrating under a scab is in a low-PO_2 environment. The PO_2 on stripped (keratin layer is removed) skin under oxygen-permeable, water-impermeable plastic membranes is proportional to that of air. The result is more rapid epithelization. PO_2 in skin diminishes when subjects are put under stress.

Injury diminishes dermal and subcutaneous tissue perfusion and oxygen concentration by damaging the microvasculature. Subsequent coagulation deepens the injury and further reduces perfusion. Inflammatory cells, primed and often activated on entering the wound, begin to consume large amounts of oxygen in their so-called respiratory burst. They convert this oxygen to superoxide and thence to other oxidants.[1] The energy for the conversion comes from aerobic glycolysis (i.e., does not require oxygen), and lactate is produced as a byproduct (Figure 10.1). The result is hypoxia in an inflamed, highly oxidative, highly lactated environment. This condition is literally a metabolic definition of a "healing wound." The extents of vascular injury and inflammation are highly variable. However, even "insignificant" wounds contain areas of ischemia where the healing cells exist in hypoxic, microscopic units of a few macrophages, a few fibroblasts, and relatively few nearby sources of oxygen.

One of the challenges to healing is to develop new vessels (i.e., angiogenesis) to provide oxygen for collagen deposition. New vessels need collagenous support. Indeed, endothelial cells eventually supply their own, but neither dermal nor endothelial collagen can be deposited in the absence of a considerable concentration of oxygen. Until new vessels acquire blood flow, the necessary oxygen for collagen deposition must diffuse a considerable distance from the last free-flowing (uninjured, uncoagulated) vessel. This requires a high arterial PO_2 so that the diffusion distance can be overcome.[4]

The PO_2 in the center of a wound can be quite low.[3] Ten to 15 mmHg has been measured in "dead spaces" of "normal" wounds. As wound spaces shrink, the PO_2 in them rises to about 40 or 50 mmHg (if the arterial PO_2 and perfusion are normal),

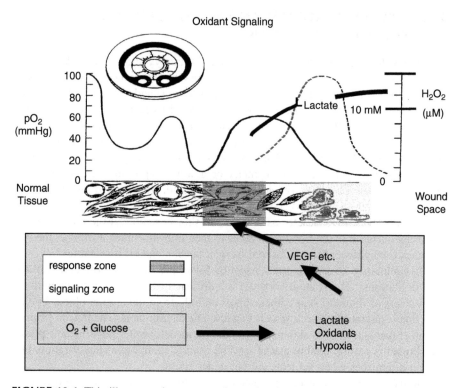

FIGURE 10.1 This illustrates the current schema for the events that occur with regard to oxygen in the healing wound. The macrophage, the sensor and activator of wounds, migrates from left to right followed by immature, replicating fibroblasts and then by budding vessels that eventually will fuse to each other, thus establishing blood flow. Glucose and oxygen diffuse in. The glucose is converted to lactate anaerobically, leading to lactate. The molecular oxygen is largely converted to oxidants and synthesized into collagen to allow its deposition. The PO_2 and lactate are shown. Both hypoxia and lactate are in position to stimulate the macrophages to secrete vascular endothelial growth factor (VEGF) and other growth factors that are not shown. The hypoxia is not necessary, as wounds with higher PO_2 than shown here (during oxygen therapy) heal faster than normal. Young fibroblasts are programmed to produce collagen by lactate. Other growth factors such as TGFbeta (that are largely of inflammatory origin) enhance its production. Oxygen is necessary for collagen deposition, which peaks in the zones of high oxygen.

a figure one can accept as an estimate of "normal, average" at the wound edge. If conditions are optimal, 100% oxygen at 1 atm raises it to the region of 150 to 200 mmHg. Hyperbaric oxygen (HBO) at 2 atm raises it to about 400 mmHg or above, with a wide variation. The PO_2 of a large dead space in well-perfused skin may rise only to 90 mmHg or so during HBO depending on its size.

A large variability in PO_2 and collagen deposition has been found in human surgical wounds 7 to 10 d postoperatively. Statistically, most of the variability is due to arterial PO_2 and vasoactivity.[2]

10.3 MECHANISMS OF OXYGEN EFFECTS

10.3.1 IMMUNITY TO INFECTION

The most direct entry to the explanation of how oxygen works in wounds is by considering immunity to infection. Immunity undoubtedly involves many mechanisms, but phagocytosis and bactericidal oxidant production by leukocytes appear to be the major ones, at least to surgeons who are concerned about the usual wound pathogens, such as *Staphylococcus aureus, Pseudomonas aeruginosa, Escherichia coli, Bacteroides* spp., and *Klebsiella.*[1,5]

Leukocytes are "activated" when they enter into wounds and then even more when they ingest bacteria. That is, they express a number of latent functions. For one, they begin to consume oxygen in large quantities by converting it to bactericidal oxidants such as superoxide and peroxide that are then inserted into the phagosomes where they kill engulfed bacteria by oxidizing their membranes. The activated enzyme is the NADPH-linked oxygenase of leukocytes (a.k.a. "phox" or "phagocytic oxygenase") that converts oxygen to oxidants in what is called the "oxidative burst." The equation is:

$$O_2 + \text{glucose} \longrightarrow \text{(phox)} \longrightarrow > O_2^- + \text{lactate} + H^+$$

The Km is about 75 mmHg.

The term "burst" comes from the fact that oxygen consumption rises as much as 50-fold within minutes of activation and stays high for several hours. About 98% of the excess oxygen consumed is converted to superoxide, which is then converted to hydrogen peroxide and other oxidants, including peroxynitrite, all bacteriocides. This large proportion of conversion is possible because the energy comes from conversion of glucose to lactate, aerobic glycolysis.

Ischemic wounds are notoriously vulnerable to infection. The Km of phox, that is, the oxygen concentration necessary to support superoxide formation at half the maximum possible rate, is about 75 mmHg. The PO_2 at the wound edge is rarely above 50 mmHg if the subject is breathing air at 1 atm. Humans benefit from significantly less than half the bactericidal potential of phox when we breathe air. Vulnerability to infection increases markedly when PO_2 is reduced. Raising PO_2 from a reduced value restores the loss and, on further elevation, is capable of adding an increment that may double the normal killing rate. Many studies show that bacteria are cleared more rapidly from hyperoxic as opposed to hypoxic wounds. It is clear that assurance of adequate oxygen tension in wounds is an excellent means of preventing wound infections in humans and some animals. It is additive to specific antibiotics and, alone, is approximately as effective.[6] Oxygen is also useful in treating established infections.

Phox is an assembly of proteins. The absence of any of their genes, a condition termed "chronic granulomatous disease," produces a susceptibility to the same organisms that infect wounds.[7] Various degrees of gene deficit impair resistance to infection from a mild to a profound degree and at worst are often fatal. As oxygen tensions fall into the 20 mmHg range, wounds in normal patients approach a severe degree of vulnerability that approaches absence of the pertinent genes. It is now generally accepted that hypoxia of the magnitude that is seen clinically in human wounds is a major source of vulnerability to infection. For example, ensuring an adequate PO_2 in wounds simply by warmth, oxygen breathing, and blood volume support decreases wound infections in surgical patients by more than half.[8,9] The effect has been proven specific to tissue hypoxia which, on occasion, may require hyperbaric oxygen to correct.

As an important aside, the lactate byproduct is also a vasodilator via a redox reaction.[10] It also has a number of other salutary effects that stimulate pertinent growth factors, angiogenesis, and collagen synthesis, also putatively by redox reactions.

Nitric oxide, NO, is also bactericidal. It is formed from arginine and molecular oxygen by nitric oxide synthetase:

$$O_2 + arginine \rightarrow NO + citrulline$$

The rate of NO production is also proportional to local oxygen concentration. The Km is uncertain and may be tissue or even cell specific, but the current estimate is about 15 mmHg for the leukocyte form.[11] NO is also a vasodilator.[12] We have looked and found no evidence of hyperoxia-induced vasoconstriction in skin and subcutaneous tissue at oxygen tension up to 600 mmHg arterial oxygen tension (PAO_2).[13] However, vasoconstriction does increases as arterial hypoxia deepens.

10.3.2 COLLAGEN SYNTHESIS

Oxygen concentration (PO_2) influences collagen synthesis, deposition, and cross-linking.[2,14] This does not, however, mean that anemia must be corrected to over packed cell volume (PCV) 30%, because, within broad limits, anemia is irrelevant to healing in well-perfused patients whose healing is unaffected by PCV within the range 15 to 35%. If anemia impairs heart function, the heart takes precedence because perfusion is so important.[15]

The reasons why local oxygen concentration are important to collagen synthesis and deposition are reasonably well understood:

First, the combination of oxygen and lactate from leukocytes together with transition metals leads to oxidant production, and this in turn stimulates collagen gene transcription.

A second path that also involves lactate involves polyadenosylribosylation, a protean regulator of protein activity that depends heavily on the NAD+ pool — as opposed to the NADH pool. Lactate converts NAD+ to NADH. This reaction determines the rate of ADPRibosylation because NAD+ is the origin of all ADPRibose, and the ADPRibose influences a number of upstream wound functions, for instance collagen gene transcription. (For a fuller explanation, see Reference 16.)

Third, oxidants are also generated by a period of hypoxia followed by restoration of oxygen, i.e., "oxidative stress." This sequence is well known to cause release of oxidants, and these oxidants induce collagen gene transcription in cultured fibroblasts. The emerging view is that, among many other ways [transforming growth factor-β (TGF-β), etc.], oxidant signaling is one of the most important enhancers of collagen transcription, and in fact, wound healing in general.[7] Oxidant signaling in wounds is an established concept, but so is oxidant damage that occurs after excessive oxidant stress. A balance exists, and wounds are more than well enough able to defend themselves against oxidant stress, since they are well protected by protein carboxylation and nitration, thiols, superoxide dismutase, and catalase, among other factors.

Fourth, collagen deposition and cross-binding require oxygen. Contrary to conventional concepts, many biologic processes other than energy metabolism depend upon PO_2. Three oxygenases (enzymes that consume oxygen as a substrate), each critically important in wound healing, regulate at least three other enzymatic steps in the pathway from collagen synthesis to extracellular cross-binding in the collagen fibril. These steps are posttranslational modification and two steps in extracellular cross-linking. The enzymes are prolyl hydroxylase, lysyl hydroxylase, and lysyl oxidase. The reasons are well understood: First, proline, not hydroxyproline, is incorporated into in the procollagen peptides as they are synthesized. Later, in a post-translational step that occurs in the endoplasmic reticulum, prolyl hydroxylase inserts an oxygen atom into selected prolines converting some of them to hydroxyprolines. The rate of hydroxylation is oxygen dependent because the oxygen atom can be obtained only from molecular oxygen. Only hydroxylated collagen can be exported from the cell. Since enzymatic reaction rates are hyperbolic with respect to the concentrations of their substrates, collagen deposition is 0 at $PO_2 = 0$, half-maximal at $PO_2 = 25$ (the Km), and maximal only at above 200 mmHg. This is the entire physiologic range of PO_2 and beyond. Second and similarly, lysines hydroxylated by lysyl hydroxylase assist extracellular cross-linking of collagen monomers into collagen fibrils. The half-maximal rate of lysyl hydroxylase also occurs at a PO_2 of approximately 25 mmHg. If this step is incomplete, collagen fibers become weak. Third, lysines in the collagen molecule that become stable covalent links in collagen fibers are condensed by lysyl oxidase, yet another oxygen-requiring enzyme, in the extracellular polymerization of collagen. The Km of lysyl hydroxylase is not well defined but appears to be higher than 25 mmHg and thus collagen cross-linking may be as susceptible to hypoxia as its deposition. If these steps are incomplete, collagen fibers are sparse and weak.

Hypoxia stimulates the release of several growth factors and cytokines that induce collagen synthesis, particularly hypoxia-inducible-factor (hif-1α), tumor necrosis factor (TNF), TGF-β, interleukin-1, and vascular endothelial growth factor (VEGF). However, this function appears to be duplicated by lactate and oxidant signaling.[7,17,18] Thus, except perhaps at its very beginnings, hypoxia is not a necessary condition for healing. The practical difference between collagen depositions in clinically relevant hyperoxia as opposed to hypoxia can be as much as threefold more than that in air breathing.

All this runs contrary to classic thought. The standard questions that arise are:

1. Should hyperoxia not decrease lactate?
2. Is hypoxia unnecessary for lactate production?

The demonstrated fact is that hyperoxygenation of wounded animals does not lower wound lactate levels.[19] This is true because lactate has at least three sources in wounds of which only one is relevant to oxygen. Furthermore, addition of lactate to fibroblasts in the presence of oxygen in culture and/or wounds in animals enhances collagen production significantly.[20]

10.3.3 ANGIOGENESIS

Macrophages are a potent source of VEGF. In turn, VEGF is the most important inducer of wound angiogenesis.[21] The logic of parsimony suggests that since macrophages, new blood vessels, and fibroblasts exist close together in wounds and act cooperatively (Figure 10.1), the mechanisms of angiogenesis should be similar and complementary to those of immune defenses, collagen synthesis, and deposition and should involve oxidants and lactate. Angiogenesis is dependent upon collagen deposition (by endothelial cells) to give physical support to growing vessels. In fact, the mechanisms of angiogenesis and collagen synthesis and deposition are strikingly similar.

It is well accepted that hypoxia leads to release of VEGF from many cell types.[22] It is not as well known, but is nevertheless also true, that lactate stimulates VEGF release from macrophages even in the presence of oxygen.[18] The mechanism currently appears to involve oxidant formation from oxygen, iron or other transition metals, and lactate.

This fact is particularly useful because the assumption that hypoxia is the single cause of VEGF release in wounds is incompatible with the fact that angiogenesis develops most rapidly in hyperoxygenated wounds. It is accelerated during hyperbaric oxygen therapy.[23] Furthermore, hypoxia truncates angiogenesis both clinically and experimentally. Hyperoxia enhances an endothelial response through oxidants. Small increases of peroxide, consistent with hyperoxia, increase release of vascular endothelial growth factor by endothelial cells.[18] Oxygen is required for vessel formation. Therefore hyperoxia secures both a release of VEGF and a response from the endothelial cells. This argues for the central importance of oxygen and lactate in healing and fits the clinical facts. Both hypoxia and hyperoxia enhance VEGF release, which is lowest at normal tissue oxygen concentrations (unpublished data).

10.3.4 EPITHELIZATION

Epithelial cells, like all others, can extract oxygen from wherever it is found, directly from air as well as blood. The rate of their growth in culture is proportional to PO_2 and is not inhibited by even very high PO_2.[24] Squamous epithelium is, however, in a peculiar position with regard to oxygen. Keratin presents a major diffusion block to oxygen that can be overcome only by heating to about 41°C.

Epithelization over first and second degree wounds or tape-stripped skin can be enhanced with oxygen administered systemically. However, when administered locally, oxygen is "shut out" by the exudate and coagulum. Inflammation also soon adds to oxygen consumption, and even systemic oxygen is used as fast as it arrives at the site of injury.[4] However, major differences in epithelization are observed in some patients during oxygen breathing and the differences in data are hard to interpret. If topical oxygen is to be used, the underlying lesion should be moist and clear of exudate.

In general, living epithelial cells are attuned to a relatively high PO_2. A period of hypoxia (the injury) followed by restoration of oxygen increases specific integrins and promotes motility.[25] Oxidants cause epithelial cells to produce VEGF release via protein kinases.[26] This seems to explain why epithelization is smooth and thin when wounds heal quickly as opposed to the continued hyperkeratosis that one sees next to chronic and inflamed wounds. This explanation seems also to explain how interleukin-1 assists epithelial healing.[27]

In summary, decreased perfusion, increased diffusion distances, and a rising demand for oxygen in wounds due to inflammation all lead to local hypoxia, an oxidative environment, and high lactate. Provision of oxygen to wounded tissue, where circulation and other conditions are sufficient, raises tissue PO_2 in wounds and profoundly influences healing. The mechanisms, as far as they are known, are strikingly similar.

10.4 CONTROLLING OXYGEN IN NORMAL AND WOUNDED TISSUE

To understand the behavior of oxygen in tissue, one needs first to understand some terminology and how tissue PO_2 is regulated.

The usual clinical use of the term "oxygen delivery," the cardiac output multiplied by the oxygen-carrying capacity of a liter of blood alone, has little reference to wounded tissue. For reference to healing wounds that, as noted above, present an obstacle to diffusion of oxygen, we need to know the arterial PO_2 as well because partial pressure, i.e., concentration, overcomes diffusion distances.

Wound "tissue PO_2" measures oxygen concentration in a given tissue — in other words, an expression of oxygen "availability." It is not equivalent to oxygen delivery. For present purposes, tissue PO_2 is usually expressed as millimeters of mercury. It can also be expressed as moles or millimoles per unit volume. The "concentration" in tissue is important because (as explained above) substrate concentrations control the rates of enzymatic reactions. PO_2 is specifically important because the relatively low PO_2 of oxygen often controls the rates of important enzymes that use it as a substrate, and, as noted, several such enzymes are critical to healing.

How much substrate a given enzyme can use in a given time depends upon the avidity, the strength, with which the enzyme and the substrate combine. The avidity is expressed as the Km for that enzyme, that is, the concentration of the substrate (oxygen in this case) that allows the enzyme to produce its end product at half the maximal rate. Mitochondrial cytochrome oxidase, one of the most avid for oxygen, produces its product (H_2O) at half-maximal rate even when PO_2 is less than 1 mmHg. That is, it is so avid for oxygen that PO_2 must fall to lethal levels before its rate is affected.

On the other hand, collagen prolyl hydroxylase (see below) is vital in healing. It has a Km of about 45 mm, i.e., 25 mmHg.[28] Its product, hydroxylated collagen, cannot be deposited into the extracellular space until it is hydroxylated. The other substrate of this enzyme is oxygen. Thus it depends on PO_2 throughout the entire physiologic range. Wound cells survive at low PO_2 by glycolysis alone but in such conditions function poorly because they become so vulnerable to infection.

Tissue PO_2 can never be higher than the arterial PO_2. Arterial blood at low PO_2 can deliver considerable oxygen if there is enough hemoglobin, but lacking concentration, it can penetrate only short distances. How much oxygen is used depends on the PO_2 at the point of use. High local tissue concentrations can be reached even in anemic subjects if arterial PO_2 and blood flow are high and oxygen extraction is relatively low, as it is in most wounds, generally about 1 ml/100 cc plasma.[15]

Tissue oxygen consumption is highly variable according to local PO_2 and the cell or organ in question. Since wounds use little oxygen, the gradient from vessel to wound space is less than might otherwise be the case, say in the heart at exercise. Infections increase the gradient. Cardiac myocytes, for example, are generously equipped with enzymes (cytochrome oxidase, for instance) that have a high affinity for oxygen; i.e., they consume oxygen and function well at low PO_2. Working muscle, with its high oxygen consumption, relies upon a high hemoglobin content and high flow as well as a relatively high PO_2. On the other hand, reparative cells, i.e., fibroblasts, endothelial cells, and inflammatory cells, have relatively few mitochondria. Their enzymes have a lower affinity for oxygen, and they function poorly at oxygen concentrations that are capable of sustaining life but not healing. For this reason, as PO_2 falls, wound healing fails well before tissue viability is in danger from simple hypoxia. Tissue dies partly because infection increases oxygen consumption until the PO_2 falls below the partial pressure that is necessary to sustain life.

10.5 CLINICAL STRATEGIES FOR OVERCOMING THE OBSTACLES

Correcting tissue hypoxia is more complex than simply breathing oxygen. Using wound oximeters, we have seen many surgical patients whose wound PO_2 is low and totally unaffected by breathing oxygen. Even in the absence of arteriosclerosis and with their arterial PO_2 significantly elevated, wound PO_2 can be low due to vasoconstriction. When given adequate fluid and warmed, such patients will then respond to oxygen administration. This emphasizes the importance of local perfusion.

Perfusion, the rate at which blood perfuses a tissue, is critical to that tissue's functions. Medicine has long been interested in cardiac output and the state of the arteries, but commonly, the perfusion of wounded and healing tissue is reduced (unnecessarily) by the vasoconstriction that occurs as a result of low blood volume, cold, pain, and vasoconstrictive drugs (i.e., sympathetic stimulation). Vessels of the skin are particularly vulnerable to sympathetic vasoconstriction. In practical terms,

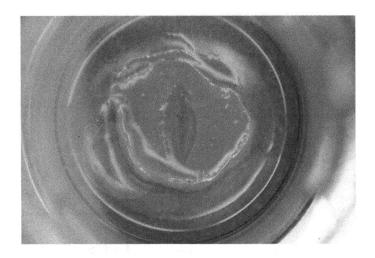

COLOR FIGURE 1.2 Appearance of wounded skin equivalents grown in organotypic culture at an air–liquid interface. An organotypic culture transferred to a second collagen gel after incisional wound is seen 6 d after wounding. The shape of the original wound is elliptical, and the wound is nearly closed in the center.

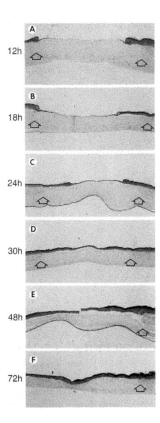

COLOR FIGURE 1.3 Morphology of skin equivalents at various points after wounding. Wounded skin equivalents were stained with hematoxylin and eosin at (A) 12 h, (B) 18 h, (C) 24 h, (D) 30 h, (E) 48 h, and (F) 72 h after wounding. Two phases of epithelial response can be seen. The first phase extends from the earliest migration of epithelium (A,B) until the wound is completely covered by a thin epithelium (C). The second phase of stratification begins at 30 h (D) and is complete when the tissue is of similar thickness to that of the unwounded epithelium at the wound margins (F). Open arrows demarcate the wound margins. (Original magnification × 10.)

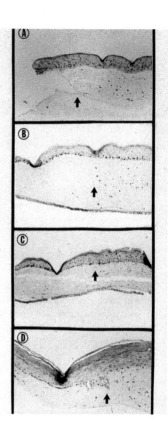

COLOR FIGURE 1.4 Proliferative activity of reepithelialized wounds at various points after wounding. Wounded skin equivalents were labeled with an 8-h pulse of BrdU, stained with a monoclonal antibody to BrdU, and counterstained with hematoxylin at (A) 8 h, (B) 24 h, (C) 48 h, and (D) 4 d after wounding. While few BrdU nuclei are seen shortly after wounding (A), a sharp increase in proliferative activity is seen in both the wound and the adjacent wound margins 24 h after wounding (B). This proliferative activity is maintained in the wound by 48 h as the tissue stratifies (C). Proliferation is considerably less at 4 d post-wounding when the reepithelialization process is complete (D). The arrows demarcate the wound margins. Labeling Index (LI) was calculated as the percentage of basal nuclei labeled with BrdU. (Original magnification × 50 for A, B, and C, and × 66 for D.)

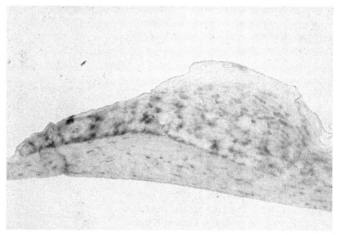

COLOR FIGURE 1.5 MMP-1 RNA expression is restricted to migrating keratinocytes covering the wound. Basal keratinocytes at the leading edge of the epithelial tongue express MMP-1 RNA, as detected by *in situ* hybridization 4 d after wounding. Keratinocytes distal from the wound edge demonstrate no MMP-1 RNA expression. Thus, only keratinocytes in contact with Type I collagen on the wound surface expressed this protease.

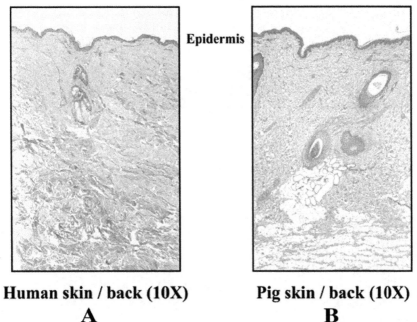

Epidermis

Human skin / back (10X)

A

Pig skin / back (10X)

B

COLOR FIGURE 6.1 Hemotoxin- and eosin-stained back skin of human (A) and swine (B).

Epidermal Migration Assessment

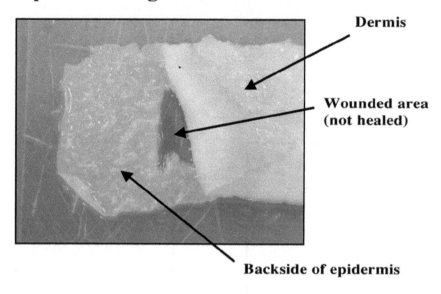

Dermis

Wounded area (not healed)

Backside of epidermis

COLOR FIGURE 6.2 Wound healing specimen from salt-split technique of Eaglstein and Mertz.

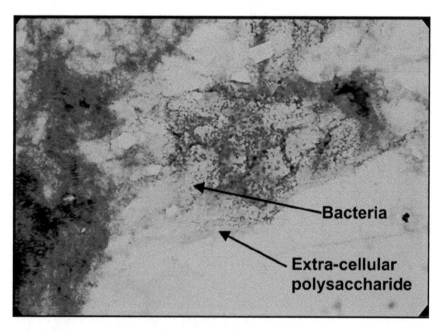

Bacteria

Extra-cellular polysaccharide

COLOR FIGURE 6.3 Modified Congo red stain of bacteria living in a biofilm matrix made up of EPS taken from a chronic wound scraping.

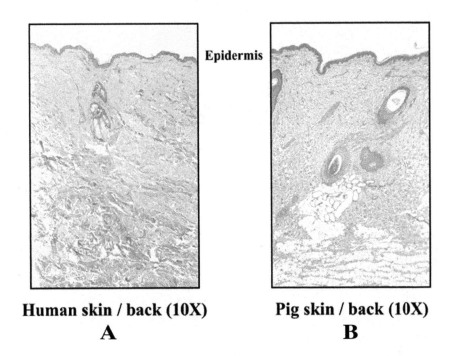

Epidermis

Human skin / back (10X)
A

Pig skin / back (10X)
B

COLOR FIGURE 6.1 Hemotoxin- and eosin-stained back skin of human (A) and swine (B).

Epidermal Migration Assessment

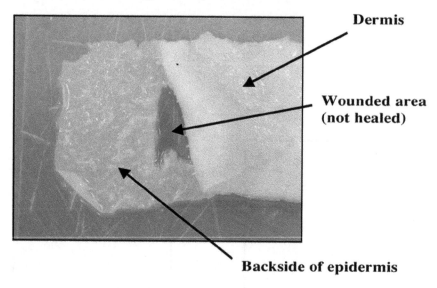

Dermis

Wounded area
(not healed)

Backside of epidermis

COLOR FIGURE 6.2 Wound healing specimen from salt-split technique of Eaglstein and Mertz.

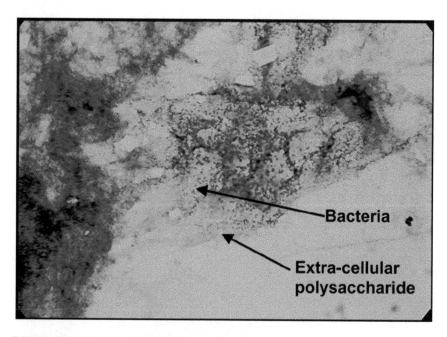

Bacteria

Extra-cellular
polysaccharide

COLOR FIGURE 6.3 Modified Congo red stain of bacteria living in a biofilm matrix made up of EPS taken from a chronic wound scraping.

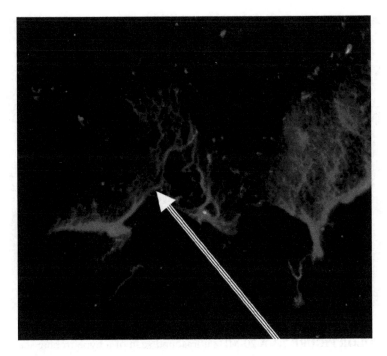

COLOR FIGURE 6.4 Calcfluor white fluorescent stain of EPS from a bacterial-induced wound biofilm from swine.

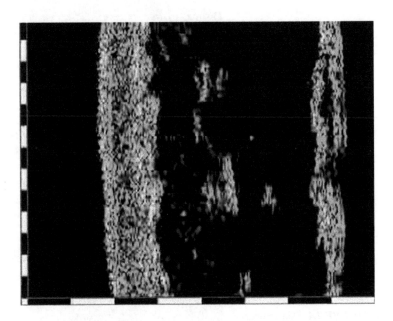

COLOR FIGURE 7.2 A 20-MHz ultrasound scan of normal skin.

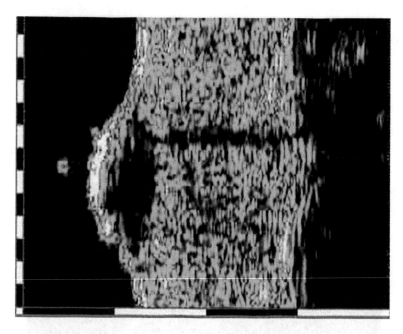

COLOR FIGURE 7.3 A 20-MHz ultrasound scan of a hypertrophic scar.

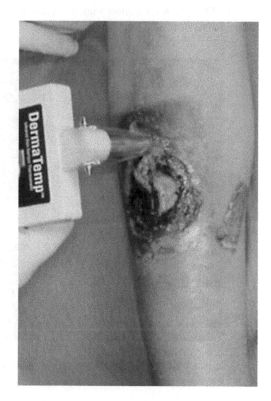

COLOR FIGURE 7.4 Skin temperature measurement on the surrounding
skin of an infected ulcer.

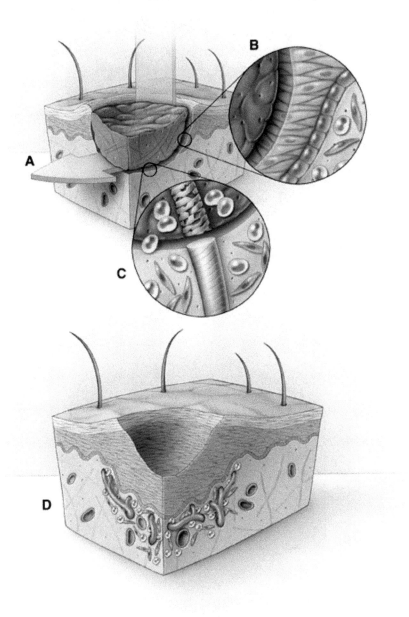

COLOR FIGURE 14.2 A proposed view of how a debriding agent (collagenase) might have beneficial effects on wound bed preparation and healing. (A) The necrotic plug is being removed by enzymatic action. (B) The collagen bundles are being cut at the necrotic–viable tissue interphase. (C) Rapid epithelialization that might occur either indirectly (as necrotic tissue is removed) or through the direct effect of collagenase on keratinocyte migration. (D) The wound, now free of necrotic tissue, has good granulation tissue and is mostly epithelialized.

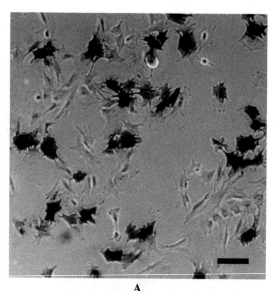

A

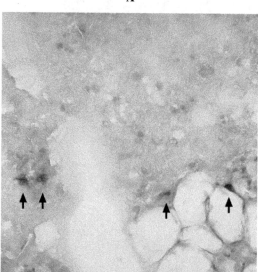

B

COLOR FIGURE 16.3 Transplantation of cultured fibroblasts to porcine full thickness skin wounds. (A) Cultured fibroblasts were transfected *in vitro* with β-galactosidase (a marker gene) prior to transplantation. Transfected cells are stained blue. (B) Transplanted transfected fibroblasts stained blue in a histological section in a wound 4 d post grafting, demonstrating integration of the grafted cells into the neodermis (granulation tissue). These wounds displayed increased numbers of keratinocyte colonies, greater reepithelialization, and thicker neoepidermis as compared to wounds seeded with keratinocytes only. Scale bar: 50 μm. (Reproduced from Svensjö et al., *Transplantation* 73 (7), 1033–1041, 2002. With permission from Lippincott Williams & Wilkins.)

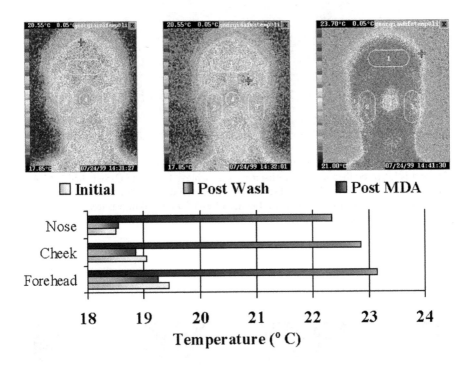

COLOR FIGURE 18.1 Skin surface thermography before and after microdermabrasion. The amount of physiological activity of the skin is measured by the amount of infrared radiation emanating from the surface using 600 lines of spatial resolution with 30° field of view at 30 frames/sec of real-time imaging. The instrument is internally referenced and self-calibrating to absolute zero with a resolution of 0.05°C at 35°C (TIP-200, Boston, MA). Scale is Temperature, °C.

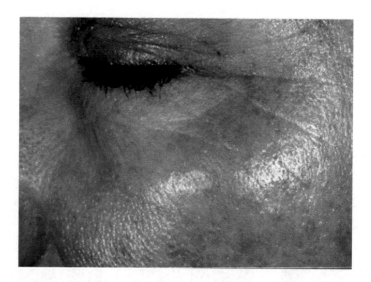

COLOR FIGURE 18.3 Immediately after 1064 nm Q-switched Nd:YAG laser treatment. The end point of erythema without blistering was achieved with the Q-Switched Nd:YAG Laser (Medlite IV, Hoya ConBio, Fremont CA) (λ = 1064 nm), for a pulse duration of 4–6 nsec, with a spot size of 6 mm at a fluence of 3–3.5 J/cm^2. Skin was treated five times over a three-month period.

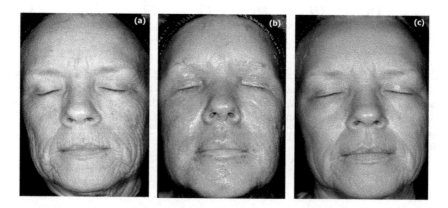

COLOR FIGURE 18.9 Epithelialization of facial skin following CO_2 laser resurfacing. Representative patient (#107) in the treatment group, treated with three passes of the UltraPulse CO_2 laser (Coherent Technologies, Palo Alto, CA) utilizing a computer pattern generator set at a density of 6 and an energy setting of 300 mJ. (a) Pretreatment image, (b) 2 d following resurfacing procedure, and (c) 4 weeks following resurfacing procedure.

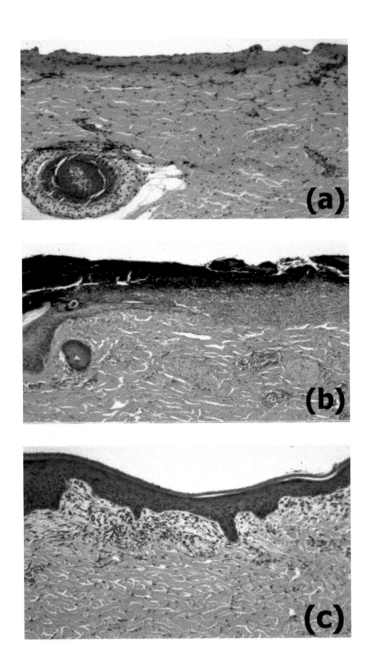

COLOR FIGURE 18.10 Histology of skin following CO_2 laser procedure. Representative section of skin treated with three passes of the UltraPulse CO_2 laser (Coherent Technologies, Palo Alto, CA) utilizing a computer pattern generator set at a density of 6 and an energy setting of 300 mJ. (a) Immediately after procedure, (b) 3 d post procedure, and (c) 5 d post-procedure. (H&E stain at 100× magnification.)

this is enormously important. As perfusion falls, the fraction of delivered oxygen that is consumed increases, and PO_2 in capillary blood and in tissue falls. The operative rule is to keep wounds moist, warm, and without evaporative heat loss to minimize pain; maintain blood volume and hydration; and to avoid alpha-adrenergic drugs. Warmth is particularly important because it can overcome the effects of most of the other vasoconstrictors. Remember, one of skin's most important properties is to regulate heat loss.

For optimal results, all of these elements must be corrected at the same time because any one is sufficient to cause maximal vasoconstriction. Think of what happens to peripheral perfusion when you are relaxed, not smoking, well fed and happy, but cold. You have pallid fingers and toes until you get warm.

Warmth has been regarded as potentially harmful to chronic wounds for many years. Sympathetic innervation (i.e., central control) is supposed to be inoperative in diabetic legs, but local reflexes and some central control often remain. Warming a cold limb to ideally about 35°C often elevates perfusion and PO_2 in cold, ischemic wounds. External warmth penetrates to the subcutaneous tissue, usually vasodilates, and increases subcutaneous tissue PO_2.[8,29] Our wound clinic has not yet seen warmth lower PO_2 around a chronic wound, but excessive warmth is a potential problem, and the detailed clinical rules are still to be written. A response to warmth predicts a therapeutic potential. Sympathetic overactivity is a frequent property of chronic wounds, and preventing cold- and pain-mediated vasoconstriction is almost always beneficial.

Similarly, pain activates vasoconstriction. It is necessary to avoid the vicious cycle of pain/vasoconstriction/more pain, etc. Beta-adrenergic blockade, diuretics, and smoking increase hypoxic problems and should be regulated or dispensed with. Their harmful effects appear to be due to limitation of oxygen supply. Beta-blockers are often necessary, but they leave unopposed alpha activity. Many postoperative patients are blood volume depleted, in pain, cold, and beta-blocked, and almost as often, these conditions are preventable.

Wound PO_2 can often be elevated through the use of the alpha antagonist Clonidine® (Boehringer Ingelheim GmbH, Germany) in the patch dosage form because blood volume changes and vasoconstriction occur very rapidly, and the need for protection is constant. Many anesthesiologists like to use this strategy, and the drug is an excellent medication for hypertension. When β-blockers are used for hypertension, they can often be safely discontinued by substituting Clonidine. (Clonidine should not be discontinued rapidly.)

Another corollary of these rules is that expansion of blood volume is more important than increasing red cell mass.[2] The reasons are given above.

These strategies can be put into place arbitrarily in most cases. Some strategies, particularly those involving chronic wounds, are best planned on the basis of transcutaneous oximetry, which should be available in all noninvasive vascular laboratories.[30]

Hyperbaric oxygen remains an unnecessarily controversial means of overcoming a major obstacle to oxygen diffusion. The most precise indication for hyperbaric therapy is a chronic wound in which periwound transcutaneous PO_2 (TcPO_2) is low and responds to oxygen breathing in a hyperbaric chamber with the ulcerated part warm and at heart level. Clearly, local perfusion should be maximized.

Hyperbaric oxygen for chronic wound healing remained a controversial issue for many years mainly due to the difficulty of effectively stratifying chronic wounds and, therefore, predicting responders. Transcutaneous oxygen measurement, while not perfect, has largely changed that.[30] From all existing data, hyperbaric oxygen stimulates neo-angiogenesis. Hyperbaric oxygen treatment for ischemic lesions of the leg does not prevent minor amputations but does prevent major amputations, often for years.[31]

As experience with oximetry has expanded, the success rate of hyperbaric therapy has risen, and indications have been clarified. Several prospective and blinded studies have recently been completed. Despite their small size, the data seems clear that if the problem is ischemia (periwound hypoxia), and oxygen breathing raises periwound PO_2, hyperbaric oxygen can save limbs.[31] On the basis of the enzyme kinetics noted above, one can predict that hyperbaric oxygen has little to offer normoxic wounds, and it does not.

One of the most fruitful applications of hyperbaric oxygen has been in osteoradionecrosis. The data are convincing.[32,33]

The usual daily therapy is short. How can such a short exposure have a significant effect? First, tissue hyperoxia due to a 90-min exposure actually lasts for about another 2 h. Second, as noted above, during the exposure, bacterial killing is increased. The effect of eliminating large numbers of bacteria has "downstream" significance just as one would expect from a bolus of antibiotic. Third, VEGF release from macrophages, angiogenesis, collagen synthesis, and epithelization are enhanced for 3 to 4 h. In fact, the very periodicity of hyperbaric administration is responsible for its success. If oxygen at that tension is continued for long, oxidants become lethal to patients.

10.6 OTHER CHRONIC WOUNDS

There are a number of sources of chronic (impeded) wounds, including trauma, arteriosclerosis, venous insufficiency, diabetes, hypertension, arteritis, osteomyelitis, pressure necrosis, radionecrosis, and tumors.

With some exceptions, chronic wounds are poorly oxygenated. Most are on the lower extremity and are associated with arterial or venous insufficiency and/or excessive inflammation. The healing potential of a lower extremity wound is directly related to its circulation and to the arterial PO_2. As noted, the circulation is currently best assessed by the $TcPO_2$ in its vicinity.[30] This measurement, however, must be carefully done in order to isolate the physiologic and vasoactive variables. It must be done with the leg warmed under a cover of a water-vapor-impermeable plastic and a cotton blanket. The skin temperature must be measured and recorded. The ideal method is to start with a well-hydrated, pain-free patient and then to obtain stability with the patient supine. One hundred percent oxygen is then breathed by mask. Once stability is again reached, the leg is raised 30 degrees. Stability is reached again, and the patient is asked to sit or stand. In this manner, artifacts due to dehydration, pain, and cold are avoided, and the effects of arterial and venous disease are to a degree isolated. A slight fall on elevation is normal; a large one is due to obstructive arterial disease. A brief rise above the supine value with standing is also normal, but a large rise followed by a fall is indicative of venous disease. Infection lowers PO_2. Cellulitic skin may have a zero PO_2 even in the presence of normal perfusion; therefore, these values should be obtained after infection is controlled as well as possible. Unfortunately, the numerical difference between "small" and "large" is still not defined. It is usually obvious.

If the baseline $TcPO_2$ is over 30 mmHg, especially if a plentiful response to oxygen occurs, the ulceration is not due to hypoxia. If it is less, hypoxia is a likely contributor. 15 mmHg or less (cold alone even with normal arteries can cause this level) without a rise due to oxygen indicates a grave prognosis unless vascular surgery can be performed. A low PO_2 that responds to oxygen breathing suggests that hyperbaric oxygen will be helpful. The capacity of oxygen to heal an ischemic wound is not fully estimated until the patient and wound are uninfected, hydrated, warm, and free of pain.

The degree of hypoxia in venous wounds has been debated, but the majority of evidence now supports the theory that chronic, intermittent ischemia and hypoxia followed by reperfusion cause tissue death via prolonged and repeated oxidant production. The ischemia is caused by poor flow during prolonged standing. The reoxygenation occurs when bringing the leg up toward heart level restores the arterio-venous (A/V) pressure gradient. The result is a brief but large production of oxidants that reach the damaging range. Prevention of stasis by pressure wrappings, the first treatment of choice, prevents the rise of venous pressure and accomplishes the same objective. Surgical interruption of venous perforators in or near the ulcer, thus preventing local ischemia/reperfusion, can be very helpful, but the healing time is still prolonged. Hyperbaric oxygen therapy is not usually a choice for venous ulcers unless they are hypoxic for other reasons as well. Chronic venous ulcers that have healed several times cause an almost ischemic scar. Therefore, debridement down to normally bleeding tissue becomes essential for rapid healing.

By far the most effective therapy for ischemic wounds is revascularization, reduction of oxygen consuming inflammation, warmth, and stopping use of (vaso-constricting) tobacco and other drugs. When all this is done, breathing oxygen can often be expected to raise wound PO_2 to recovery levels. Few hyperbaric units observe all these conditions.

One of the best uses of transcutaneous oximetry is in proving (or disproving) the efficacy of such therapies, since it is a system in which failure can be detected in hours or days rather than waiting weeks in vain for a result.

10.7 CONCLUSIONS

Hypoxia is the most common deficiency found in failed skin wounds, and restoration of oxygen concentration in tissue allows wound cells to deposit collagen, to resist infection, to epithelize, and to develop new vasculature.

Although tissue hypoxia can stimulate the assembly of many mechanisms of healing, it frustrates each of them in the end. Lactate accumulation mimics hypoxia in most closed if not all wounds, and leaves the clinician in a position to increase oxygen concentration (PO_2) in both acute and chronic ischemic wounds with benefits to almost all aspects of healing as well as resistance to infection.

PO_2 in wounds is profoundly influenced by the rate at which blood perfuses them. Perfusion is reduced by vasoconstriction. Vasoconstriction is a response to low blood volume, pain, fear, smoking, cold, etc. All can be corrected in most cases.

Vasoconstriction can almost always be overcome using warmth, fluids, or medications, even in the hyperbaric chamber.

Wound PO_2 also varies with arterial PO_2 and falls as the distance that oxygen has to diffuse to get to the healing wound cells increases.

Surgical debridement, infection control, and hyperbaric oxygen are useful to overcome diffusion obstacles and excessive demand for oxygen due to inflammation.

Breathing oxygen is often helpful, but delivery to tissue is uncertain unless perfusion is adequate. It is helpful to measure the PO_2 in the area of the wound.

REFERENCES

1. Allen, D.B. et al., Wound hypoxia and acidosis limit neutrophil bacterial killing mechanisms, *Arch. Surg.*, 132, 991, 1997.
2. Jonsson, K. et al., Tissue oxygenation, anemia and perfusion in relation to wound healing in surgical patients, *Ann. Surg.*, 214, 605, 1991.
3. Hunt, T.K., Zederfeldt, B.H., and Goldstick, T.K., Oxygen and healing, *Am. J. Surg.*, 118, 521, 1969.
4. Silver, I.A., Oxygen tension and epithelialization, in *Epidermal Wound Healing*, Maibach, H.I. and Rovee, D.T., Eds., Year Book Medical Publishers, Chicago, 1972, p. 291.
5. Jonsson, K., Hunt, T.K., and Mathes, S.J., Oxygen as an isolated variable influences resistance to infection, *Ann. Surg.*, 208, 783, 1988.
6. Knighton, D.R., Halliday, B., and Hunt, T.K., Oxygen as an antibiotic: the effect of inspired oxygen on infection, *Arch. Surg.*, 119, 199, 1984.
7. Sen, C.K. et al., Oxygen, oxidants, and antioxidants in wound healing: an emerging paradigm, *Ann. N.Y. Acad. Sci.*, 957, 239, 2002.
8. Kurz, A. et al., Perioperative normothermia to reduce the incidence of surgical-wound infection and shorten hospitalization, *N. Engl. J. Med.*, 334, 1209, 1996.
9. Hunt, T.K. and Hopf, H.W., Wound healing and wound infection: what surgeons and anesthesiologists can do, *Surg. Clin. North Am.*, 77, 587, 1997.
10. Mori, K. et al., Lactate-induced vascular relaxation in porcine coronary arteries is mediated by Ca^{2+}-activated K^+ channels, *J. Mol. Cell Cardiol.*, 30, 349, 1998.
11. Albina, J.E. et al., HIF-1 expression in healing wounds: HIF-1α induction in primary inflammatory cells by TNF-α, *Am. J. Physiol. Cell Physiol.*, 281, C1971, 2001.
12. Zabel D.D., Hopf, H.W., and Hunt, T.K., The role of nitric oxide in subcutaneous and transmural gut tissue oxygenation, *Shock*, 5, 341, 1996.
13. Rollins, M.D., Tissue Oxygen Physiology, thesis, University of California Medical Center, San Francisco, 1999.
14. Hussain, M.Z., Ghani Q.P., and Hunt, T.K., Inhibition of prolyl hydroxylase by poly [ADP-ribose] and phosphoribosyl-AMP. Possible role of ADP-ribosylation in intracellular prolyl hydroxylase regulation, *J. Biol. Chem.*, 264, 7850, 1989.
15. Jonsson, K. et al., Tissue oxygenation, anemia and perfusion in relation to wound healing in surgical patients, *Ann. Surg*, 214, 605, 1991.

16. Ghani, Q.P. et al., Control of procollagen gene transcription and prolyl hydroxylase activity by poly [ADP-ribose], in *ADP-Ribosylation Reactions,* Poirier, G. and More-aer, A., Eds., Springer Verlag, New York, 1992, p. 111.

17. Constant, J.S. et al., Lactate elicits vascular endothelial growth factor from macrophages: a possible alternative to hypoxia, *Wound Repair Regen.,* 8, 353, 2000.

18. Cho, M., Hunt, T.K., and Hussain, M.Z., Hydrogen peroxide stimulates macrophage vascular endothelial growth factor release, *Am. J. Physiol. Heart Circ. Physiol.,* 280, H2357, 2001.

19. Hunt T.K. et al., Anaerobic metabolism and wound healing: an hypothesis for the initiation and cessation of collagen synthesis in wounds, *Am. J. Surg.,* 135, 328, 1978.

20. Green, H. and Goldberg, B., Collagen and cell protein synthesis by established mammalian fibroblast line, *Nature,* 204, 347, 1964.

21. Nissen, N.N. et al., Vascular endothelial growth factor mediates angiogenic activity during the proliferative phase of wound healing, *Am. J. Pathol.,* 152, 1445, 1998.

22. Ferrara, N. and Davis-Smyth, T., The biology of vascular endothelial growth factor, *Endocrine Rev,,* 18, 4, 1997.

23. Sheikh, A.Y. et al., Effect of hyperoxia on vascular endothelial growth factor levels in a wound model, *Arch. Surg.,* 135, 1293, 2000.

24. Medawar, P.B., The cultivation of adult mammalian skin epithelium, *Q. J. Micr. Sci.,* 89, 187, 1948.

25. Daniel, R.J. and Groves, R.W., Increased migration of murine keratinocytes under hypoxia is mediated by induction of urokinase plasminogen activator., *J. Invest. Dermatol.,* 119, 1304, 2002.

26. Korn, H.N., Wheeler, E.S., and Miller, T.A., Effect of hyperbaric oxygen on second-degree burn wound healing, *Arch. Surg.,* 112, 732, 1977.

27. Sauder, D.N. et al., Interleukin-1 enhances epidermal wound healing, *Lymphokine Res.,* 9, 465, 1990.

28. Myllyla, R., Tuderman, L., and Kivirikko, K.I., Mechanism of the prolyl hydroxylase reaction. 2. Kinetic analysis of the reaction sequence, *Eur. J. Biochem.,* 80, 349, 1977.

29. Rabkin, J.M. and Hunt, T.K., Local heat increases blood flow and oxygen tension in wounds, *Arch. Surg.,* 122, 221, 1987.

30. Wütschert, R. and Bounameaux, H., Determination of amputation level in ischemic limbs. Reappraisal of the measurement of $TcPO_2$, *Diabetes Care,* 20, 1315, 1997.

31. Faglia, E. et al., Adjunctive systemic hyperbaric oxygen therapy in treatment of severe prevalently ischemic diabetic foot ulcer. A randomized study, *Diabetes Care,* 19, 1338, 1996.

32. Marx, R.E. et al., Relationship of oxygen delivery to angiogenesis in irradiated tissue, *Am. J. Surg.,* 160, 519, 1990.

33. Marx, R.E. et al., Prevention of osteoradionecrosis: a randomized prospective clinical trial of hyperbaric oxygen versus penicillin, *J. Am. Dent. Assoc.,* 111, 49, 1985.

11 Nutrition and Wound Healing

Robert H. Demling

CONTENTS

11.1 INTRODUCTION

Optimum nutrition is now recognized to be a key factor in maintaining all phases of wound healing, especially if a catabolic state and/or an element of protein–energy malnutrition (PEM) exists. It has long been recognized that a wound dramatically increases metabolic state and that increased nutrients must be provided to the wound for healing.[1-6] Hunter in 1794,[3] followed by Cuthbertson and Moore[1,2] in the 1950s identified the fact that an acute wound takes priority for available nutrients in order to heal. As a result, some degree of body protein loss occurs to provide the necessary amino acids for energy.

0-8493-1561-1/04/$0.00+$1.50

Normal healthy humans can tolerate some loss of body protein or more specifically a loss of lean body mass (LBM), without complications, in order to heal an acute wound. However, this is not the case if a hypercatabolic state characteristically seen with large wounds, infection, or superimposed trauma exists. Catabolism, a characteristic of the stress response to any injury, will result in a net tissue and protein breakdown with the use of amino acids for fuel, unless nutritional support is provided.[7-22] The same can be said for patient populations with PEM and wounds, a common situation in the elderly or disabled.[9-13] The host will preferentially use nutrients to restore lean body mass and shunt nutrients away from the wound. The reason is that lost body weight in a catabolic state is in large part lean mass, and resulting morbidity directly corresponds with the degree of lean mass loss (Figure 11.1).

Any wound activates the stress response, leading to a hypermetabolic catabolic state. The energy or caloric demands correspond with the degree of injury and are greatest for burns (Table 11.1). The percent increase in metabolic rate corresponds with the increase in caloric demands. The degree of catabolism or lean mass loss correlates with the degree of morbidity and mortality (Table 11.2).[9-16]

Conditions associated with a risk of protein-energy malnutrition and a resulting decrease in wound healing are shown in Table 11.3. Populations with ongoing catabolism or those who already have involuntary weight loss are at the highest risk for decreased healing.[5-8,24-36] It is well recognized that the chronic wound population frequently suffers from coexisting PEM. Weight loss, particularly loss of lean mass, corresponds with the development of pressure ulcers and other chronic wounds.

Anabolic strategies need to be developed very early in the course of wound treatment to produce an environment conducive to healing.[10-13]

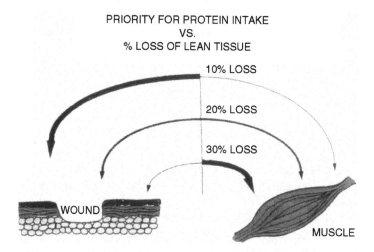

PRIORITY FOR PROTEIN INTAKE
VS.
% LOSS OF LEAN TISSUE

10% LOSS

20% LOSS

30% LOSS

WOUND

MUSCLE

FIGURE 11.1 The wound takes priority for available nutrients as long as LBM loss does not exceed 10% of total. With greater losses, more nutrients are used to restore lean mass while wound healing rate decreases. Lost lean mass needs to be in part restored before optimum healing rate can resume.

TABLE 11.1
Effect of Injury on Metabolic Demands

Illness	Increase Above Basal (%)
Starvation	−10 to 0
Elective operation	0 to 10
Major infection	25 to 50
Long bone fracture	25 to 50
Multiple blunt trauma	50 to 70
Large wound	
Thermal injury	
10% BSA[a]	25
20% BSA	50
40% BSA	75
50% BSA	100

[a] BSA = body surface area.

TABLE 11.2
Complications Related to Loss of Lean Body Mass[a]

IWL (% of Total)	Complications (Related to Lost Lean Mass)	Associated Mortality (%)
10	Impaired immunity, increased infection	10
20	Decreased healing, weakness, infection	30
30	Too weak to sit, pressure sores, pneumonia, no healing	50
40	Death, usually from pneumonia	100

Note: IWL = involuntary weight loss.

[a] A major component of IWL is lean mass; in the presence of a catabolic state, lean mass is lost.

TABLE 11.3
Conditions Associated with Development of Protein-Energy Malnutrition and Impaired Healing

- Catabolic illness: the stress response, e.g., trauma, surgery, wounds, infection, corticosteroids
- Involuntary weight loss exceeding 10% of ideal body weight
- Chronic illnesses: e.g., diabetes, cancer, mental impairment, arthritis, renal failure

11.2 NUTRITIONAL ASSESSMENT

It is essential to determine the macro- and micronutrient needs of the patient with a wound. The presence of any significant wound increases energy demands by 30 to 50% and protein demands by at least 50% above normal needs.[18–22] These increased demands are the result of the systemic metabolic changes associated with an injury and the increased nutrient demands of the wound.[33–37] The presence of a systemic hypercatabolic state, as described in Table 11.1, results in a further increase in nutrient demands. In addition, management of any moderate-to-severe protein-energy malnutrition (PEM) requires at least a 50% increase in calories and doubling of protein intake in order to restore previously lost lean mass and body weight.[30–36]

Assessment tools include a variety of standard nutritional formulas and also the use of indirect calorimetry, where the amount of oxygen consumed is converted into calories burned. This assessment can be performed by a nutritionist. Of course, anyone managing wounds should also be able to determine nutrient needs.[33–38]

Assessment of the degree of PEM, if present, is outlined in Table 11.4. A prealbumin level is considered to be the most sensitive biochemical indicator, as it has a very short half-life of about 48 h.[33–38] Albumin has a half-life of over 20 d and is therefore not a very sensitive marker of nutritional status.

11.3 GENERAL NUTRITIONAL SUPPORT

Optimum nutrition should be initiated immediately in the presence of any hypercatabolic state, such as an injury or infection. The same is true for an already compromised host with preexisting malnutrition or chronic illness, especially the frail elderly.

The standard caloric and protein intake guidelines are presented in Table 11.5. The guidelines are based on increases over and above the recommended daily allowance (RDA), which is used to define needs for the normal healthy population. The ideal distribution of calories is shown in Table 11.6.[31,32,40,41]

The status of protein intake corresponds best with the rate of wound healing. An intake of 1.5 g/kg/d appears to be the ideal value, according to recent wound healing studies.[40–45] Proteins with increased concentrations of essential and conditionally essential amino acids have a higher biologic value, which means more nitrogen is retained.[43–45]

TABLE 11.4
Markers of Malnutrition

Index	Normal	Mild	Moderate	Severe
% ideal body weight	100 to 110	80 to 90	70 to 80	≤70
% weight loss relative to total	0	5 to 15	15 to 25	≥25
Albumin (g/dl)	3.8 to 4.5	2.6 to 3.5	2.1 to 2.7	≤2.1
Prealbumin (mg/dl)	18 to 24	10 to 15	5 to 10	≤5

TABLE 11.5
Daily Nutritional Requirements

Condition	Calories (cal/kg)	Protein (g/kg)
Normal	25 to 30	0.8
Wound alone	30 to 35	1.3
Hypercatabolic state	35 to 40	1.5 to 2.0
PEM and wound	35 to 40	1.5

TABLE 11.6
Caloric Mix

Macronutrient	% of Calories
Carbohydrate (complex form)	55 to 60%
Fat (polyunsaturated)	25%
Protein (high biologic value)	20%

TABLE 11.7
Protein Intake

- Essential macronutrient for all healing phases
- Deficiency leads to impairment in all healing phases
- Certain amino acids are more important, namely cysteines, the essential and conditionally essential amino acids, glutamine, and arginine
- Recommended dose is 1.5 g/kg/d for injured or compromised person, especially with a significant wound

Nutrient supplements are often required to meet the nutritional goals. High calorie, high protein supplements are available in very palatable liquid forms as well as in candy bar form.

11.4 SPECIFIC NUTRIENT NEEDS

The wound, in addition to requiring energy and protein, has specific nutrient needs, both macro- and micronutrient. The micronutrients used by the wound are especially important. An added provision of increased quantities is often needed to avoid a deficiency state. These specific nutrients will be discussed.[46–51]

11.4.1 Arginine and Glutamine

Arginine and glutamine are nitrogen-rich amino acids that are important in wound healing. The levels of both these amino acids rapidly decrease with injury.[46–48] The advantages of these compounds in wound healing are described in Tables 11.8 and 11.9. Both arginine and glutamine are considered to be conditionally essential amino acids as endogenous production does not appear to be sufficient to keep up with demands during the stress response to injury.[46–51] Supplementation has been recommended, although a deficiency-induced impairment in wound healing has not been well documented.

11.4.2 Carbohydrates and Lactate

Carbohydrates are utilized in a number of aspects of healing in addition to their role as an energy source. Matrix is composed of proteoglycans and glycosaminoglycans, which are made from polysaccharide chains linked to protein. Glucose is also used to glycosylate hydroxyproline, a necessary step in collagen synthesis.[52,53]

Lactate is a metabolic byproduct of glucose. This two-carbon compound appears to have many very important wound healing effects (Table 11.10). The increase in lactate, which is produced by all wound cells, activates the genetic expression of many key healing pathways.[54,55]

TABLE 11.8
Arginine

- Promotes wound healing
- Precursor for proline in collagen
- Precursor for nitric oxide
- Increases hydroxyproline production
- Stimulates release of anabolic hormones, insulin, and human growth hormone and insulin-like growth factor
- Local immune stimulant of lymphocytes
- Considered a conditionally essential amino acid
- Large doses recommended: 15 to 25 g/d

TABLE 11.9
Glutamine

- Direct fuel for epithelial cells, fibroblasts, and macrophages
- Lymphyocyte fuel
- Improves neutrophils' killing
- Anticatabolic agent, preserving lean mass
- Stimulates release of growth hormone
- Potent antioxidant in form of glutathione
- Considered a conditionally essential amino acid
- Large doses recommended: 10 to 30 g/d in divided doses, b.i.d. to t.i.d.

TABLE 11.10
Wound Lactate

- Produced by wound cells, especially macrophages
- Required for macrophage release of angiogenesis factors
- Stimulates collagen synthesis by fibroblasts
- Energy source

11.4.3 FATTY ACIDS

The essential omega-6 fatty acids, linoleic and linolenic acid, are required for both cell membrane formation and prostaglandin production and therefore must be provided in adequate doses. A deficiency is difficult to produce unless one is using a fat-free diet. Although omega-3 fatty acids appear to be protective of cardiovascular function, recent data would indicate that replacing omega-6 fatty acids with omega-3 fatty acids may impair healing.[56]

11.4.4 VITAMIN C (ASCORBIC ACID)

The water-soluble vitamin ascorbic acid has long been known to be essential for healing; a severe deficiency state leads to symptoms of scurvy.[57] Descriptions of markedly abnormal wound healing in sailors suffering from scurvy are evident in the writings of physicians and explorers beginning in the sixteenth century.

A number of investigators have reported ascorbic acid to be essential for overall collagen synthesis.[58–60] A deficiency leads to a decrease in total collagen. Others have clearly shown that the hydroxylation of proline and lysine is dependent on molecular oxygen, ascorbic acid, and Fe^{++}. Ascorbic acid appears to activate prolyl and lysyl hydroxylases. This process is required to stabilize the triple-helix structure of collagen. A vitamin C deficiency state impairs immune function. Vitamin C is also an important intracellular antioxidant.[39]

The recommended daily allowance in normal humans, to maintain body vitamin C levels, is 30 to 60 mg/d. However, after injury, vitamin C levels rapidly decrease. The process is felt to be due to increased usage in the injured area. An intake of 2 g/d is necessary to maintain plasma levels after severe burns. However, for a moderate wound, an intake of 200 mg/d is recommended (Table 11.11).[58–61]

11.4.5 VITAMIN A

The fat-soluble vitamin A is also recognized as an essential prohealing agent. Like all vitamins, it has multiple actions. The most important appears to be the promotion of the key early inflammatory reaction to wounding. In fact, vitamin A supplementation, systemic or topical, has been shown to reverse the antiinflammatory impairment of healing by corticosteroids (Table 11.12).[62–65]

Vitamin A is also involved in angiogenesis and the differentiation of cells, especially keratinocytes. Supplementation with vitamin A has also been reported to increase wound collagen content. One theory as to the mechanism of action is that

---

TABLE 11.11
Vitamin C — Ascorbic Acid

- Collagen synthesis
- Hydroxylation of proline and lysine
- Neutrophils' antibacterial activity
- Complement activation
- Water soluble intracellular antioxidant
- Essential micronutrient
- Increased losses after injury
- Recommended dose with wounds: 200 mg/d

TABLE 11.12
Vitamin A

- Promotes the early inflammatory reaction to wounding
- Increases angiogenesis
- Increases hydroxyproline and collagen accumulation
- Involved in cell differentiation, especially epithelial keratinization
- Necessary for cell mediated and humoral immune defenses
- An essential micronutrient
- Increased losses of vitamin A seen with injury
- Recommended daily dose with injury or malnutrition: 10,000 to 25,000 IU

---

the vitamin influences cellular phenotypes by directly affecting gene expression. Vitamin A also affects cell surface glycoproteins involved in cell adherence, intracellular communication, and interaction with growth factors.

Vitamin A is also important for immune function, both cell mediated immunity and humoral defense mechanisms, with a deficiency leading to increased risk of infections. As is the case with vitamin C, vitamin A levels decrease after injury. Increased metabolism and increased urinary losses are known to occur.[66,67]

Since large amounts of vitamin A are stored in the liver, rapid depletion is not likely in healthy humans. However, malnourished patients are likely to already be deficient, and injured patients have increased losses. Replacement therapy in these groups is indicated at a daily dose of 10,000 to 25,000 IU.[66,67]

11.4.6 VITAMIN E

There is currently no evidence that vitamin E has a specific role in normal wound healing.[68] No deficiency state of this fat-soluble vitamin with injury has been recognized. However, its potent antioxidant values make this compound systemically highly important, and therefore it is often supplemented in critical illness.

11.4.7 MICROMINERALS: ZINC, COPPER, IRON

11.4.7.1 Zinc

Although zinc has been considered an essential micromineral for centuries, its specific importance, especially in wound healing, has only been recognized in the last 50 years. If zinc levels are low, healing is slowed; healing is restored with replacement (Table 11.13).

Zinc has many metabolic roles. It is a critical cofactor for many metallo-enzymes, including deoxyribonucleic acid (DNA) and ribonucleic acid (RNA) polymerases, for protein synthesis, and for matrix metalloproteinases. Zinc stimulates cell proliferation, thereby stabilizing cell membranes. Zinc has an important role in immune function, recognized by the fact that a deficiency leads to increased infection. Its specific role in healing is not yet clear.[69–73]

Zinc loss in the urine increases after injury. As with other micronutrients, the proper replacement therapy is undefined. The recommended dose for a stable wound patient is 3 to 4 mg/d, and for a catabolic patient, 5 to 6 mg/d. As zinc is quite insoluble and difficult to absorb, a standard replacement is in the form of zinc sulfate 220 mg twice a day.[74,75]

11.4.7.2 Copper

Copper is also a key micromineral involved in collagen crosslinking thru hydroxylation of proline and hydroxyproline. Copper is essential for erythropoesis and for the action of the antioxidant superoxide dismutase. The recommended intake is 1 to 1.5 mg/d.

11.4.7.3 Iron

Iron, especially Fe^{++}, is required for hydroxylation of lysine and proline, a fundamental step in collagen synthesis. An iron deficiency also leads to anemia and impaired leukocyte killing, both of which could affect healing.[75,76] Standard iron replacement is used to prevent or correct a deficiency.

TABLE 11.13
Effect of Zinc on the Wound

- An essential component of DNA, RNA polymerase, metalloproteinase activity
- Involved with DNA synthesis, protein synthesis, mitosis, cell proliferation
- Cell membrane stability by inhibition of lipid peroxidation
- Host defenses
- An essential micronutrient
- Increased losses in urine after injury
- Dose for wounds 5 to 6 mg/d, although higher doses are often used

---

11.5 USE OF ANABOLIC AGENTS

Increasing anabolic activity, with the use of anabolic hormones, has been demonstrated to decrease the catabolic response to injury. Preserving lean body mass improves all aspects of wound healing. These agents can be seen as providing added benefit to nutritional support. Anabolic hormones, most notably human growth hormone, insulin-like growth factors (IGFs), and synthetic testosterone analogs, can also directly increase wound healing.

11.5.1 HUMAN GROWTH HORMONE

Human growth hormone (HGH) increases total body protein synthesis.[77–80] However, endogenous HGH levels decrease with severe injury, impairing net anabolism. Growth hormone is also reported to have anticatabolic properties through an effect on cortisol receptors.

A large number of studies have demonstrated the wound healing properties of HGH as well as its anticatabolic properties. Skin is a target tissue for HGH both directly, through its growth factor effect on human fibroblasts, and indirectly, through increasing circulating insulin-like growth factor (IGF-1), a known wound growth factor.[77–80] Side effects include hyperglycemia and an overall stimulation of inflammation and metabolic rate.[81,82] Antiinsulin properties and the need to give HGH parenterally have limited its use in the wound population.

11.5.2 INSULIN-LIKE GROWTH FACTOR

IGF-1 is a known growth factor in wounds, acting on all phases of healing. A number of clinical trials have also demonstrated its anabolic properties. IGF-1 levels decrease in severely injured or infected patients.[83–85] Hypoglycemia is a complication of IGF-1 infusion, making glucose monitoring essential. IGF-1 is usually provided parenterally. However, there is increasing interest in topical use, thereby limiting systemic complications.[85]

11.5.3 ANABOLIC STEROID (OXANDROLONE)

Anabolic steroids have been recognized for decades as potent anabolic agents.[86] Anabolic steroids act on androgenic receptors in lean mass, especially on the skin fibroblast. A number of studies have demonstrated their ability to preserve lean mass after injury, thereby improving local healing.[89–91] In addition, several recent studies have demonstrated direct wound healing properties. One mechanism is the increase in the messenger RNA for collagen synthesis.[92] However, in other studies, all aspects of healing appear to be increased.

Currently, the safest such agent, and the only anabolic steroid which is approved in the U.S. to treat weight loss and catabolism, is oxandrolone (BTG, Iselin, New Jersey).[87,89] This anabolic steroid is given orally, is excreted by the kidney, and has no effects on aspects of metabolism other than protein synthesis. A number of clinical trials in burn, trauma, and experimental wounds have demonstrated its efficacy in restoring lean mass and increasing wound healing rate (Table 11.14).[87–91] Like all

---

TABLE 11.14
Effect of an Anabolic Strategy on Wound Healing

WOUND plus:
  Catabolic state
  Protein degradation
  Protein-energy malnutrition
  Leads to
    IMPAIRED HEALING
WOUND plus:
  Anabolic strategy
  Optimum nutrition
  Anabolic environment
  Leads to
    IMPROVED HEALING

---

other anabolic agents, oxandrolone is to be used only when optimum nutrition has been achieved.

11.6 SUMMARY

Nutrition is a major factor in all phases of the wound healing process. Adequate energy, protein, and micronutrients delivered to the wound are necessary to maintain an adequate rate of new tissue synthesis.

The need for an aggressive anabolic strategy is accentuated if the wound population is already hypercatabolic or has any significant underlying involuntary weight loss or protein–energy malnutrition. Of course, the presence of a wound itself leads to a catabolic state with additional injury, accentuating the process. The anabolic strategy includes providing increased caloric and protein intake as well as increased micronutrients. The addition of an anabolic hormone may also be of benefit.

REFERENCES

1. Cuthbertson, D., Inter-relationships of metabolic changes consequent to injury, *Br. Med. Bull.*, 10, 33–37, 1954.
2. Moore, F.D., Getting well. The biology of surgical convalescence, *Ann. N.Y. and Sci.*, 73, 387–390, 1958.
3. Hunter, J., *Treatise on the Blood, Inflammation and Gunshot Wounds,* Nicol, London, 1794.
4. Moore, F.D. and Brennan, M., Surgical injury, body composition, protein metabolism and neuro-endocrinology, in Ballinger, W. and Collins, J., *Manual of Surgical Nutrition,* W.B. Saunders, Philadelphia, 1975, pp. 169–202.
5. Kobak, M., Benditt, E., Wissler, B. et al., The relationship of protein deficiency to experimental wound healing, *Surg. Gynecol. Obstet.*, 85, 751–756, 1947.
6. Levinson, S., Parani, C., and Braasch, J., The effect of thermal burns on wound healing, *Surg. Gynecol. Obstet.*, 99, 77–82, 1954.

7. Haines, E., Briggs, H., Shea, R. et al., Effect of complete and partial starvation on the rate of fibroplasias in the healing wound, *Arch. Surg.,* 27, 846–858, 1933.

8. Thompson, W., Randin, I., and Frank, I., Effect of hypoproteinemia on wound disruption, *Arch. Surg.,* 36, 500–518, 1938.

9. Wallace, J.I., Schwartz, R.S., LaCroix, A.Z., Uhlmann, R.F., and Pearlman, R.A., Involuntary weight loss in older outpatients: incidences and clinical significance, *J. Am. Geriatr. Soc.,* 43. 329–337, 1995.

10. McCamsh, M., Malnutrition and nutrition support interventions: costs, benefits, outcomes, *Nutrition,* 4, 556–557, 1993.

11. Mouve, M. and Bokmor, T., The prevalence of undiagnosed protein caloric under nutrition in a population of hospitalized elderly patients, *J. Am. Geriatr. Soc.,* 13, 202–205, 1991.

12. Ek, A., Unosson, M., Larsson, J. et al., The development and healing of pressure sores related to the nutritional state, *Clin. Nutr.,* 10, 245–250, 1991.

13. Warren, M. and Morgan, D., Malnutrition in surgical patients: an unrecognized problem, *Lancet,* 1, 689–692, 1977.

14. Coats, K., Morgan, S., Bartolucci, A., and Weinsier, R., Hospital associated malnutrition: a re-evaluation 12 years later, *J. Am. Diet. Assoc.,* 93, 27–33, 1993.

15. Haydock, D. and Hill, G., Impaired wound healing in surgical patients with varying degrees of malnutrition, *JPEN,* 10, 550–554, 1986.

16. Pinchcofsky-Devin, G. and Kaminski, M., Correlation of pressure sores and nutritional status, *J. Am. Geriatr. Soc.,* 39, 435–440, 1986.

17. Demling, R., Endocrine changes with illness, in *Current Surgical Therapy,* Cameron, J., Ed., Mosby, Philadelphia, 1998, pp. 113–114.

18. Bessy, J., Stress response to injury: endocrinologic and metabolic, in *Current Practice of Surgery,* Greenfield, L., Ed., Churchill, New York, 1995 pp. 1–12.

19. Wolfe, R., Relation of metabolic studies to clinical nutrition: the example of burn injury, *Am. J. Clin. Nutr.,* 64, 800–808, 1996.

20. Wolfe, R., An integrated analysis of glucose, fat and protein metabolism in severely traumatized patients, *Ann. Surg.,* 209, 63–72, 1989.

21. Demling, R., Anticatabolic and anabolic strategies in critical illness: a review of current treatment modalities, *Shock,* 10, 155–160, 1998.

22. Bissey, P.Q., Metabolic response to critical illness, in Wilmore, D., Ed., *Pre- and Postoperative Care of the Surgical Patient, Vol. 1, Critical Care,* Scientific American, New York, 1996, p. 11.

23. Bergstrom, N., Lack of nutrition in AHCPR preventive guidelines, *Decubitus,* 6, 4–6, 1993.

24. Weingarten, M., Obstacles to wound healing, *Wounds,* 5, 238–244, 1993.

25. Shizgal, H., Nutritional assessment and skeletal muscle function, *Am. J. Clin. Nutr.,* 44, 761–771, 1986.

26. Levenson, S. and Seifter, E., Dysnutrition, wound healing and resistance to infection, *Clin. Plast. Surg.,* 4, 375–385, 1977.

27. Kotler, D., Tierney, A.R., Wang, J., and Pierson, R.N., Jr., Magnitude of cell body mass depletion and timing of death from wasting in AIDS, *Am. J. Clin. Nutr.,* 40, 444–447, 1989.

28. Windsor, J. and Hill, G.L., Weight loss with physiologic impairment: a basic indication of surgical risk, *Ann. Surg.,* 207, 290–296, 1988.

29. Wallace, J.L. and Schwartz, R.S., Involuntary weight loss in elderly outpatients: recognition, etiologies and treatment, *Clin. Geriatr. Med.,* 113, 717–735, 1997.

30. Torun, B. and Cherv, F., Protein-energy malnutrition, in Shels, M., Ed., *Modern Nutrition in Health and Disease,* Lea & Febiger, Philadelphia, 1994, p. 950.

31. DeBiasse, M. and Wilmore, D., What is optimum nutritional support? in *New Horizons,* vol. 1, Williams & Wilkins, Baltimore, 1994, pp. 122–135.

32. Lipschitz, D., Approaches to the nutritional support of the older patient, *Clin. Geriatr. Med.,* 11, 715–730, 1995.

33. American Dietetic Association, Nutrition assessment in the adult, in *Manual of Clinical Dietetics,* The American Dietetic Association, Chicago, 1996, p. 3.

34. Klipstein-Grobusch, K. and Reilly, J., Energy intake and expenditure in elderly patients admitted to the hospital with acute illness, *Br. J. Nutr.,* 73, 323–324, 1995.

35. Rodriguez, D., Nutrition in patients with severe burns: state of the art, *J. Burn Care Rehab.,* 17, 62–70, 1996.

36. Barrocas, A., Nutritional assessment. Practical approaches, *Clin. Geriatr. Med.,* 11, 675–683, 1995.

37. Evans, W. and Campbell D., Nutrition, exercise and healthy aging, *J. Am. Diet. Assoc.,* 97, 632–638, 1997.

38. Lukaski, H., Methods for the assessment of human body composition, *Am. J. Clin. Nutr.,* 46, 163–175, 1987.

39. Haydock, D. and Hill, G., Impaired wound healing in surgical patients with varying degrees of malnutrition, *JPEN,* 10, 550–554, 1986.

40. Haydock, D. and Hill, G., Improved wound healing response to surgical patients receiving intravenous nutrition, *Br. J. Surg.,* 74, 320–323, 1987.

41. Demling, R.H., Stasik, L., and Zagoren, A.J., *Protein–Energy Malnutrition and Wounds: Nutritional Intervention.* Treatment of Chronic Wounds Number 10, Curative Health Services, Hauppauge, NY, 2000.

42. Bergstrom, N., Bennett, M.A., Carlson, C.E. et al., Treatment of Pressure Ulcers. Clinical Practice Guideline, No. 15, AHCPR Publication No. 95–0652, Agency for Health Care Policy and Research, Rockville, MD, December 1994.

43. Demling, R. and DeSanti, L., Increased protein intake during the recovery phase after severe burns increases body weight gain and muscle function, *J. Burn Care Rehab.,* 17, 151–168, 1998.

44. Breslow, R. and Hallfrisch, J., The importance of dietary protein in healing pressure ulcers, *J. Am. Geriatr. Soc.,* 41, 357–362, 1993.

45. Volpi, E., Ferrando, A., Yeckel, W. et al., Exogenous amino acids stimulate net muscle protein synthesis in the elderly, *J. Clin. Invest.,* 101, 2000–2007, 1998.

46. Barbul, A., Lazarou, S., Efron, B. et al., Arginine enhances wound healing and lymphocyte immune responses in humans, *Surgery,* 108, 331–337, 1990.

47. Furst, P., Abers, S., and Stehle, P., Evidence for nutritional need for glutamine in catabolic patients, *Kidney Int.,* 36, 287–291, 1989.

48. Caldwell, M., Local glutamine metabolism in wounds and inflammation, *Metabolism,* 38, 34–39, 1989.

49. Roth, E., Karner, J., and Collenschlager, G., Glutamine: an anabolic effector, *JPEN,* 14, 130–136, 1990.

50. Barbul, A., Arginine: biochemistry, physiology and therapeutic implications, *JPEN,* 10, 227–237, 1986.

51. Visek, W., Arginine and disease states, *J. Nutr.,* 115, 532–541, 1985.

52. Linker, A., Structure of heparin sulfate oligosaccharides and their degradation by exo-enzymes, *J. Biochem.,* 183, 711–720, 1979.

53. Weitzhander, M. and Bernfield, M., Proteoglycan glycoconjugates, in *Wound Healing: Biochemical and Clinical Aspects,* Cohen, C., Ed. W.B. Saunders, Philadelphia, 1992, p. 195.

54. Jensen, J. and Hunt, T.K., Effect of lactate, pyruvate and pH on secretion of angiogenesis and mitogenesis factors by macrophases, *Lab. Invest.,* 54, 574–578, 1986.

55. Hunt, T.K. and Hussain, Z., Wound microenvironment, in *Wound Healing: Biochemical and Chemical Aspects,* Cohen, C., Ed., W.B. Saunders, Philadelphia, 1992, p. 274.

56. Halsey, T., O'Neill, J., and Nebleth, W., Experimental wound healing in essential fatty acid deficiency, *J. Pediatr. Surg.,* 15, 505–508, 1980.

57. Lanman, T., Vitamin C deficiency and wound healing, *Ann. Surg.,* 165, 616–622, 1937.

58. Schorah, C., Total vitamin C and dehydroascorbic acid concentration in plasma of critically ill patients, *Am. J. Clin. Nutr.,* 63, 760–765, 1996.

59. Hornig, D. et al., Ascorbic acid, in *Modern Nutrition in Health and Disease,* Shels, M., Olson, J., and Shike, M., Eds., Lea & Febiger, Philadelphia, 1988, p. 417.

60. Gross, R., The effect of ascorbate on wound healing, *Int. Opthalmol. Clin.,* 40, 51–57, 2000.

61. Lund, C., Levenson, S., and Green, R., Ascorbic acid, thiamine, riboflavin and nicotinic acid in relation to acute burns in man, *Arch. Surg.,* 55, 557–583, 1947.

62. Erlich, H., Effect of beta carotene, vitamin A and glucocarotenoids on collagen synthesis in wounds, *Proc. Soc. Exp. Biol. Med.,* 137, 936–938, 1971.

63. Kinsky, N., Antioxidant functions of carotenoids, *Free Rad. Biol. Med.,* 7, 617–635, 1989.

64. Weinzwieg, J., Weinzweig, B., and Levenson, S., Supplemental vitamin A prevents the tumor induced defect in wound healing, *Ann. Surg.,* 211, 269–276, 1990.

65. Olson, J., Vitamin A, retinoids and carotinoids, in *Modern Nutrition in Health and Disease,* Shils, M. and Young, V., Eds., Lea & Febiger, Philadelphia, 1988, p. 328.

66. Durin, M. and Tannock, I., Influence of vitamin A on immunologic response, *Immunology,* 23, 283–287, 1972.

67. Cohen, B., Gell, G., and Cullen, P., Reversal of postoperative immunosuppression in man by vitamin A, *Surg. Gynecol. Obstet.,* 179, 658–662, 1979.

68. Erhlich, P., Tarver, H., and Hunt, T.K., Inhibiting effects of vitamin E on collagen synthesis and wound repair, *Ann. Surg.,* 175, 235–240, 1972.

69. Demling, R., Micronutrients in critical illness, in *Crit. Care Clin.,* 11, 651–670, 1995.

70. Gottschlich, M., Vitamins supplementation in the patient with burns, *JBCR,* 11, 273–280, 1990.

71. Chesters, J., Biochemistry of zinc in cell division and tissue growth, in *Zinc in Human Biology,* International Life Science Institute, London, 1989, pp. 109–118.

72. Prasad, A., Zinc: an overview, *Nutrition,* 11, 93–100, 1995.

73. Berger, M. et al., Copper, zinc, and selenium balances and status after major trauma, *J. Trauma,* 40, 103–109, 1996.

74. Berger, M., Cavadine, C., Cheolero, R. et al., Influence of large intakes of trace elements on recovery after major burns, *Nutrition,* 10, 327–334, 1994.

75. Demling, R. and De Santi, L., Use of anticatabolic agents for burns, *Curr. Opin. Crit. Care,* 2, 482–491, 1996.

76. Demling, R., Anticatabolic and anabolic strategies in critical illness, *Shock,* 10, 155–160, 1998.

77. Ziegler, T. and Wilmore, D., Strategies for attenuating protein-catabolic responses in the critically ill, *Am. Rev. Med.,* 45, 459–463, 1994.

78. Sherman, S., Demling, R. et al., Growth hormone enhances re-epithelialization of human split thickness skin graft donor sites, *Surg. Forum,* 40, 37, 1989.

79. Manson, J., Smith, R., and Wilmore, D., Growth hormone stimulates protein synthesis during hypocaloric parenteral nutrition, *Ann. Surg.,* 208, 136–149, 1988.

80. Gatzen, C., Scheltinga, M.R., Kimbrough, T.D.D., Jacobs, D.O., and Wilmore, D.W., Growth hormone attenuates the abnormal distribution of body water in critically ill surgical patients, *Surgery,* 112, 181, 1992.

81. MacGorman, L., Rizza, R., and Gerbsh, J., Physiologic concentration of growth hormone exert insulin-like and insulin-antagonistic effect on both hepatic and extra-hepatic tissues in man, *J. Clin. Endocrin. Metab.,* 53, 556–559, 1981.

82. Kappel, M., Hansen, M., Diamant, M., and Pedersen, B., *In vitro* effects of human growth hormone on the proliferative responses and cytokine production of blood mononuclear cells, *Horm. Metab. Res.,* 26, 612–614, 1994.

83. Lieberman, S., Butterfield, G., Harrison, D., and Hoffman, A., Anabolic effects of insulin-like growth factor-1 in cachectic patients with acquired immunodeficiency syndrome, *J. Clin. Endocrinol. Metab.,* 78, 404–410, 1994.

84. Bondy, C., Underwood, L., and Clemmons, D., Clinical uses of insulin like growth factor-1, *Ann. Intern. Med.,* 120, 593–601, 1994.

85. Abribat, T., Brazeau, P., Davingnon, L., and Garrell, D., Insulin-like growth factor-1 blood levels in severely burned patients: effect of time post injury, age of patient and burn severity, *Clin. Endocrinol.,* 39, 583–589, 1993.

86. Tennenbaum, R. and Shkear, G., Effect of anabolic steroid on wound healing, *Oral Surg.,* 30, 834–835, 1970.

87. Karim, A., Ranney, E., Zagarella, B.A. et al., Oxandrolone disposition and metabolism in man, *Clin. Pharmacol. Ther.,* 14, 862–866, 1973.

88. Fox, M. and Minot, A., Oxandrolone, a potent anabolic steroid, *J. Clin. Endocrinol.,* 22, 921–926, 1962.

89. Demling, R. and Orgill, D., The anticatabolic and wound healing effects of the testosterone analog, oxandrolone, after severe burn injury, *J. Crit. Care,* 15, 12–18, 2000.

90. Demling, R. and DeSanti, L., Oxandrolone, an anabolic steroid, significantly increases the rate of weight gain in the recovery phase after burn injury, *J. Trauma,* 43, 47–50, 1997.

91. Demling, R., Oxandrolone, an anabolic steroid, enhances the healing of a cutaneous wound in the rat, *Wound Repair Regen.,* 8, 97, 2000.

92. Erlich, P., The influence of the anabolic agent oxandrolone upon the expression of procollagen types I and II in RNA in human fibroblasts cultured on collagen or plastic, *Wounds,* 13, 66–70, 2001.

12 Wound Dressings

Stephen Thomas

CONTENTS

12.1 INTRODUCTION

When Winter published his seminal paper in 1962 on the effect of occlusion upon the rate of epithelialization of superficial wounds in the young domestic pig,[1] he began a new chapter in our understanding of the mechanisms by which wounds heal and the influence that dressings have upon this process. Based upon the results of this and later work, he subsequently identified 18 features that he believed characterized a good surgical dressing.[2]

In the intervening period, many sophisticated new products have been developed, made from a wide range of materials including polyurethane, salts of alginic acid, and other gelable polysaccharides such as starch and carboxymethylcellulose. These materials are used alone or in combination to form films, foams, fibrous products, beads, hydrogels, or adhesive gel-forming wafers more commonly called hydrocolloid dressings, all of which possess some of the key attributes identified by Winter.

Successful wound management involves the use of these dressings to control the moisture content of a wound and its local environment while preventing or combating infection and reducing to a minimum pain or trauma during dressing removal. Other features such as odor control or the ability to neutralize proteolytic enzymes in wound fluid can also be important in some instances. Sometimes, however, dressings are applied purely for cosmetic reasons, for example when used to cover or conceal an extensive fungating tumor.[3]

Despite the best efforts of the medical device industry, however, no single product has been developed that combines all the required features in an effective manner, so problems encountered in wound management are often addressed by the use of a dressing "system," which consists of a number of individual components, each of which fulfills a specific function. There are in fact significant benefits to be gained by adopting this approach, as it provides the clinician with greater flexibility when managing a particular wound at a given stage in the healing cycle.

Although much attention is given to the choice of a wound contact layer, the important contribution made by secondary dressings is often overlooked, even though this can be vital in determining the success or otherwise of a particular treatment, especially when using products such as hydrogels or alginate sheets.[4]

The aim of the current chapter is to briefly review the types of dressings that are available and illustrate how these may be used to facilitate wound healing or otherwise improve patients' quality of life. In most dressing reviews, it is customary to classify products according to their structure or composition. In the current review, however, an alternative approach has been adopted in which products are brought together according to their function. This approach requires a basic understanding of different wound types and the conditions that each requires in order to heal at the optimum rate. A simple wound classification system such as that shown below forms a useful starting point in this process. Within this system, wounds are not classified according to etiology but are divided into four basic types according to their appearance and condition:

- *Necrotic wounds* — covered with devitalized epidermis, frequently black in color, and generally very dry.
- *Sloughy wounds* — containing viscous adherent slough and generally yellow in color. These wounds, which vary from relatively dry to heavily exuding, can become infected and/or malodorous.
- *Granulating wounds* — containing significant amounts of highly vascularized granulation tissue and generally red or deep pink in color. Such wounds frequently produce significant amounts of exudate in the early stages. They also can become infected and malodorous.
- *Epithelializing wounds* — having a pink margin or isolated pink islands on the surface of granulation tissue. Such wounds frequently produce little or no exudate and generally show little tendency to become infected or malodorous.

These descriptions relate not only to different types of wounds but also to the various stages through which a single wound may pass as it heals.

12.2 MANAGEMENT OF NECROTIC AND DRY SLOUGHY WOUNDS

Under favorable conditions, devitalized tissue in a wound such as a pressure sore separates spontaneously from the healthy tissue beneath by a process of autolysis. If this tissue becomes dehydrated, however, autolytic activity is inhibited and the dead tissue shrinks and progressively darkens until it eventually becomes olive green or black and hard and dry to the touch. The contractile forces produced during this process stimulate pain receptors in the healing tissue around the wound margin.

Other wounds, irrespective of etiology, can develop a glutinous yellow covering commonly referred to as "slough." This varies in consistency from a viscous semi-solid, resembling custard, to hard dry eschar. Slough is not dead tissue, but a complex mixture of fibrin, deoxyribonucleoprotein, serous exudate, leukocytes, and bacteria. A thick layer of slough can build up rapidly on the surface of a previously clean wound, but this should not be confused with the thin pale yellow fibrinous coating that sometimes develops on granulating wounds.

Both necrotic tissue and slough inhibit the healing process and predispose a wound to infection by acting as a bacteriological culture medium. Removal of slough and necrotic tissue forms an important part of the preparation of the wound bed, a key stage in the wound healing process.[5]

If surgical intervention is not an option, debridement can be achieved by the application of a dressing that delays or reverses the process of dehydration and facilitates autolysis. One commonly used technique involves the use of amorphous hydrogels — products that share a common structure consisting of about 2 to 3% of a hydrophilic gel-forming polymer such as sodium carboxymethylcellulose, modified starch, or sodium alginate dispersed in an aqueous medium that often contains 20% propylene glycol as a humectant and preservative. In this technique, a layer of gel is applied to the wound and covered with an appropriate secondary dressing to reduce the loss of moisture from the gel by evaporation. Suitable secondary dressings include absorbent pads covered with a perforated plastic film or a vapor-permeable polyurethane film or foam.

When the dressing is applied in this way, water is donated from the gel to the dead tissue and further evaporative loss is prevented, causing the tissue to become rehydrated and thus more easily removed. Although most gels are similar in appearance, laboratory tests have indicated that their fluid-donating properties can vary considerably.[6] A further advantage of the amorphous hydrogels is that they may be introduced into narrow wounds or sinuses using an applicator or syringe fitted with a quill. The gel is subsequently removed by irrigation with water or sterile saline.

Numerous early papers described the successful use of hydrogels as debriding agents in a variety of wound types including sternal wounds,[7] a large infected wound following a radical vulvectomy,[8] multiple necrotic wounds on an arm,[9] an infected amputation wound,[10] pressure ulcers,[11] three surgical wounds,[12] Fournier's gangrene,[13] extensive areas of necrotic tissue on the abdomen of a baby,[14] necrotic wounds on the limbs of a infant suffering from homozygous protein C deficiency (a rare condition that affects the clotting cascade causing extensive tissue damage),[15] and a degloving injury of the leg.[16]

In 1987, the use of an amorphous hydrogel in the management of extravasation injuries in neonates,[17] a condition that can result in severe scarring or loss of function if managed inappropriately, was described. The gel was applied liberally to the affected area, and the entire area was enclosed in a sterile plastic bag, specially shaped to form a boot or glove. It was reported that the treatment offered a number of significant advantages over more traditional techniques: the gel is painless to apply and remove and, because it is transparent, it permits the wound to be examined at all times. The high moisture content of the gel means that dehydration and further loss of viable tissue are prevented, resulting in a healed wound with a highly acceptable cosmetic appearance. This technique has since been widely adopted and is now regarded as a standard treatment for this condition.[18] A similar approach was subsequently used with advantage in the treatment of necrotic lesions associated with meningococcal septicemia.[19] It is in situations such as this, when the gels are applied inside plastic bags or beneath relatively impermeable plastic films, that their ability to promote rehydration without inducing maceration becomes important.

A number of clinical studies have been published in which hydrogel dressings were compared with other products in the treatment of sloughy or necrotic wounds. The first of these, published in 1993, compared the original formulation of IntraSite™ gel (Scherisorb) with a polysaccharide bead dressing, Debrisan® paste, in the management of sloughy pressure ulcers.[20] The results of this investigation suggested that the gel, which contained 78% water, was more effective than the Debrisan paste, which contained 5.5% water, at promoting debridement. Similar results were achieved in a larger multicenter, parallel-group, prospective randomized clinical trial involving 135 patients with pressure ulcers, in which IntraSite gel was compared with Debrisan paste.[21]

An unnamed amorphous hydrogel was compared with a conventional treatment (wet saline compress) in the treatment of 32 pressure ulcers.[22] All patients were followed for 12 weeks or until the ulcer had healed. Relative volumes of hydrogel-dressed wounds at the end of the study period were significantly less than those of saline-treated wounds (26 and 64%, respectively, $p < 0.02$).

Hydrogel dressings are very widely used and well tolerated by patients, rarely causing any adverse effects. The most common problem tends to be maceration of the peri-wound skin, which can occur if the dressings are left in place too long on heavily exuding wounds. There is also a possibility that propylene glycol, which is present in most amorphous hydrogels, may cause skin reactions in some patients,[23] although this problem is not commonly encountered in clinical practice.

An alternative method of rehydrating necrotic or dry sloughy tissue involves the use of a hydrocolloid dressing. These dressings are virtually impermeable to moisture vapor in their intact state, so when they are placed on a necrotic wound they form a physical barrier, preventing the loss of moisture vapor through the dead tissue, causing it to accumulate within the necrotic layer. Numerous brands of hydrocolloids are available, but as with the hydrogels, despite superficial similarities in appearance, significant differences exist in the fluid-handling properties of the various products.[24] Early reports of this ability of hydrocolloids to promote wound debridement were made by Tracy et al.[25] in 1977 and Johnson[26] in 1984; since that time, hydrocolloids have become widely used for this purpose, especially for the management of pressure ulcers on heels of bedridden patients.

Other products used for the management of sloughy and necrotic wounds include honey[27] and sugar, both of which are well described in the literature. Although ordinary granulated or icing sugar has been used successfully,[28] it is more commonly used in the form of a paste containing polyethylene glycol 400 and hydrogen peroxide.[29,30]

A significant development in the area of wound cleansing is the renewed interest in the use of larval therapy (maggots) for the rapid removal of slough and necrotic tissue from wounds such as leg ulcers, pressure ulcers, and lesions on the feet of diabetic patients.[31] It has also been reported that maggots are of value in burns and in plastic surgery for cleansing wounds prior to grafting.[32] This somewhat unusual form of therapy, reintroduced into America by Sherman and coworkers,[33,34] has also become widely used throughout Europe. The larvae used are those of the common greenbottle *Lucilia sericata,* and the ability of these creatures to remove necrotic tissue and combat infection, including that caused by methicillin-resistant *Staphylococcus aureus* (MRSA),[35,36] is quite remarkable. The history and scientific basis for the use of this technique has been reviewed previously.[37]

12.3 MANAGEMENT OF MOIST OR EXUDING WOUNDS

Some wounds, especially those containing significant quantities of soft slough, produce copious volumes of exudate, which is further increased in the presence of infection. Hard data on the amount of fluid produced by different wound types is limited, but in one study, Lamke et al.[38] measured evaporative water loss from burns and reported values on the order of 5 g/10 cm^2/24 h, a figure that is in close agreement with values for leg ulcers published by Thomas et al.[39]

Over the years, manufacturers have spent a considerable amount of time and effort designing dressings capable of dealing with large volumes of tissue fluid, with varying degrees of success. The simplest products consist of dressing pads made from cellulose fibers or absorbent polyurethane foam, which function by simple absorption. Others incorporate a semipermeable membrane that allows the aqueous component of exudate to evaporate through the back of the dressing to the external environment. A third group of products contains gel-forming agents or superabsorbents that take up liquid and retain it within the body of the dressing in the form of a gel. Many dressings combine two or more of these functions to maximize their fluid-handling capabilities.

One group of commonly used gel-forming agents consists of the salts of alginic acid, which have a long history in the management of wounds. Large quantities are used each year for the treatment of exuding wounds, such as leg ulcers, pressure ulcers, and infected surgical wounds. Alginates are extracted from seaweed, where they occur naturally as mixed salts of alginic acid and are found primarily as the sodium form. The yield varies with the species but is typically of the order of 20 to 25%. They consist of a three-dimensional network of long-chain molecules held together at junctional sites.[40] The alginate molecule is a polysaccharide formed from homopolymeric regions of β-D-mannuronic (M) and α-L-guluronic (G) acids, called M-blocks and G-blocks, respectively, interspersed with regions of mixed sequence (MG-blocks). The relative proportions and arrangement of these blocks have a marked effect upon the chemical and physical characteristics of the alginate and therefore any fiber made from it. These properties are determined by the botanical source of the seaweed from which the alginate is extracted.

Originally, alginate fibers were presented in the form of a loose fleece formed primarily from fibers of calcium alginate, but more recently dressings have been developed in which the fibers have been entangled to form a product with a more cohesive structure to increase the strength of the fabric when soaked with exudate or blood. Some products also contain a significant proportion of sodium alginate to improve the gelling properties of the dressing in use, and other dressings made from freeze-dried alginate have also been produced.

On contact with wound exudate, an ion exchange reaction takes place between the calcium ions in the dressing and sodium ions in serum or wound fluid. Once a significant proportion of the calcium ions present in the fiber have been replaced by sodium, the fiber swells and partially dissolves, forming a gel-like mass, although the degree of swelling is determined principally by the chemical composition of the alginate as determined by its botanical source.

Calcium ions present in high-M alginates are less firmly attached to the molecule than those in high-G alginates, and as a result are more easily replaced by sodium ions, resulting in increased fluid uptake and fiber swelling and faster gel formation. High-M alginates are therefore more absorbent on a gram-for-gram basis, and form softer gels than those rich in high-G. They are also more readily soluble in saline solution.

The variations in gel structure and rheology caused by the differences in chemical structure have important implications for the clinical use of the products. The soft gel residues from products made from high-M alginates can be washed off the wound or irrigated out of sinuses or cavities with a jet of saline, but the fibers in dressings made from high-G alginates swell only slightly in the presence of wound fluid and may appear relatively unchanged even after an extended period. Such dressings are therefore usually removed in one piece using a forceps or gloved hand.

Several reviews have been published on alginates[40] and alginate dressings,[41–44] and the literature also contains numerous references to their use in the management of toxic epidermal necrolysis,[45] dehisced surgical abdominal wounds,[8,46–48] leg ulcers,[49] burns and donor sites,[50–55] and pressure ulcers,[43,56–59] and for foot care following surgery for ingrown toenails.[60–62] When used in the form of a ribbon or rope, alginates have been shown to offer advantages over conventional treatments for packing cavities after surgery.[63–65]

Although it is recognized that differences between the various brands of dressings may influence their handling characteristics, particularly when wet, it is generally assumed that these differences are of limited relevance to the performance of the dressings clinically or at a cellular level. There is some evidence to suggest, however, that these assumptions may not be correct and that alginates may influence wound healing in a number of ways not yet fully understood.[66]

More recently, dressings have been produced from chemically modified carboxymethylcellulose, hyaluronan (hyaluronidase),[67] and chitin and chitosan.[68] These newer dressings, although similar in their physical characteristics to the alginates, are claimed to offer additional benefits to a healing wound. Despite these theoretical benefits, dressings made from hyaluronan and chitin or chitosan have yet to make a significant impact on the wound care market.

Alginates should not be regarded as wound dressings as such but as gel-forming wound contact materials that require the application of an appropriate secondary dressing if they are to function correctly. This may be illustrated by a simple example. It is not uncommon to see publications that state that alginates are suitable for the management of heavily exuding wounds because they absorb up to 20 times their own weight of fluid. Although it is true that alginates are capable of taking up many times their own weight of fluid, a standard 10×10 cm alginate dressing only weighs about 1 to 2 g, and therefore the total amount of fluid that it can absorb is limited. To put this into context, leg ulcers have typically been found to produce up to 0.5 ml of exudate/cm^2/24 h,[39] but in the presence of infection this may double. For a wound 20 cm^2 in area that could be dressed with a single piece of alginate dressing measuring 10×10 cm, this would equate to the production of 10 to 20 ml of fluid per day.

The fluid-handling capacity of alginate dressings ranges from about 15 to 25 g/100 cm^2, but under compression this may be reduced to somewhere between 5 and 10 ml. A standard 10×10 cm dressing would therefore be unable to cope with the exudate produced from a 20 cm^2 wound for more than about 12 h unless additional capacity was provided in the form of an absorbent pad. The application over an alginate sheet of a standard film dressing, which has a maximum moisture vapor transmission rate of approximately 1000 g/m^2/24 h,[69] would in practice allow the loss of about a further 5 g of fluid in 24 h, making a total fluid handling capacity for an alginate/film dressing combination of 10 to 15 ml in the first day. This is still less than the volume of fluid produced by a heavily exuding leg ulcer or donor site. On the second day, however, the alginate dressing, which is fully saturated, would be unable to absorb any further exudate, and therefore fluid would rapidly accumulate beneath the dressing, resulting in leakage and/or maceration of the surrounding skin.

The application of a so-called intelligent film dressing over a sheet of alginate might partially resolve the problems described above. In the presence of liquid, such films have a moisture vapor transmission rate (MVTR) of 5000 to 10,000 g/m^2/24 h, which would greatly enhance the ability of the dressing to cope with exudate production. As the wound begins to dry, the MVTR of the film would decrease and thus help to preserve moisture in the alginate fiber. Such a combination could prove particularly valuable in the treatment of donor sites, where a simple absorbent pad left in place for an extended period would allow the dressing to dry out, leading to problems of adherence and secondary trauma.

The properties of alginate dressings are such that they are only suitable for use in the treatment of moderately exuding wounds. There is little point in using these dressings on very dry wounds, as they require the presence of wound fluid to form a protective gel. In such situations, the use of an alternative product such as a hydrocolloid may be considered.

As previously discussed, hydrocolloid dressings tend to be impermeable to water vapor in their intact state, but in the presence of wound fluid they absorb liquid and begin to gel, rendering the dressing progressively more permeable to water vapor. This process that can take a few hours or a couple of days depending upon the product concerned. The ability of the hydrocolloids to change their physical properties in this way means that they are suitable for a wider range of applications than the alginates, ranging from very dry to lightly or moderately exuding wounds.

When hydrocolloid dressings were originally introduced, many clinicians were initially concerned that the relatively occlusive environment produced by the dressing would tend to promote wound infections, particularly those caused by anaerobic bacteria. In clinical practice, this has not proven to be the case. Mulder et al.[70] examined the effects of different types of dressings on bacterial growth in 48 ulcers of different etiology and found that bacterial proliferation was significantly lower in wounds dressed with a hydrocolloid compared with wounds dressed with gauze or a polyurethane film. They concluded that although there was evidence to suggest that increased bacterial growth delays wound closure, the mere presence of bacteria in a wound does not indicate the potential for infection, as the pathogenicity of the organism must also be considered.

Although heavy colonization by skin and wound flora is often seen under certain types of occlusion, clinical infection is not a frequent occurrence and is most often found in wounds compromised by devitalized tissue, drains, or sutures, which can facilitate bacterial proliferation. Hutchinson et al. have addressed this issue in detail.[71-74] In a retrospective review, Hutchinson examined 69 papers in which occlusive dressings (polyurethane films, hydrocolloids, hydrogel sheets, etc.) were compared with other, more traditional dressings such as gauze or low-adherent dressings, including paraffin gauze. He found that overall the infection rate with conventional dressings was 7.1%, compared with 2.6% for occlusive dressings, and proposed that the low rate of infection beneath the occlusive products resulted from normal activity of the host defenses.[71]

The use of hydrocolloids have been described in a variety of wound types, including the treatment of leg ulcers of all descriptions. An early assessment of the value of hydrocolloids for this purpose was made in 1984 by Cherry et al.,[75] who reported that 51% of 54 patients included in this study had their ulcers healed by the application of the hydrocolloid. The following year Mulder et al.[76] successfully treated 18 patients with ulcers which had failed to respond to conventional treatments.

In a larger multicenter study[77] involving 152 ulcers from seven centers in six countries, 62% of ulcers healed in an average of 51 ± 5 days when dressed with Granuflex. A reduction of pain was reported by 79% of patients, and no cases of wound infection were recorded despite the fact that a wide variety of organisms were cultured from the ulcers. Other studies reported that hydrocolloids gave improved healing rates in comparison with povidone–iodine[78] and saline-soaked gauze,[79] although a comparison with a zinc oxide paste bandage produced no statistically significant difference between the two treatment groups at any point in the study.[80]

Hydrocolloids have also been compared with paraffin gauze[81-83] and an alginate dressing, Kaltostat®,[84] in other, smaller studies. The results of these investigations suggested that the use of hydrocolloids appeared to enhance healing rates, reduce pain, or offer other advantages over conventional dressings, but these observations were either not tested or not found to be significant statistically.

The value of occlusive dressings in the treatment of chronic venous ulcers was questioned by Backhouse et al.,[85] who compared Granuflex® with a simple textile primary dressing (N-A Dressing) in a trial involving 56 patients. In all cases, the dressing was covered with a multilayer bandage system. Complete healing occurred by 12 weeks in 21 out of 28 (75%) of patients dressed with occlusive dressings and 22 out of 28 (78%) of patients dressed with N-A Dressings. The authors concluded that careful graduated compression bandaging achieves healing in the majority of venous ulcers, and little is gained by applying occlusive dressings. The ulcers in this study were very small, with an average area of less than 3.5 cm^2, as wounds larger than 10 cm^2 were specifically excluded even though it is these larger wounds that are most difficult to heal in normal clinical practice. The effect of hydrocolloid dressings on the healing rates of more extensive wounds was investigated by Moffat et al.[86] in a subsequent study in which they compared Comfeel® ulcer dressing with N-A Dressing in 60 patients with ulcers that had previously failed to respond to high compression therapy. The study was conducted over a 12-week period with time to healing as the primary outcome variable. Despite a relatively short follow-up period, seven ulcers (23%) in the nonadherent group and 13 (43%) in the hydrocolloid group healed completely. This just failed to achieve statistical significance ($p = 0.077$). The authors concluded that hydrocolloids might prove of great benefit to this small, difficult group of patients who fail to respond satisfactorily to other treatments. This often-overlooked investigation calls into question the validity of the frequently expressed view that the choice of primary dressing is irrelevant in the treatment of venous leg ulcers provided with adequate sustained compression.

Another important indication for hydrocolloid dressings is the management of pressure ulcers. Early uncontrolled preliminary investigations[26,87-89] were later supported by more structured randomized trials in which the dressings compared favorably with more conventional treatments such as Dakin's solution[90] or saline-soaked gauze,[91-94] once a standard treatment for this condition.

Probably the most contentious indication for the use of hydrocolloid dressings is the treatment of the diabetic foot. The relatively limited bulk of the adhesive wafers would tend to suggest that they should be of value for this purpose, but some workers have expressed reservations about their use for this indication because of the rate with which infection can develop in such wounds if they are not regularly monitored. Foster et al.[95] have suggested that hydrocolloid dressings should never be used on deep, infected, or discharging wounds on the diabetic foot or in circumstances that preclude frequent dressing changes and wound inspection, but Laing[96] argued that accurate diagnosis of the underlying cause is the first step towards successful treatment, and while patients with severe ischemia may require vascular reconstruction, neuropathic ulcers respond well to less-invasive procedures. If adequate pressure relief is provided and any necrotic material is removed, the wounds may safely be dressed with a hydrocolloid. If signs of a clinical infection are present and/or bone is exposed, osteomyelitis should be suspected, in which case aggressive surgical debridement and systemic antibiotics may be required to prevent amputation, the most serious complication of these wounds. The use of hydrocolloid dressings in the treatment of the diabetic foot has been comprehensively reviewed by Gill.[97]

Hydrocolloid dressings also have a role in the management of surgical wounds. Some early reports described the use of Granuflex following a range of surgical procedures including excision of perianal hidradenitis suppurative[98] and colorectal surgery.[99] Additionally, they have been used as an alternative to island dressings for immediate postoperative wounds following clean elective surgery[100] and as a dressing for partial and total nail avulsions.[101]

Alsbjorn et al.[102] compared healing rates achieved with a hydrocolloid (Comfeel) and paraffin gauze on drainage wounds in 21 patients who had undergone cardiac surgery, each of whom had two drains introduced through incisional wounds in the infrasternal area. Improved healing was reported with the hydrocolloid, and no increase in wound infection was detected. The benefits of a moist wound-healing environment with particular reference to the use of hydrocolloid dressings were discussed in a review published by Field and Kerstein in 1994.[103]

Other products that have made a significant impact in the management of exuding wounds are the foam dressings. These are generally made from polyurethane, either alone or as part of a multicomponent structure such as Allevyn™, which consists of a hydrophilic polyurethane layer sandwiched between a low-adherent wound contact layer and a semipermeable membrane to control moisture vapor loss and prevent strikethrough. Also available in a self-adhesive form, Allevyn was for a long time one of the most absorbent dressings available. Other foam products such as Lyo-foam® and Tielle™ do not have the same absorbent capacity as Allevyn but have a much higher moisture vapor permeability, which enables them to be used in the treatment of quite heavily exuding wounds.

Both Allevyn and Tielle have been compared with a hydrocolloid dressing, Granuflex, in clinical studies. In one large investigation involving 100 community patients with leg ulcers and 99 patients with pressure ulcers,[104] statistically significant differences in favor of Tielle dressing were detected for dressing leakage and odor production, but no statistically significant differences were recorded in the number of patients with either leg ulcers or pressure ulcers who healed in each treatment group. Similar results were reported after several studies in which Allevyn was compared with Granuflex in the treatment of various wound types. No significant differences were detected in healing rate, but the foam tended to be preferred because of ease of use and patient comfort.[105–107]

12.4 MANAGEMENT OF EPITHELIALIZING WOUNDS

The ability to remove a dressing without traumatizing the wound or the surrounding skin or causing pain to the patient was shown in a large international survey to be regarded as a major feature of the dressing's performance.[108] According to Winter,[1] the main cause of adherence of a dressing to the surface of a wound is "the mechanical key formed by proteinaceous exudate, which on drying becomes a good glue." He also recognized a secondary mechanism of adherence in which new tissue grows into the structure of the dressing and thus incorporates some of the components into the healing wound.

Unless they become infected, epithelializing wounds, whether superficial abrasions or large wounds in the final phase of healing by secondary intention, tend not to produce significant volumes of exudate and as such are prone to adhere to many types of dressings. There are therefore two principal ways of reducing adherence. The first of these depends upon the use of an intrinsically low-adherent wound contact layer, the second the application of a dressing that maintains a moist environment and thereby prevents the formation of the adhesive bond between the dressing and the tissue beneath.

Over the years, dressings with a variety of different types of wound contact layers have been developed that aim to reduce adherence to a drying wound; these have been described as "nonadherent" or more accurately, "low-adherent." These include simple fabrics impregnated with white soft paraffin, nonwoven fabric coated with metallic aluminum, and products faced with a perforated plastic film or impregnated with silicone. It is important to recognize that the term low-adherent relates only to the interaction that takes place between the dressing and the wound itself; it takes no account of possible trauma caused to the surrounding skin by removal of moisture-retentive adhesive products such as hydrocolloids, adhesive films, and self-adhesive foams. It has recently been proposed, therefore, that the term "atraumatic dressings" be adopted to describe products that do not cause trauma either to newly formed tissue or to the periwound skin.[109]

Recently, however, a new family of dressings has been introduced that are claimed to overcome the twin problems of adherence to the wound and damage to the surrounding skin caused by excessive adhesion. They rely upon an adhesive technology involving the use of "soft" silicone, a material that adheres readily to intact dry skin but does not stick to the surface of a moist wound and does not cause damage upon removal.[110] Mepitel®, the first product of this category to be introduced, is a porous, semitransparent wound contact layer consisting of a flexible polyamide net coated with soft silicone. Although Mepitel is nonabsorbent, it contains numerous pores, which allow the passage of exudate from the wound into a secondary absorbent dressing. The dressing has been used in the treatment of skin grafts,[111,112] extensive wounds resulting from wide local excision of skin tumors,[113] burns,[114,115] and a variety of other superficial injuries, where it compared favorably with conventional treatments. The literature relating to this group of products has formed the subject of an earlier review.[109]

The second approach to overcoming problems of adherence — maintaining the surface of the wound in a moist condition — can be achieved by using a variety of different dressing materials. Simple polyurethane films have been used historically, but as these are permeable to moisture vapor there remains the possibility that the wound surface will dry out if exudate production is very low. Similar problems occur with foam dressings unless these have some form of relatively occlusive backing layer.

As previously discussed, the most occlusive dressings are the hydrocolloid sheets, some which are virtually impermeable to liquid in their intact state. As a result, these materials rarely adhere to the wound surface but, in common with all adhesive products, they can cause superficial damage to the periwound skin in some patients, particularly the elderly or those receiving steroid therapy. It has been reported that healing rates of burns dressed with hydrocolloids compare favorably with those dressed with silver sulfadiazine or human allografts[116,117] or chlorhexidine-impregnated paraffin gauze.[118]

Similar benefits have been reported in the treatment of donor sites, where the use of hydrocolloids reduced healing times from approximately 13 to 7 d compared with conventional treatments[119–122] and produced healed wounds with a better cosmetic result. Healed donor sites were said to be soft and supple and ready for reharvesting, in marked contrast to the dry sensitive areas that formed beneath conventional dressings.

Porter[123] compared hydrocolloid dressings with alginate dressings in 65 patients with split skin graft donor sites. The alginate dressings were applied to the raw donor areas and held in place by layers of dry gauze, plaster wool, and a crepe bandage. The mean time from operation to the observation of complete healing was 10.0 d for the donor areas dressed with the hydrocolloid and 15.5 d for wounds dressed with alginate; this difference was found to be statistically significant. The relatively poor performance of alginates in this study was probably due the use of an inappropriate secondary dressing system that caused the alginate to dry out during the later stages of the treatment, as described previously.

Numerous papers have been published that describe the successful use hydrocolloids in the treatment of superficial traumatic wounds and sport-related injuries such as superficial lacerations, abrasions, and gravel rash.[124–128] Where comparisons were undertaken with conventional treatments, it was reported that the hydrocolloids appeared to promote more rapid healing and improve patient comfort. Military personnel have used hydrocolloid dressings to protect their feet during violent or prolonged physical exercise,[129] and a review of the pathophysiology, prevention, and treatment of blisters that appeared in the journal *Sports Medicine*[130] recommended the use of hydrocolloids for treating deroofed blisters.

The relatively pain-free removal of hydrocolloid dressings makes them particularly suitable for use in pediatric wound management in the management of burns and donor sites and grazes.[131] They have even been used to achieve skin closure in minor postoperative wounds.[132,133] For this application, it was claimed that the dressing "minimized the physical and psychological trauma to the infant or child and reduced the disruption to the child's and the parents' daily routines."

Hydrocolloids have also been used to treat moist skin desquamation following radiotherapy,[134,135] but for this particular indication, alternative dressings may be preferred given the fragile nature of the skin and the possibility of traumatic injury on removal. One group of products that may be used for this purpose are the hydrogel sheets. A number of these are now available, but the first to be used in wound management was Geliperm®, which was introduced in 1977. This has a copolymer structure consisting of agar and polyacrylamide and is available in the form of a hydrated sheet, which contains about 96% water. Other hydrogels have since been developed, made from a number of different gel-forming agents. These materials have potential value as a delivery system for antibiotics, antiseptic agents, and growth factors. One early study[136] showed that Geliperm could take up solutes with a molecular weight of up to about one million, although the rate of diffusion of these materials into and out of the gel was inversely proportional to their molecular weight. The principal factors that influence the acceptability of a hydrogel sheet dressing when used as a skin substitute are water vapor permeability, adherence to the excised wound surface, oxygen permeability, mechanical properties, impermeability to microorganisms and the ability to absorb exudate.[137]

Provided that they are not allowed to dry out, hydrogel dressings in sheet form can be applied and removed without causing pain and trauma. If required, in appropriate cases the dressings may be refrigerated before use, producing a cooling effect that further alleviates pain and irritation. Once in place they are said to reduce pain and therefore have a high degree of patient acceptability. As retention of the non-adhesive gel sheets can be a problem, it is sometimes an advantage to use the material in conjunction with a piece of an adhesive retention sheet (such as Mefix® or

Hypafix™). Queen et al.,[138] in a laboratory study, showed that the use of the adhesive sheet also reduced evaporative loss from the gel by 60 to 65% to a more clinically appropriate level of around 4000 g/m²/24 h. Some hydrogel sheets have such films as an integral part of their structure.

Because the ability of occluded hydrogels to cope with large volumes of fluid is limited, they are best used on low-exudate wounds, such as dermabrasions, minor burns, donor sites, and superficial pressure areas. Small pieces of gel sheet are sometimes applied to the eyes of unconscious patients in intensive care units to keep the eyes closed and prevent them from becoming excessively dry.

It might be supposed that hydrogel sheets, which are largely composed of water, should be of value in the treatment of relatively dry epithelializing wounds or extensive superficial skin injuries, provided that evaporation from the outer surface is controlled. This has proven to be the case, and gels have gained considerable support following hair transplantations, 10 dermabrasions, and 42 excisional surgeries.[139,140] Their high moisture content also been shown to impart reasonable cooling properties in the treatment of superficial burns.

Strunk et al.[141] described the successful use of Vigilon for painful, slough-filled lesions in a patient undergoing radiotherapy for esophageal carcinoma and concomitant corticosteroid therapy for cicatricial pemphigoid.

Early studies with hydrogel dressings suggested that they might have value as a coupling agent for ultrasound in the treatment of fractures[142] and soft tissue injuries,[143] providing a sterile environment and physical protection to the skin while preventing problems of pin track infections.

According to a survey published in 1998 by Duke et al., hydrogel sheets are used extensively both pre- and post-laser resurfacing for photodamaged skin, rhytides, and acne scarring.[144] In one study, Newman et al.[145] compared a hydrogel sheet, 2nd Skin® (Primskin), with three other "closed" (semipermeable) dressings in a randomized controlled trial in 40 patients who had undergone laser resurfacing of the face. They reported that although patients preferred not to continue with any of the dressings longer than necessary, usually stopping after 2 to 3 days, the use of all of the materials examined in the study decreased pain and reduced crust formation and pruritus compared with historical controls. There were no complications, such as scarring, hyperpigmentation, or prolonged erythema, after treatment.

The moist environment provided by the hydrogel sheets also appears to be of value in the treatment of hypertrophic scars. Ricketts et al.[146] compared a hydrogel sheet (ClearSite®) with a silicone gel sheet (Silastic®) in the side-by-side treatment of 15 scars, using both clinical and biochemical criteria. They showed that silicone is not a necessary component of occlusive dressings used for the treatment of hypertrophic scars and demonstrated that the hydrogel functioned by augmenting collagenolysis via promotion of the inflammatory process.

According to Corkhill et al.,[147] hydrogel sheet dressings appear to possess many of the properties of an ideal dressing; they are flexible, nonantigenic, and permeable to water vapor and metabolites, but impermeable to bacteria. Despite these theoretical benefits, as a family the hydrogel sheets have failed to make a significant impact on clinical practice. At least part of the reason for this may be found in the results of the fluid handling studies described previously, which suggest that these dressings probably have limited applications in mainstream wound management. In view of their unique tactile properties, however, they may have advantages over conventional materials for specialist applications, reducing pain or discomfort in certain types of problem wounds. For more general applications such as the treatment of leg ulcers and pressure ulcers, hydrocolloids, foams, and alginates are generally preferred. It is also possible, however, that they may become more widely used in the future as carriers for water-soluble growth-promoting agents, but this remains to be seen

12.5   MANAGEMENT OF INFECTED WOUNDS

Given the vast numbers of bacteria carried by a normal healthy individual, it is perhaps inevitable that some will find their way into any defects in the epidermis irrespective of their cause or location. The consequences of bacterial contamination depend upon a number of factors, including the number of organisms, their pathogenicity (potential to cause disease), and the ability of the patient's own defense system to combat any possible infection. The latter, in turn, may depend upon the patient's age, general health, and nutritional status, as well as other factors such as the administration of immunosuppressive drugs. The number of organisms that might be considered to constitute an infection in a wound was discussed by Lawrence,[148] who considered that the level of 10^5/g formed a useful guide — provided it was recognized that the bacteriological picture of a wound could change as the condition of the wound itself changes. For example, burns covered with wet slough frequently contain an abundance of Gram-negative bacilli — including *Pseudomonas aeruginosa, Proteus mirabilis, Klebsiella* spp., and *Escherichia coli* — together with *Streptococcus faecalis, Staphylococcus aureus,* and *Streptococcus pyogenes.* As the slough separates, however, the number of Gram-negative organisms decreases, and the Gram-positive bacteria predominate. Of all these organisms, Lowbury and Cason[149] have identified *S. pyogenes* and *P. aeruginosa* as being among the most serious pathogens in a burn. *Streptococcus pyogenes* will cause the total failure of a skin graft if present at the time of operation, and *P. aeruginosa* has been found to be an important cause of systemic infections in patients with severe burns, although other organisms may also cause serious problems from time to time.

The isolation of microorganisms from a wound is not, of itself, a cause for concern, as many lesions heal uneventfully despite the presence of relatively large number of bacteria. It is generally acknowledged, therefore, that systemic antimicrobial therapy should only be administered to patients who show the classical symptoms of infection — redness and swelling with heat and pain — or to immunocompromised individuals and others who, by virtue of their general health, are prone to development of a clinical infection that may result in a life-threatening septicemia.

The role of topical antimicrobial therapy in the form of medicated dressings is rather more contentious. These materials are generally reserved for the treatment of wounds that show some signs of local infection or that fail to heal at the expected rate. In any event, the use of topical antibiotics is not generally encouraged, as it may cause sensitivity reactions or lead to the emergence of antibiotic-resistant strains of bacteria. Dressings containing antiseptic agents such as iodine or silver salts are to be preferred in most instances.

The use of iodine preparations has been criticized in the past because of the potential problems resulting from the topical application of antiseptics, which are claimed to delay or impair wound healing.[150] It has, however, been suggested that these concerns are unfounded.[151,152] More recent scientific studies designed specifically to assess the cellular effects of one formulation, cadexomer iodine, have shown that iodine is released in quantities that are nontoxic to human cells *in vitro* and that the appropriate use of cadexomer iodine *in vivo* does not lead to cellular toxicity.[153] Cadexomer iodine was originally presented in the form of small free-flowing beads, which were subsequently formed into a paste (Iodosorb®) that was subsequently impregnated into a fabric carrier to form a medicated paste dressing (Iodoflex®). In an early randomized trial involving the treatment of 38 decubitus ulcers,[154] it was found that cadexomer iodine beads were superior to standard treatments in removing pus and debris from the surface of the ulcer; wound healing rates, as measured by a decrease in wound area, were also significantly improved. The major indication for the use of Iodosorb, however, is in the management of leg ulcers, and numerous studies have been reported that describe its use for this indication.[155,156] These and other studies involving cadexomer iodine have been critically reviewed in two earlier publications by Bradley et al. in 1999[157] and Bianchi in 2001,[158] who concluded that, with one exception, most papers on cadexomer iodine were over 10 years old and of limited relevance because of study design or the choice of comparator.

Recently, there has been considerable renewed interest in the use of dressings containing silver. The antimicrobial properties of metallic silver have been used empirically for thousands of years, long before the existence of microorganisms was first suspected. For example, Aristotle advised Alexander the Great (335 B.C.) to store his water in silver vessels and boil it before use. Several excellent reviews have been published on the antimicrobial properties of silver, which include information on the mechanism of action, development of bacterial resistance, toxicity, clinical indications, and the historical background to its use.[159–162]

The first silver-containing dressing to make a commercial impact was Actisorb® Plus (now Actisorb Silver 220), which consists primarily of silver-impregnated activated charcoal cloth. Charcoal cloth without the addition of silver was shown by Frost et al.[163] in experimental studies to adsorb bacteria from suspension, an effect that was claimed to have potential benefits within an infected wound. Further tests showed that although these organisms were held firmly by the dressing, they still remained viable, so silver was added to the cloth prior to carbonization to provide a degree of antimicrobial activity.

Within the last few years, numerous other dressings have been introduced that contain silver in a variety of different forms. Acticoat™ is an absorbent dressing bearing a silver-coated high-density polyethylene membrane[164] that has a wide spectrum of activity,[165] with the potential to provide significant clinical benefits in the treatment of infected burns,[166–168] although less positive results were obtained when the dressing was used as a skin graft donor site dressing.[169]

Other recent entrants to the silver-dressing market include Avance™ and Contreet-H. Avance is an absorbent polyurethane foam containing a silver compound and is marketed for the treatment of most types of exuding wounds, including leg ulcers and pressure sores. Contreet consists of a well-established hydrocolloid dressing, Comfeel, to which has been added an unnamed silver salt.

The antimicrobial properties of a selection of silver-containing dressings were compared in a laboratory study,[170] which showed that the silver content and hence the antimicrobial activity of the various dressings varied considerably, a finding that has important implications for the use of the products concerned.

12.6 MANAGEMENT OF MALODOROUS WOUNDS

Wounds such as leg ulcers or fungating tumors produce noxious odors, which even in moderate cases can cause significant distress or embarassment to patients and their relatives. In extreme cases, this odor can become so overpowering that it may cause an individual to withdraw from social contacts, even with family and close friends.[171]

Wounds most commonly associated with odor production include leg ulcers and fungating (cancerous) lesions of all types. The smell from these wounds is caused by a cocktail of volatile agents that includes short-chain organic acids (n-butyric, n-valeric, n-caproic, n-heptanoic, and n-caprylic) produced by anaerobic bacteria,[172] together with a mixture of amines and diamines, such as cadaverine and putrescine, that are produced by the metabolic processes of other proteolytic bacteria.

Organisms frequently isolated from malodorous wounds include anaerobes, such as *Bacteroides* and *Clostridium* species, and numerous aerobic bacteria including *Proteus, Klebsiella,* and *Pseudomonas* spp. Recent research has shown that the wound odor produced by some bacteria is specific to that species and that this may be analyzed electrochemically to identify the presence of organisms such as β-hemolytic streptococci.[173]

The most effective way of dealing with malodorous wounds is to prevent or eradicate the infection responsible for the odor. This may be achieved in a number of ways. The administration of systemic antibiotics or antimicrobial agents may be effective in some cases, but often the nature of the wound is such that it is not possible to achieve an effective concentration of the antibiotic at the site of infection by this method, particularly in the presence of slough or necrotic tissue. Most topical antiseptics are also likely to be of limited value, and many of these have been shown to have adverse effects on wound healing.[174,175]

One preparation that has been found to be effective in certain situations is a hydrogel containing a suitable concentration of metronidazole, typically about 0.8% w/v. Research has shown despite the fact that metronidazole is traditionally associated with the treatment of anaerobic infections, in the concentrations used topically it may also have an effect upon a range of aerobic organisms,[176] although the clinical evidence for the widespread use of this material has been questioned in the past.[177]

Less conventional methods of treating malodorous wounds include the use of honey,[27] some varieties of which contain potent antimicrobial agents, and sugar,[28] either alone or in the form of a paste. The hyperosmotic environment produced by high concentrations of sugar is believed to inhibit bacterial growth[178] and thus prevent odor formation. Live yogurt is also sometimes applied in an attempt to encourage overgrowth of pathogenic organisms by lactic acid bacteria such as *Lactobacillus bulgaricus* and *Streptococcus thermophilus.*

More recently, larval therapy has been shown to be an extremely effective way of eliminating wound infection and odor from extensive necrotic wounds.[179,180]

If for some reason, however, it is not possible to eliminate the bacteria responsible for the production of the odor, it may be possible to deal with the problem by some other means. Historically, wound odors were masked by burning incense, and in more recent times by the use of aerosols or air fresheners. Obviously, although these do not resolve the underlying problem, they may make life a little more bearable for patients and their families.

In 1976, a more scientific approach to the control of odor was reported by Butcher et al.,[181] who described the use of a charcoal cloth developed by the Chemical Defence Establishment in Porton Down, U.K. This material was incorporated into pads containing surgical gauze and a layer of a water-repellant fabric. When these pads were used in the treatment of fungating breast cancer, gangrene, and immediate postoperative colostomies, the associated odors were said to be totally suppressed.

Activated charcoal cloth is produced by carbonizing a suitable cellulose fabric by heating it under carefully controlled conditions. During this process, the surface of the carbon breaks down to form small pores. These greatly increase the effective surface area of the fibers and hence their ability to remove unpleasant smells, as it is believed that the molecules that are responsible for the production of the odor are attracted to the surface of the carbon and are held there (adsorbed) by electrical forces. In the main, these molecules are small and detected by the nose in low concentrations in the air. A single dressing, which, by virtue of the large surface area of the carbon, is capable of taking up very large numbers of molecules should therefore prove capable of removing odor over prolonged periods.

Since 1976, a number of odor-absorbing dressings containing activated charcoal have been produced commercially. The first of these was Actisorb (Johnson & Johnson). In laboratory studies, it was found that if the dressing was shaken with a suspension of bacteria, the organisms became firmly attached to the charcoal fabric and thus removed from the solution, although they still remained viable. A modified version of this dressing was therefore developed (Actisorb Plus), which contains 0.15% silver chemically bound onto the carbon. This imparts pronounced antibacterial activity to the dressing, killing the bacteria that are bound to the cloth.

Since the introduction of Actisorb Plus, a number of dressings containing activated charcoal have been developed. Some of these, like Actisorb itself, are intended to be placed in direct contact with the wound. These products vary in structure and composition and hence in their ability to cope with wound exudate, often an important feature of malodorous wounds. Other products are designed as secondary dressings, which are placed over a primary dressing but beneath the retaining dressing or bandage. Examples include CliniSorb (CliniMed) and Denidor (Jeffreys, Miller & Co).

12.7 CONCLUSIONS

Many sophisticated dressings are available to the wound care practitioner, which may be used alone or in combination to absorb exudate, combat odor and infection, relieve pain, promote autolytic debridement (wound cleansing), or provide and maintain a moist environment at the wound surface to facilitate the production of granulation tissue and the process of epithelialization.

Some dressings simply absorb exudate or wound fluid and may therefore be suitable for application to a variety of different wound types. Others have a very clearly defined specialist function and as such have a more limited range of indications. This may mean that they are only suitable for the treatment of specific types of wounds or for the management of a wider range of wounds during a particular phase of the healing cycle. Wound healing is a dynamic process, and the performance requirements of a dressing can change as the wound progresses towards healing.

Consider, for example, a black necrotic pressure sore on a heel. If surgical debridement is not an option, a dressing that increases the moisture content of the dead tissue will facilitate rehydration and autolytic debridement of the affected area. If this initial treatment is successful, removal of the necrotic cap may reveal a heavily discharging sloughy wound, the treatment of which will almost certainly involve the use of a dressing with a significant absorbent capacity. If the wound is also judged to be infected, a product with proven antimicrobial activity may be indicated for a limited period. Assuming the infection is brought under control and sufficient granulation tissue is produced to fill the resulting cavity, at some stage the wound may require a further change in therapy to conserve liquid once again and provide the moist wound-healing environment required for rapid epithelialization.

Effective wound management requires an understanding of the process of tissue repair and knowledge of the properties of the dressings available. Only when these two factors are considered together can the process of dressing selection be undertaken in a logical and informed fashion. In most instances, dressings are applied to absorb tissue fluid from exuding wounds such as leg ulcers, pressure ulcers, or donor sites, but in other situations dressings are used to conserve or donate moisture to promote autolysis or facilitate epithelialization. While some dressings can perform both functions with varying degrees of success, some products tend to fulfill only one or other of these requirements. This means that it may be necessary to use different dressings at various stages in the life cycle of a wound if optimum rates of healing are to be achieved.

REFERENCES

1. Winter, G.D., Formation of the scab and the rate of epithelization of superficial wounds in the skin of the young domestic pig, *Nature*, 193, 293–294, 1962.
2. Winter, G.D., Methods for the biological evaluation of dressings, in Turner, T.D. and Brain, K.R., Eds., *Surgical Dressings in the Hospital Environment*, Surgical Dressings Research Unit, UWIST, Cardiff, 1975, pp. 47–81.
3. Thomas, S., A structured approach to the selection of dressings, *World Wide Wounds*, http://www.worldwidewounds.com/1997/july/Thomas-Guide/Dress-Select.html, 1997.
4. Thomas, S., The importance of secondary dressings in wound care, *J. Wound Care*, 7, 189–192, 1998.
5. Falanga, V., Classifications for wound bed preparation and stimulation of chronic wounds, *Wound Repair Regen.*, 8, 347–352, 2001.

6. Thomas, S. and Hay, P., Fluid handling properties of hydrogel dressings, *Ostomy Wound Manage.,* 41, 54–56, 58–59, 1995.
7. Regan, M.B., The use of intrasite gel in healing open sternal wounds, *Ostomy Wound Manage.,* 38, 15, 18–21, 1992.
8. Roberts, K.J., Rowland, C.M., and Benbow, M.E., Managing a patient's infected wound site after a radical vulvectomy, *J. Wound Care,* 1(4), 14–17, 1992.
9. Benbow, M., The treatment of a patient with infected arm wounds, *J. Wound Care,* 2, 326–329, 1993.
10. Platt, L. and Benbow, M., Care of a patient's foot after amputation of toes, *J. Wound Care,* 1(4), 18–20, 1992.
11. Spooner, R., Managing a patient's multiple pressure sores, *J. Wound Care,* 2, 139–141, 1993.
12. Krasner, D., Treating postoperative wounds with an amorphous hydrogel, *J. Wound Care,* 2, 148–150, 1993.
13. Cooper, L. and Benbow, B.A., Management of a patient with Fournier's gangrene, *J. Wound Care,* 2, 266–268, 1993.
14. Riggs, R.L. and Bale, S., Management of necrotic wounds as a complication of histiocytosis X, *J. Wound Care,* 2, 260–261, 1993.
15. Benbow, M. and Pearce, C., The care of an infant with homozygous protein C deficiency, *J. Wound Care,* 3, 21–24, 1994.
16. Price, A. and Thomas, S., Care of a patient after a degloving of the leg injury, *J. Wound Care,* 3, 129–130, 1994.
17. Thomas, S., A new approach to the management of extravasation injury in neonates, *Pharm. J.,* 239, 584–585, 1987.
18. Irving, V., Managing extravasation injuries in preterm neonates, *Nurs. Times,* 97, 40–46, 2001.
19. Thomas, S., Humphreys, J., and Fear-Price, M., The role of moist wound healing in the management of meningococcal skin lesions, *J. Wound Care,* 7, 503–507, 1998.
20. Thomas, S. and Fear, M., Comparing two dressings for wound debridement; results of a randomised trial, *J. Wound Care,* 2, 272–274, 1993.
21. Colin, D., Kurring, P.A., Quinlan, D., and Yvon, C. Managing sloughy pressure sores, *J. Wound Care,* 5, 444–446, 1996.
22. Matzen, S., Peschardt, A., and Alsbjorn, B., A new amorphous hydrocolloid for the treatment of pressure sores: a randomised controlled study, *Scand. J. Plast. Reconstr. Surg. Hand Surg.,* 33, 13–15, 1999.
23. Gallenkemper, G., Rabe, E., and Bauer, R., Contact sensitization in chronic venous insufficiency: modern wound dressings, *Contact Dermatitis,* 38, 274–278, 1998.
24. Thomas, S. and Loveless, P., A comparative study of the properties of 12 hydrocolloid dressings, *World Wide Wounds,* http://www.worldwidewounds.com/1997/july/Thomas-Hydronet/hydronet.html.
25. Tracy, G.D., Lord, R.S., Kibel, C., Martin, M., and Binnie, M., Varihesive sealed dressing for indolent leg ulcers, *Med. J. Aust.,* 1(21), 777–780, 1977.
26. Johnson, A., Towards rapid tissue healing, *Nurs. Times,* 80, 39–43, 1984.
27. Keast-Butler, J., Honey for necrotic malignant breast ulcers, *Lancet,* ii, 809, 1980.
28. Thomlinson, R.H., Kitchen remedy for necrotic malignant breast ulcers, *Lancet,* ii, 594, 1980.
29. Archer, H.G., Barnett, S., Irving, S., Middleton, K.R., and Seal, D.V., A controlled model of moist wound healing: comparison between semi-permeable film, antiseptics and sugar paste, *J. Exp. Pathol. (Oxford),* 71, 155–170, 1990.

30. Topham, J., Sugar paste and povidone–iodine in the treatment of wounds, *J. Wound Care,* 5, 364–365, 1996.
31. Thomas, S., Jones, M., Shutler, S., and Andrews, A., Wound care. All you need to know about... maggots, *Nurs. Times,* 92, 63–66, 68, 70 passim, 1996.
32. Namias, N., Varela, J.E., Varas, R.P., Quintana, O., and Ward, C.G., Biodebridement: a case report of maggot therapy for limb salvage after fourth-degree burns, *J. Burn Care Rehabil.,* 21, 254–257, 2000.
33. Sherman, R.A., Wyle, F., and Vulpe, M., Maggot therapy for treating pressure ulcers in spinal cord injury patients, *J. Spinal Cord Med.,* 18, 71–74, 1995.
34. Stoddard, S.R., Sherman, R.M., Mason, B.E., and Pelsang, D.J., Maggot debridement therapy — an alternative treatment for nonhealing ulcers, *J. Am. Podiatr. Med. Assoc.,* 85, 218–221, 1995.
35. Thomas, S. and Jones, M., Maggots can benefit patients with MRSA, *Practice Nurse,* 20, 101–104, 2000.
36. Thomas, S. and Jones, M., *Maggots and the Battle against MRSA,* SMTL, Bridgend, UK, 2000.
37. Sherman, R.A., Hall, M.J., and Thomas, S., Medicinal maggots: an ancient remedy for some contemporary afflictions, *Annu. Rev. Entomol.,* 45, 55–81, 2000.
38. Lamke, L.O., Nilsson, G.E., and Reithner, H.L., The evaporative water loss from burns and water vapour permeability of grafts and artificial membranes used in the treatment of burns, *Burns,* 3, 159–165, 1977.
39. Thomas, S., Fear, M., Humphreys, J., Disley, L., and Waring, M.J., The effect of dressings on the production of exudate from venous leg ulcers, *Wounds,* 8, 145–149, 1996.
40. Gacesa, P., Alginates, *Carbohydrate Polym.,* 8, 1–22, 1988.
41. Morgan, D., Alginate dressings, *J. Tissue Viabil.,* 7, 4–14, 1996.
42. Thomas, S., Alginates, *J. Wound Care,* 1(1), 29–32, 1992.
43. Young, M.J., The use of alginates in the management of exudating, infected wounds: case studies, *Dermatol. Nurs.,* 5, 359–363, 356, 1993.
44. Gensheimer, D., A review of calcium alginates, *Ostomy Wound Manage.,* 39, 34–38, 42–43, 1993.
45. Imamura, Y., Fujiwara, S., Sato, T., Katagiri, K., and Takayasu, S., Successful treatment of toxic epidermal necrolysis with calcium sodium alginate fiber, *Int. J. Dermatol.,* 35, 834–835, 1996.
46. Cannavo, M., Fairbrother, G., Owen, D., Ingle, J., and Lumley, T., A comparison of dressings in the management of surgical abdominal wounds, *J. Wound Care,* 7, 57–62, 1998.
47. Berry, D.P., Bale, S., and Harding, K.G., Dressings for treating cavity wounds, *J. Wound Care,* 5, 10–17, 1996.
48. Eagle, M., The care of a patient after a Caesarean section, *J. Wound Care,* 2, 330–336, 1993.
49. Thomas, S. and Tucker, C.A., Sorbsan in the management of leg ulcers, *Pharm. J.,* 243, 706–709, 1989.
50. Groves, A.R. and Lawrence, J.C., Alginate dressing as a donor site haemostat, *Ann. Roy. Coll. Surg. Engl.,* 68, 27–28, 1986.
51. Attwood, A.I., Calcium alginate dressing accelerates split skin graft donor site healing, *Br. J. Plast. Surg.,* 42, 373–379, 1989.
52. Basse, P., Siim, E., and Lohmann, M., Treatment of donor sites—calcium alginate versus paraffin gauze, *Acta Chir. Plast.,* 34, 92–98, 1992.

53. O'Donoghue, J.M., O'Sullivan, S.T., Beausang, E.S., Panchal, J.I., O'Shaughnessy, M., and O'Connor, T.P., Calcium alginate dressings promote healing of split skin graft donor sites, *Acta Chir. Plast.,* 39, 53–55, 1997.

54. Cihantimur, B., Kahveci, R., and Ozcan, M., Comparing Kaltostat with Jelonet in the treatment of split-thickness skin graft donor sites, *Eur. J. Plast. Surg.,* 20, 260–263, 1997.

55. Rives, J.M., Pannier, M., Castede, J.C., Martinot, V., LeTouze, A., Romana, M.C. et al., Calcium alginate versus paraffin gauze in the treatment of scalp graft donor sites, *Wounds Compend. Clin. Res. Pract.,* 9, 199–205, 1997.

56. Sayag, J., Meaume, S., and Bohbot, S., Healing properties of calcium alginate dressings, *J. Wound Care,* 5, 357–362, 1996.

57. Chapuis, A. and Dollfus, P., The use of a calcium alginate dressing in the management of decubitus ulcers in patients with spinal cord lesions, *Paraplegia,* 28, 269–271, 1990.

58. McMullen, D., Clinical experience with a calcium alginate dressing, *Dermatol. Nurs.,* 3, 216–219, 270, 1991.

59. Motta, G.J., Calcium alginate topical wound dressings: a new dimension in the cost-effective treatment for exudating dermal wounds and pressure sores, *Ostomy Wound Manage.,* 25, 52–56, 1989.

60. Burrow, B.A. and Lindsay, A., A limited evaluation of alginates and a small scale comparison between Kaltostat and a standard non-adherent dressing, Ultraplast alginate, in the treatment of nail avulsion by matrix phenolisation, *Chiropodist,* October 1989, pp. 211–218.

61. Smith, J., Comparing Sorbsan and polynoxylin/Melolin dressings after toenail removal, *J. Wound Care,* 1(3), 17–19, 1992.

62. Foley, G.B. and Allen, J., Wound healing after toenail avulsion, *The Foot,* 4, 88–91, 1994.

63. Gupta, R., Foster, M.E., and Miller, E., Calcium alginate in the management of acute surgical wounds and abscesses, *J. Tissue Viability,* 1, 115–116, 1991.

64. Dawson, C., Armstrong, M.W., Fulford, S.C., Faruqi, R.M., and Galland, R.B., Use of calcium alginate to pack abscess cavities: a controlled clinical trial. *J. Roy. Coll. Surg. Edinb.,* 37, 177–179, 1992.

65. Ingram, M., Wright, T.A., and Ingoldby, C.J., A prospective randomized study of calcium alginate (Sorbsan) versus standard gauze packing following haemorrhoidectomy, *J. Roy. Coll. Surg. Edinb.,* 43, 308–309, 1998.

66. Thomas, S., Alginate dressings in surgery and wound management — part 3, *J. Wound Care,* 9, 163–166, 2000.

67. Chen, J.W.Y. and Abatangelo, G., Functions of hyaluronan in wound repair, *Wound Repair Regen.,* 7, 79–89, 1999.

68. Biagini, G., Bertani, A., Muzzarelli, R., Damadei, A., DiBenedetto, G., Belligolli, A. et al., Wound management with N-carboxybutyl chitosan, *Biomaterials,* 12, 281–286, 1991.

69. Thomas, S., Loveless, P., and Hay, N.P., Comparative review of the properties of six semipermeable film dressings, *Pharm. J.,* 240, 785–789, 1988.

70. Mulder, G., Kissil, M., and Mahr, J.J., Bacterial growth under occlusive and non-occlusive wound dressings, *Wounds,* 1, 63–69, 1989.

71. Hutchinson, J.J., Prevalence of wound infection under occlusive dressings: a collective survey of reported research, *Wounds,* 1, 123–133, 1989.

72. Hutchinson, J.J. and McGuckin, M., Occlusive dressings: a microbiologic and clinical review, *Am. J. Infect. Control,* 18, 257–268, 1990.

73. Hutchinson, J.J. and Lawrence, J.C., Wound infection under occlusive dressings, *J. Hosp. Infect.,* 17, 83–94, 1991.

74. Hutchinson, J.J., Infection under occlusion, *Ostomy Wound Manage.,* 40, 28–30, 32–33, 1994.

75. Cherry, G.W., Ryan, T., and McGibbon, D., Trial of a new dressing in venous leg ulcers, *Practitioner,* 288, 1175–1178, 1984.

76. Mulder, G.D., Albert, S.F., and Grimwood, R.E., Clinical evaluation of a new occlusive hydrocolloid dressing, *Cutis,* 35, 396–397, 400, 1985.

77. van Rijswijk, L., Brown, D., Friedman, S., Degreef, H., Roed-Petersen, J., Borglund, E. et al., Multicenter clinical evaluation of a hydrocolloid dressing for leg ulcers, *Cutis,* 35, 173–176, 1985.

78. Groenewald, J.H., Comparative effects of HCD and conventional treatment on the healing of venous ulcers, in *An Environment for Healing: The Role of Occlusion,* Ryan, T.J., Ed., Royal Society of Medicine, London, 1985, 105–109.

79. Ohlsson, P., Larsson, K., Lindholm, C., and Moller, M., A cost-effectiveness study of leg ulcer treatment in primary care. Comparison of saline-gauze and hydrocolloid treatment in a prospective, randomized study, *Scand. J. Prim. Health Care,* 12, 295–299, 1994.

80. Eriksson, G., Comparison of two occlusive bandages in the treatment of venous leg ulcers, *Br. J. Dermatol.,* 114, 227–230, 1986.

81. Handfield-Jones, S.E., Grattan, C.E., Simpson, R.A., and Kennedy, C.T., Comparison of a hydrocolloid dressing and paraffin gauze in the treatment of venous ulcers, *Br. J. Dermatol.,* 118, 425–427, 1988.

82. Winter, A. and Hewitt, H., Testing a hydrocolloid, *Nurs. Times,* 86, 59–61, 1990.

83. Arnold, T.E., Stanley, J.C., Fellows, E.P., Moncada, G.A., Allen, R., Hutchinson, J.J. et al., Prospective, multicenter study of managing lower extremity venous ulcers, *Ann. Vasc. Surg.,* 8, 356–362, 1994.

84. Rainey, J., A comparison of two dressings in the treatment of heavily exuding leg ulcers, *J. Wound Care,* 2, 199–200, 1993.

85. Backhouse, C.M., Blair, S.D., Savage, A.P., Walton, J., and McCollum, C.N., Controlled trial of occlusive dressings in healing chronic venous ulcers, *Br. J. Surg.,* 74, 626–627, 1987.

86. Moffatt, C.J., A trial of a hydrocolloid dressing in the management of indolent ulceration, *J. Wound Care,* 1(3), 20–22, 1992.

87. Yarkony, G.M., Kramer, E., King, R., Lukanc, C., and Carle, T.V., Pressure sore management: efficacy of a moisture reactive occlusive dressing, *Arch. Phys. Med. Rehabil.,* 65, 597–600, 1984.

88. Tudhope, M., Management of pressure ulcers with a hydrocolloid occlusive dressing: results in twenty-three patients, *J. Enterostom. Ther.,* 11, 102–105, 1984.

89. van Rijswijk, L., Full-thickness pressure ulcers: patient and wound healing characteristics, *Decubitus,* 6, 16–21, 1993.

90. Gorse, G.J. and Messner, R.L., Improved pressure sore healing with hydrocolloid dressings, *Arch. Dermatol.,* 123, 766–771, 1987.

91. Alm, A., Hornmark, A.M., Fall, P.A., Linder, L., Bergstrand, B., Ehrnebo, M. et al., Care of pressure sores: a controlled study of the use of a hydrocolloid dressing compared with wet saline gauze compresses, *Acta Dermatol. Venereol. Suppl. (Stockh.),* 149, 1–10, 1989.

92. Colwell, J.C., Foreman, M.D., and Trotter, J.P., A comparison of the efficacy and cost-effectiveness of two methods of managing pressure ulcers, *Decubitus,* 6, 28–36, 1993.

93. Xakellis, G.C. and Chrischilles, E.A., Hydrocolloid versus saline-gauze dressings in treating pressure ulcers: a cost-effectiveness analysis, *Arch. Phys. Med. Rehabil.,* 73, 463–469, 1992.

94. Chang, K.W., Alsagoff, S., Ong, K.T., and Sim, P.H., Pressure ulcers — randomised controlled trial comparing hydrocolloid and saline gauze dressings, *Med. J. Malaysia,* 53, 428–431, 1998.

95. Foster, A.V.M., Spencer, S., and Edmonds, M.E., Deterioration of diabetic foot lesions under hydrocolloid dressings, *Pract. Diabetes Int.,* 14, 62–64, 1997.

96. Laing, P., Diabetic foot ulcers, *Am. J. Surg.,* 167, 31S–36S, 1994.

97. Gill, D., The use of hydrocolloids in the treatment of diabetic foot, *J. Wound Care,* 8, 204–206, 1999.

98. Michel, L., Use of hydrocolloid dressing following wide excision of perianal hidradenitis suppurativa, in *An Environment for Healing: The Role of Occlusion,* Ryan, T.J., Ed., Royal Society of Medicine, London, 1985, pp. 143–148.

99. Hulten, L., Wound dressing after colorectal surgery, in *An Environment for Healing: The Role of Occlusion,* Ryan, T.J., Ed., Royal Society of Medicine, London, 1985, pp. 149–151.

100. Young, R.A.L. and Weston-Davies, W.H., Comparison of a hydrocolloid dressing and a conventional island dressing as a primary surgical wound dressing, in *An Environment for Healing: The Role of Occlusion,* Ryan, T.J., Ed., Royal Society of Medicine, London, 1985, pp. 153–156.

101. Ashford, R.L. and Fullerton, C., The use of Granuflex Extra Thin (hydrocolloid) dressing on partial and total nail avulsions — clinical observations, *JBPM,* 190–192, October 1991.

102. Alsbjorn, B.F., Ovesen, H., and Walther-Larsen, S., Occlusive dressing versus petroleum gauze on drainage wounds, *Acta Chir. Scand.,* 156, 211–213, 1990.

103. Field, F.K. and Kerstein, M.D., Overview of wound healing in a moist environment, *Am. J. Surg.,* 167, 2S–6S, 1994.

104. Thomas, S., Banks, V., Bale, S., Fear-Price, M., Hagelstein, S., Harding, K.G. et al., A comparison of two dressings in the management of chronic wounds, *J. Wound Care,* 6, 383–386, 1997.

105. Bale, S., Squires, D., Varnon, T., Walker, A., Benbow, M., and Harding, K.G., A comparison of two dressings in pressure sore management, *J. Wound Care,* 6, 463–466, 1997.

106. Bale, S., Hagelstein, S., Banks, V., and Harding, K.G., Costs of dressings in the community, *J. Wound Care,* 7, 327–330, 1998.

107. Seeley, J., Jensen, J.L., and Hutcherson, J., A randomized clinical study comparing a hydrocellular dressing to a hydrocolloid dressing in the management of pressure ulcers, *Ostomy Wound Manage.,* 45, 39–44, 46–47, 1999.

108. Moffatt, C., The principles of assessment prior to compression therapy, *J. Wound Care,* 7, suppl 6–9, 1998.

109. Thomas, S., Atraumatic dressings, *World Wide Wounds,* 2003, http://www.worldwidewounds.com/2003/january/Thomas/Atraumatic-Dressings.html.

110. Dykes, P.J., Heggie, R., and Hill, S.A., Effects of adhesive dressings on the stratum corneum of the skin, *J. Wound Care,* 10, 7–10, 2001.

111. Vloemans, A.F. and Kreis, R.W., Fixation of skin grafts with a new silicone rubber dressing (Mepitel), *Scand. J. Plast. Reconstr. Surg. Hand Surg.,* 28, 75–76, 1994.

112. Platt, A.J., Phipps, A., and Judkins, K., A comparative study of silicone net dressing and paraffin gauze dressing in skin-grafted sites, *Burns,* 22, 543–545, 1996.

113. Dahlstrøm, K.K., A new silicone rubber dressing used as a temporary dressing before delayed split skin grafting. A prospective randomised study, *Scand. J. Plast. Reconstr. Surg. Hand Surg.,* 29, 325–327, 1995.

114. Gotschall, C.S., Morrison, M.I., and Eichelberger, M.R., Prospective, randomized study of the efficacy of Mepitel on children with partial-thickness scalds, *J. Burn Care Rehabil.,* 19, 279–283, 1998.

115. Bugmann, P., Taylor, S., Gyger, D., Lironi, A., Genin, B., Vunda, A. et al., A silicone-coated nylon dressing reduces healing time in burned paediatric patients in comparison with standard sulfadiazine treatment: a prospective randomized trial, *Burns,* 24, 609–612, 1998.

116. Hermans, M.H.E. and Hermans, R.P., Preliminary report on the use of a new hydro-colloid dressing in the treatment of burns, *Burns Incl. Therm. Inj.,* 11, 125–129, 1984.

117. Wyatt, D., McGowan, D.N., and Najarian, M.P., Comparison of a hydrocolloid dressing and silver sulfadiazine cream in the outpatient management of second-degree burns, *J. Trauma,* 30, 857–865, 1990.

118. Wright, A., MacKechnie, D.W., and Paskins, J.R., Management of partial thickness burns with Granuflex "E" dressings, *Burns,* 19, 128–130, 1993.

119. Biltz, H., Comparison of hydrocolloid dressing and saline gauze in the treatment of skin graft donor sites, in *An Environment for Healing: The Role of Occlusion,* Ryan, T.J., Ed., Royal Society of Medicine, London, 1985, pp. 125–128.

120. Madden, M.R., Nolan, E., Finkelstein, J.L., Yurt, R.W., Smeland, J., Goodwin, C.W. et al., Comparison of an occlusive and a semi-occlusive dressing and the effect of the wound exudate upon keratinocyte proliferation, *J. Trauma,* 29, 924–930, discussion 930–931, 1989.

121. Doherty, C., Lynch, G., and Noble, S., Granuflex hydrocolloid as a donor site dressing, *Care Crit. Ill,* 2, 193–194, 1986.

122. Leicht, P., Siim, E., Dreyer, M., and Larsen, T.K., Duoderm application on scalp donor sites in children, *Burns,* 17, 230–232, 1991.

123. Porter, J.M., A comparative investigation of re-epithelialisation of split skin graft donor areas after application of hydrocolloid and alginate dressings, *Br. J. Plast. Surg.,* 44, 333–337, 1991.

124. Knapman, L. and Bache, J., Hydrocolloid dressings in accident and emergency, *Nurs. Stand. Spec. Suppl.,* 6, 8–11, 1989.

125. Andersson, A.P., Puntervold, T., and Warburg, F.E., Treatment of excoriations with a transparent hydrocolloid dressing: a prospective study, *Injury,* 22, 429–430, 1991.

126. Hermans, M.H., Hydrocolloid dressing versus tulle gauze in the treatment of abrasions in cyclists, *Int. J. Sports Med.,* 12, 581–584, 1991.

127. Hazen, P.G., Grey, R., and Antonyzyn, M., Management of lacerations in sports: use of a biosynthetic dressing during competitive wrestling, *Cutis,* 56, 301–303, 1995.

128. Heffernan, A. and Martin, A.J., A comparison of a modified form of Granuflex (Granuflex Extra Thin) and a conventional dressing in the management of lacerations, abrasions and minor operation wounds in an accident and emergency department, *J. Accid. Emerg. Med.,* 11, 227–230, 1994.

129. Hedman, L.A., Effect of a hydrocolloid dressing on the pain level from abrasions on the feet during intensive marching, *Mil. Med.,* 153, 188–190, 1988.

130. Knapik, J.J., Reynolds, K.L., Duplantis, K.L., and Jones, B.H., Friction blisters. Pathophysiology, prevention and treatment, *Sports Med.,* 20, 136–147, 1995.

131. Forshaw, A. Hydrocolloid dressings in paediatric wound care, *J. Wound Care,* 2, 209–212, 1993.
132. Schmitt, M., Vergnes, P., Canarelli, J.P., Gaillard, S., Daoud, S., Dodat, H. et al., Evaluation of a hydrocolloid dressing, *J. Wound Care,* 5, 396–399, 1996.
133. Rasmussen, H., Larsen, M.J., and Skeie, E., Surgical wound dressing in outpatient paediatric surgery. A randomised study, *Dan. Med. Bull.,* 40, 252–254, 1993.
134. Margolin, S.G., Breneman, J.C., Denman, D.L., LaChapelle, P., Weckbach, L., and Aron, B.S., Management of radiation-induced moist skin desquamation using hydro-colloid dressing [published erratum appears in *Cancer Nurs.,* 13, 267, 1990], *Cancer Nurs.,* 13, 71–80, 1990.
135. Mak, S.S., Molassiotis, A., Wan, W.M., Lee, I.Y., and Chan, E.S., The effects of hydrocolloid dressing and gentian violet on radiation-induced moist desquamation wound healing, *Cancer Nurs.,* 23, 220–229, 2000.
136. Butcher, G. and Woods, H.F., Geliperm as a molecular carrier, in Woods, H.F. and Cottier, D., Eds., *Geliperm: A Clear Advance in Wound Healing, Proceedings of a Conference,* Oxford, 1983, pp. 77–87.
137. Gilbert, E.C. and Schenk, W.N., Hydrogel dressings 1: physical attributes of a new absorbent wound dressing with unique fluid management characteristics, *Wounds,* 1, 198–208, 1989.
138. Queen, D., Evans, J.H., Gaylor, J.D., Courtney, J.M., and Reid, W.H., The physical effects of an adhesive dressing top layer on burn wound dressings, *Burns Incl. Therm. Inj.,* 12, 351–356, 1986.
139. Mandy, S.H., A new primary wound dressing made of polyethylene oxide gel, *J. Dermatol. Surg. Oncol.,* 9, 153–155, 1983.
140. Smith, R., Dermabrasion. Is it an option? *Aust. Fam. Phys.,* 26, 1041–1044, 1997.
141. Strunk, B. and Maher, K., Collaborative nurse management of multifactorial moist desquamation in a patient undergoing radiotherapy, *J. ET Nurs.,* 20, 152–157, 1993.
142. Breuton, R.N., The effect of ultrasound on the repair of a rabbit's tibial osteotomy held in rigid external fixation, *Bone Joint Surg.,* 69, 494, 1987.
143. Breuton, R.N. and Campbell, B., The use of Geliperm as a sterile coupling agent for therapeutic ultrasound, *Physiotherapy,* 73, 653–654, 1987.
144. Duke, D. and Grevelink, J.M., Care before and after laser skin resurfacing. A survey and review of the literature, *Dermatol. Surg.,* 24, 201–206, 1998.
145. Newman, J.P., Koch, R.J., and Goode, R.L., Closed dressings after laser skin resur-facing, *Arch. Otolaryngol. Head Neck Surg.,* 124, 751–757, 1998.
146. Ricketts, C.H., Martin, L., Faria, D.T., Saed, G.M., and Fivenson, D.P., Cytokine mRNA changes during the treatment of hypertrophic scars with silicone and non-silicone gel dressings, *Dermatol. Surg.,* 22, 955–959, 1996.
147. Corkhill, P.H., Hamilton, C.J., and Tighe, B.J., Synthetic hydrogels. VI. Hydrogel composites as wound dressings and implant materials, *Biomaterials,* 10, 3–10, 1989.
148. Lawrence, J.C., The effect of bacteria and their products on the healing of skin wounds, in *A Biological Approach to the Wound Healing Process, Proceedings of a Symposium, Royal College of Physicians, 5 June 1987,* Rue, Y., Ed., Medifax, London, 1987, pp. 9–21.
149. Lowbury, E.J.L. and Cason, J.S., Aspects of infection control and skin grafting in burned patients, in *Wound Care,* Westaby, S., Ed., Heinemann Medical, London, 1985, pp. 171–189.
150. Close-Tweedie, J., The role of povidone–iodine in podiatric chronic wound care, *J. Wound Care,* 10, 339–342, 2001.

151. Gilchrist, B., Should iodine be reconsidered in wound management? *J. Wound Care,* 6, 148–150, 1997.

152. Iodine-containing Pharmaceuticals: A Reappraisal, Proceedings of the 6th European Conference on Advances in Wound Management, Macmillan Magazines, 1997.

153. Zhou, L.H., Nahm, W.K., Badiavas, E., Yufit, T., and Falanga, V., Slow release iodine preparation and wound healing: *in vitro* effects consistent with lack of *in vivo* toxicity in human chronic wounds, *Br. J. Dermatol.,* 146, 365–374, 2002.

154. Moberg, S., Hoffman, L., Grennert, M., and Holst, A., A randomised trial of cadexomer iodine in decubitus ulcers, *Am. Geriatr. Soc.,* 31, 462–465, 1983.

155. Skog, E., Arnesjö, B., Troëng, T., Gjöres, J.E., Bergljung, L., Gundersen, J., Hallböök, T., Hessmann, Y., Hillström, L., Månsson, T., Eilard, U., Eklöff, B., Plate, G., and Norgren, L., A randomized trial comparing cadexomer iodine and standard treatment in the out-patient management of chronic venous ulcers, *Br. J. Dermatol.,* 109, 77–83, 1983.

156. Hansson, C., The effects of cadexomer iodine paste in the treatment of venous leg ulcers compared with hydrocolloid dressing and paraffin gauze dressing. Cadexomer Iodine Study Group, *Int. J. Dermatol.,* 37, 390–396, 1998.

157. Bradley, M., Cullum, N., and Sheldon, T., *The Debridement of Chronic Wounds: A Systematic Review,* Core Research, Alton, UK, 1999.

158. Bianchi, J., Cadexomer–iodine in the treatment of venous leg ulcers: what is the evidence? *J. Wound Care,* 10, 225–229, 2001.

159. Russell, A.D. and Hugo, W.B., Antimicrobial activity and action of silver, in *Progress in Medicinal Chemistry,* Ellis, G.P. and Luscombe, D.K., Eds., Elsevier Science, Amsterdam, 1994, pp. 351–369.

160. Lansdown, A.B., Silver. 1: its antibacterial properties and mechanism of action, *J. Wound Care,* 11, 125–130, 2002.

161. Lansdown, A.B. Silver. 2: toxicity in mammals and how its products aid wound repair, *J. Wound Care,* 11, 173–177, 2002.

162. White, R.J., An historical overview of the use of silver in modern wound management, *Br. J. Nurs.,* 10, 3–8, 2002.

163. Frost, M., Jackson, S., and Stevens, P., Adsorption of bacteria onto activated charcoal cloth: an effect of potential importance in the treatment of infected wounds, *Microbios Lett.,* 13, 135–140, 1980.

164. Tredget, E.E., Shankowsky, H.A., Groeneveld, A., and Burrell, R., A matched-pair, randomized study evaluating the efficacy and safety of Acticoat silver-coated dressing for the treatment of burn wounds, *J. Burn Care Rehabil.,* 19, 531–537, 1998.

165. Wright, J.B., Lam, K., and Burrell, R.E., Wound management in an era of increasing bacterial antibiotic resistance: a role for topical silver treatment, *Am. J. Infect. Control,* 26, 572–577, 1998.

166. Burrell, R.E., Heggers, J.P., Davis, G.J., and Wright, J.B., Efficacy of silver-coated dressings as bacterial barriers in a rodent burn sepsis model, *Wounds Compend. Clin. Res. Pract.,* 11, 464–471, 1999.

167. Wright, J.B., Lam, K., Hansen, D., and Burrell, R.E., Efficacy of topical silver against fungal burn wound pathogens, *Am. J. Infect. Control,* 27, 344–350, 1999.

168. Yin, H.Q., Langford, R., and Burrell, R.E., Comparative evaluation of the antimicrobial activity of ACTICOAT antimicrobial barrier dressing, *J. Burn Care Rehabil.,* 20, 195–200, 1999.

169. Innes, M.E., Umraw, N., Fish, J.S., Gomez, M., and Cartotto, R.C., The use of silver coated dressings on donor site wounds: a prospective, controlled matched pair study, *Burns,* 27, 621–627, 2001.

170. Thomas, S. and McCubbin, P., An *in vitro* analysis of the antimicrobial properties of ten silver-containing dressings, *J. Wound Care,* 12(8), 305–308, 2003.

171. Harding, K.G., Cherry, G., Dealey, C., and Turner, T.D., Eds., Psychological consquences arising from the malodours produced by skin ulcers, *Proceedings of 2nd European Conference on Advances in Wound Management,* Harrogate. Macmillan Magazines Ltd., Harrogate, UK, 1992.

172. Moss, C.W., Dees, S.B., and Guerrant, G.O., Gas chromatography of bacterial fatty acids with a fused silica capillary column, *J. Clin. Microbiol.,* 28, 80–85, 1974.

173. Parry, A.D., Chadwick, P.R., Simon, D., Oppenheim, B., and McCollum, C.N., Leg ulcer odour detection identifies beta-haemolytic streptococcal infection, *J. Wound Care,* 4, 404–406, 1995.

174. Brennan, S.S., Foster, M.E., and Leaper, D.J., Antiseptic toxicity in wounds healing by secondary intention, *J. Hosp. Infect.,* 8, 263–267, 1986.

175. Brennan, S.S. and Leaper, D.J., The effect of antiseptics on the healing wound: a study using the rabbit ear chamber, *Br. J. Surg.,* 72, 780–782, 1985.

176. Thomas, S. and Hay, N.P., The antimicrobial properties of two metronidazole medicated dressings used to treat malodorous wounds, *Pharm. J.,* 264–266, Mar. 2, 1991.

177. Hampson, J.P., The use of metronidazole in the treatment of malodorous wounds, *J. Wound Care,* 5, 421–426, 1996.

178. Chirife, J., *In-vitro* study of bacterial growth inhibition in concentrated sugar solutions: microbiological basis for the use of sugar in treating infected wounds, *Antimicrob. Agents Chemother.,* 23, 766–773, 1983.

179. Thomas, S., Jones, M., Shutler, S., and Jones, S., Using larvae in modern wound management, *J. Wound Care,* 5, 60–69, 1996.

180. Evans, H., A treatment of last resort, *Nurs. Times,* 93, 62–64, 65, 1997.

181. Butcher, G., Butcher, J.A., and Maggs, F.A.P., The treatment of malodorous wounds, *Nurs. Mirror,* 142, 76, 1976.

Part V

New Approaches to Understanding and Treating Wounds

13 Gene Therapy of Wounds

Jeffrey M. Davidson

CONTENTS

13.1 INTRODUCTION

Genetic manipulation of cells and tissues shows enormous promise for correcting a myriad of metabolic disorders. Many of the concerns about this medical approach arise from strategies in which permanent genetic alterations are made in the target cell. Gene therapy of wounds, on the other hand, can be in the form of *gene medicine*, in which short-term and/or highly regulated expression occurs from genes specifically targeted to the wound site. Given the local and transitory nature of the wound, gene medicine has the potential to fulfill several unmet needs in wound care.

This chapter will address a number of important aspects of the use of genes in tissue repair, including different technologies for gene introduction, transient versus stable expression, control of expression, selection of candidate genes for clinical applications, and the merger of gene transfer techniques with tissue engineering.

No human clinical data exist on the effect of gene medicine on wound repair, though a U.S. National Institutes of Health (NIH)-sponsored clinical trial is scheduled to begin in 2003.[1] This study will be based on the use of the most potent expression vector, adenovirus, and the only gene product shown to be clinically effective in wound healing, platelet-derived growth factor (PDGF).[2] The development of these studies is founded on a considerable amount of information obtained from animal models using a variety of vectors and cDNAs.

13.2 GENE TRANSFER STRATEGIES

The simplest approach for gene transfer is the administration of naked plasmid DNA that encodes a growth factor cDNA, in which transcription from the cDNA is driven by a strong (viral) promoter that would be predicted to be active in most somatic cells. Early studies in skeletal muscle had suggested that persistent expression might be possible. However, neither the dermis not the epidermis will readily take up and express naked DNA using normal doses. Success has nevertheless been obtained by loading experimental wounds with repeated microgram doses of plasmid DNA-encoding genes such as fibroblast growth factor-2 (FGF-2).[3] The efficiency of the uptake is very low. Others have reported an enhancement of DNA uptake by incorporating the DNA into liposomes that act as carriers to bring DNA in association with the plasma membrane where uptake is facilitated.[4–6] This is a common approach for delivering DNA to cultured cells, but the efficiency is quite low. Only a few studies have adopted this strategy.

A technology for introducing DNA into plant cells — the gene gun — was devised to overcome the presence of a durable cell wall.[7] This device is essentially a micro-shotgun that uses an explosive discharge to propel DNA bound to dense gold microparticles inside of cells. Two groups used this device to show that when the propulsion was optimized to target the basal keratinocyte layer of the epidermis, biological effects were maximized. Success in wound repair was initially obtained with epidermal growth factor (EGF),[8] and later with transforming growth factor-β (TGF-β) and PDGF.[9,10] These genes brought about more rapid wound closure or increasing wound strength, depending on the models. They also showed that remarkably little protein was needed to create these effects when it came from an internal source rather than a topical application. Gene transfer to wounds is probably 1000-fold more efficient than protein therapy.

Since these initial reports, a number of other genes have been applied with the gene gun. The advantages of the technology are that the preparation of the loaded particles is very simple and rapid. A candidate gene can be tested *in vivo* very shortly after its cloning. Thus, the cost of vector development and preparation — aside from the initial investment in the gene gun device — is low. Expression in the basal keratinocytes that are targeted by the gene gun is short lived. This is due to the use of naked DNA, which is rapidly degraded in the target cell and to the fact that nearly all the target cells proceed through differentiation and transit through the upper epidermal layers to be shed in a matter of days from the stratum corneum. From the perspective of gene medicine, this is a desirable feature, because the dose is relatively short lived. However, the target area in the present configuration of the gene gun is relatively small, so multiple applications might be needed for large wounds. In addition, the propulsion of the gold particles does cause some transient tissue damage. The significant limitations of the gene gun are its targeting efficiency (about 10% of basal keratinocytes) and the loss of efficiency with deeper penetration because of the relative sparseness of cells in the dermis. Because of the low efficiency, the gene gun functions best for expression of secreted molecules that can then diffuse away to reach other targets. Development of the device for DNA vaccination has continued. However, it has permitted us to screen dozens of candidate genes for wound healing in a relatively short time.

The natural system for introducing DNA into cells is the virus. These infectious organisms have developed a DNA packaging and delivery system without equal. In addition, various viral types have evolved to usurp various aspects of the cellular machinery. Adenovirus has been at the forefront of gene delivery for many years

TABLE 13.1
Gene Delivery Methods

	Advantages	Disadvantages	Persistence Time	Method of Introduction
Naked DNA	Low cost	Low efficiency	Up to 14 days	Injection or implantation
Liposomes	Moderate cost	Low efficiency	Up to 14 days	Injection
Gene gun	Moderate cost	Moderate efficiency; tissue damage; area of coverage	Up to 6 days	Surface shot
Electroporation	Moderate cost	Few examples with skin	Up to 14 days	Injection plus electrical pulse
Adenovirus	High efficiency; transient expression; no chromosomal integration	Immune response; lower DNA capacity; theoretical potential for recombination	Up to 2 weeks	Injection or topical application
Adeno-associated virus	Good efficiency and infects nondividing and dividing cells	Low insert size capacity; stable integration not optimal for transient therapy	Months	Injection
Retrovirus	Stable expression	Only infects dividing cells; stable integration not optimal for transient therapy	Months	Injection
Nanoparticles	Targets phagocytes as well as tissue cells; sustained release	Complex formulation; slow release may not be desired	Weeks to months	Injection

because of its ability to infect a wide variety of cell types independent of their replicative state. In its current configuration for gene therapy applications, the virus that is introduced is engineered to be incapable of replication, and its genome is "gutted" to the extent that only genes essential for viral gene expression are packaged into the viral particles. Thus, new viral particles can only be produced in "packaging" cells that contain additional viral genes necessary to assemble the viral core and envelope into infectious particles. The adenoviral system has high infective efficiency because its surface is decorated with envelope proteins that specifically interact with cell surface receptors, and the binding reaction triggers internalization into a nonlysosomal pathway. This mechanism assures that the viral DNA and proteins will not be rapidly degraded. Indeed, incorporation of adenoviral coat proteins into DNA-containing liposomes can also enhance uptake markedly. Virally expressed genes from adenovirus will continue to be expressed for 7 to 14 d in the usual cellular environment. This property of limited duration is also consistent with the gene medicine approach.

Adenoviral gene delivery has been shown to be a potent delivery system for wound repair. PDGF delivery produces a remarkably strong response in the rabbit ear ulcer model, for example.[11,12] The adenoviral system is not without drawbacks. Viral coat proteins are strong antigens that can provoke a primary inflammatory response and possible immune reactivity. Systemic delivery of adenoviral vectors, even of the most sophisticated design, can cause undesirable reactions. However, the viral load likely needed for efficacy in human clinical studies should not result in a large systemic effect. In addition, the wound site is inherently an inflammatory region, so the small increment induced by adenovirus may not be harmful in comparison to the large effects exerted by the target gene.[13] Although the chances of adenoviral genes becoming integrated into the genome is low, there is a theoretical possibility that genetic recombination could occur anytime DNA is introduced into cells, not only between the viral and host genomes, but also between the therapeutic virus and a wild-type adenoviral infection.

In an effort to overcome collateral effects of (systemic) adenoviral therapy, adeno-associated virus (AAV) has been under investigation as a gene delivery system.[14,15] The inflammatory response to these vectors is much lower than that to adenovirus; however, these virions can only accept a small load of foreign DNA, and their propagation requires the presence of a helper virus. Unlike adenovirus genes, which are not incorporated into host DNA, AAV viral DNA does undergo site-specific integration into human chromosome 19. Thus, AAV-inserted genes will be expressed for extended amounts of time. It might be argued that chronic defects in angiogenesis, such as seen in diabetes, might benefit from sustained expression of a transgene. Technical challenges to the use of this virus include the efficient removal of the more toxic helper adenovirus and the small amount of genetic information that can be stuffed into the viral genome.

Another potential candidate for gene delivery in skin might be herpes virus, which contains a very large viral genome, making it potentially able to deliver very large or multiple genes.[16,17] Initial studies on skin transfection reported some undesirable inflammatory responses. Herpes virus exposure leads to a lifelong latent infection of target cells, largely neuronal. Recent innovations in the development of herpes vectors that do not express viral proteins and do not replicate may offer another means of introducing foreign DNA into selected cells at the wound site.

Retroviruses have been advocated as gene therapy agents, particularly for situations in which permanent transformation of the local genome is desired. In this system, the viral genome is a single-stranded ribonucleic acid (RNA) molecule that is reverse-transcribed to yield cellular DNA-containing sequences (long terminal repeats) that promote integration of the viral genome into the host DNA. In wild-type virus, further replication and packaging of virions may be directed from newly integrated host DNA sequences. Since this type of infection can, in theory, be used for stable transformation of the genome, it is more important as an approach to correct inborn errors of metabolism due to a null allele. However, viral gene expression is often silenced within several months, possibly by methylation and other mechanisms that alter DNA structure and function. With respect to wound healing, this could be advantageous. As with the adenoviral vectors, retroviral genomes can be radically trimmed to restrict genomic recombination to the gene of interest. The most commonly used vector has been the Moloney murine leukemia virus.[18-20]

The lentiviruses are a subset of retroviruses that include the simian and human immunodeficiency viruses.[20] These have recently been developed into useful gene vectors by using a two-plasmid transfection system together with 293T cells that contain the viral packaging genes. Lentivirus has the potential advantage of no requirement for dividing cells. These virions appear to have a much lower inflammatory activity than adenovirus does. Although stable expression should not be needed for wound therapy, modified lentiviral vectors with regulatory elements could be a useful gene delivery system.

If one has a permanently embedded gene, how could it be eliminated or controlled to avoid excess repair or even malignant changes? Several possibilities exist. Perhaps the simplest is to control the expression of the target gene with a molecule that does not exist in the host. The insect hormone ecdysone is useful for experimental systems. A key issue for the skin is to be able to use a stimulus that can penetrate the epidermis. Other investigators have developed regulatory systems with progesterone.[21] It is also possible to engineer genes that can be forced to undergo a rearrangement that either activates or inactivates their expression. Tetracycline response systems show promise in this application.[22–24] The challenge is to control the "leakiness" of the regulation. Depending on the application, one may require 10^2, 10^3, or 10^4-fold differential expression between the on and off states of a therapeutic gene.

There are other novel methods of gene introduction. Electroporation relies upon one or more electrical pulses to produce temporary holes or pores in the plasma membrane of targeted cells.[24] It is a technique commonly used with single cells, but instrumentation has been adapted to living tissue. The technique can significantly enhance the extent of uptake of naked DNA in the liver. While the method would not be effective on skin with an intact epidermal barrier, open wounds should certainly be amenable to the technique.

Nanoparticles are structures composed of a variety of polymers that have subcellular dimensions. For this reason, they can be readily engulfed by cells. Furthermore, nanoparticles can be coated with molecules that enhance cell/receptor mediated uptake. Recent findings from this laboratory have shown that plasmid uptake is prolonged by nanoparticle encapsulation, and even adenoviral uptake is enhanced.

Microseeding is another physical technique that functions much like a multi-headed tattoo gun to introduce DNA into target tissues.[25,26] Unlike the gene gun, this device has the potential of delivering DNA solutions more deeply into the skin, and no particulate carrier is required. The efficiency may be comparable to other physical techniques, and the localization of therapy could be quite precise because of the mechanical nature of the delivery system.

13.3 GENES WITH WOUND-HEALING EFFECTS

The first wave of effector genes that was validated with gene therapy techniques consisted of well-defined growth factors whose action had already been established by protein therapy. These were all secreted proteins. Even if transfection efficiency (proportion of cells expressing the transgene product) is low, these products would be expected to act in a paracrine fashion on nearby untransfected cells. Among these

TABLE 13.2
Genes with Wound Healing Activity

	Model	Effects	Vector	Method of Introduction
Epidermal growth factor	Porcine excision	Wound resurfacing	DNA plasmid	Gene gun
Transforming growth factor-β1	Rat incisions and sponge implants	Increased tensile strength and collagen content	DNA plasmid	Gene gun
Fibroblast growth factor (acidic)	Rat incisions	Increased tensile strength	DNA plasmid	Repeated injection
Platelet derived growth factor	Rat incisions	Increased tensile strength	DNA plasmid	Gene gun
	Rabbit ear excisions	Granulation tissue, wound closure, and reepithelization	Adenovirus	Injection
	Ischemic rabbit ear excision	Granulation tissue, wound closure, and reepithelization	DNA plasmid	Collagen matrix
Insulin-like growth factor- I	Rat thermal burns	Reepithelization	DNA plasmid	Liposome injection
Hepatocyte growth factor/scatter factor	Mouse excisional wounds	Wound closure and reepithelization	DNA plasmid	Injection of virus-conjugated liposomes
Vascular endothelial growth factor	Ischemic flap	Increased survival	DNA plasmid	Arterial injection of liposomes
	Rabbit ear ischemic incisions	Increased granulation tissue	Retrovirus	Dermal equivalent with stably transformed fibroblasts
	Diabetic mouse excisions	Wound closure	Adenovirus	Direct injection
	Laparotomy closure	Increased strength	Adenovirus	Microfiber collagen sponges
Inducible nitric oxide synthase	Rat sponge implants	Increased collagen content	DNA plasmid	Injection into sponge ± liposomes
EPS-8 (signal transduction)	Rat incisions and sponges	Increased collagen and tensile strength	DNA plasmid	Gene gun
	Rabbit excisions	Increased granulation, epithelization, closure	Adenovirus	Injection
Cardiac ankyrin repeat protein	Rabbit ear excision	Increased blood flow, granulation tissue	Adenovirus	Injection
Early growth response factor-1	Rat excision	Increased collagen, wound closure	DNA plasmid	Gene gun

activities were EGF,[8] PDGF,[10,19] TGF-β1,[9] and FGF-2.[3] More recently, this list has expanded to include vascular endothelial growth factor,[14,15,27,28] hepatocyte growth factor/scatter factor, insulin-like growth factor-1,[5,29] and keratinocyte growth factor.[4,30] In some cases, physiologically significant levels of protein produced by the transgene have been measured in the wound environment.

Gene therapy is certainly not limited to soluble mediators. Intracellular pathways can be modulated by gene transfer, and if the transfection method is efficient many cells in the target tissue will be affected. For example, it is possible to potentiate the effect of endogenous EGF ligands and exogenous EGF on porcine wound healing by transfecting skin cells with the corresponding EGF receptor.[31] Intracellular signal molecules such as transcription factors can also have positive effects.[32] This includes elements in the signal transduction pathway leading to activation of new genes. This effect can be elicited in the cytoplasm by gene transfer of epidermal growth factor receptor pathway substrate (EPS)-8 or early growth response factor-1. Nuclear signals can also have dramatic effects on tissue repair. We have recently determined that the transcription co-factor cardiac ankyrin repeat protein is a potent angiogenic agent in a variety of wound healing models.

In some cases, it may be desirable to attenuate rather than enhance gene expression. Several strategies for gene inhibition are available: antisense cDNA, dominant negative cDNA, antisense oligonucleotides, ribozymes, and most recently, small interfering RNA. With the exception of oligonucleotides and ribozymes, these forms can be expressed as gene products that are produced by the typical range of vector systems. Another strategy is the expression of soluble forms of receptors that compete for binding with the authentic cellular receptors.

A further application of gene transfer extends to the area of tissue engineering. This very much broadens the range of therapeutic possibilities, since defined cells can be transformed *ex vivo* under controlled conditions. One can thus develop engineered tissues in which every cell contains and expresses a transgene of choice. As with *in vivo* transfer technologies, this foreign gene can be placed under regulation by exogenous factors. Depending on the design of the tissue equivalent, implanted cells can be designed as permanent transplants or as temporary grafts. These tissue-engineered devices have great potential as delivery systems since single or multiple genes can be placed under precise control mechanisms. It is likely that a future generation of skin substitutes will consist of cell populations that express factors favorable to improved wound healing.[33–37] The technology for propagation of keratinocyte sheets is quite mature, and stable transformation of these cells has been accomplished by several different techniques. The two commercially available dermal equivalents (Dermagraft™ and Apligraf™) are likewise obvious candidates as platforms for delivery of beneficial, therapeutic gene products.[38–40] This list could also include peptides with broader therapeutic application, such as insulin and erythropoietin. An advantage of a skin implant would be the ability to excise the implant if needed.

ACKNOWLEDGMENT

Supported by NIH grant AG06528 and the Department of Veterans Affairs.

REFERENCES

1. Margolis, D.J., Crombleholme, T., and Herlyn, M., Clinical protocol: Phase I trial to evaluate the safety of H5.020CMV.PDGF-B for the treatment of a diabetic insensate foot ulcer, *Wound Repair Regen.,* 8, 480–493, 2000.

2. Ladin, D., Becaplermin gel (PDGF-BB) as topical wound therapy. Plastic Surgery Educational Foundation DATA Committee, *Plast. Reconstr. Surg.,* 105, 1230–1231, 2000.

3. Sun, L., Xu, L., Chang, H., Henry, F.A., Miller, R.M., Harmon, J.M., and Nielsen, T.B., Transfection with aFGF cDNA improves wound healing, *J. Invest. Dermatol.,* 108, 313–318, 1997.

4. Jeschke, M.G., Richter, G., Hofstadter, F., Herndon, D.N., Perez-Polo, J.R., and Jauch, K.W., Non-viral liposomal keratinocyte growth factor (KGF) cDNA gene transfer improves dermal and epidermal regeneration through stimulation of epithelial and mesenchymal factors, *Gene Ther.,* 9, 1065–1074, 2002.

5. Spies, M., Nesic, O., Barrow, R.E., Perez-Polo, J.R., and Herndon, D.N., Liposomal IGF-1 gene transfer modulates pro- and anti-inflammatory cytokine mRNA expression in the burn wound, *Gene Ther.,* 8, 1409–1415, 2001.

6. Yu, W.H., Kashani-Sabet, M., Liggitt, D., Moore, D., Heath, T.D., and Debs, R.J., Topical gene delivery to murine skin, *J. Invest. Dermatol.,* 112, 370–375, 1999.

7. Johnston, S.A. and Tang, D.C., The use of microparticle injection to introduce genes into animal cells *in vitro* and *in vivo, Genet. Eng.,* 15, 225–236, 1993.

8. Andree, C., Swain, W.F., Page, C.P., Macklin, M.D., Slama, J., Hatzis, D., and Eriksson, E., *In vivo* transfer and expression of a human epidermal growth factor gene accelerates wound repair, *Proc. Natl. Acad. Sci. U.S.A.,* 91, 12,188–12,192, 1994.

9. Benn, S.I., Whitsitt, J.S., Broadley, K.N., Nanney, L.B., Perkins, D., He, L., Patel, M., Morgan, J.R., Swain, W.F., and Davidson, J.M., Particle-mediated gene transfer with transforming growth factor-beta 1 cDNAs enhances wound repair in rat skin, *J. Clin. Invest.,* 98, 2894–2902, 1996.

10. Eming, S.A., Whitsitt, J.S., He, L., Krieg, T., Morgan, J.R., and Davidson, J.M., Particle-mediated gene transfer of PDGF isoforms promotes wound repair, *J. Invest. Dermatol.,* 112, 297–302, 1999.

11. Liechty, K.W., Nesbit, M., Herlyn, M., Radu, A., Adzick, N.S., and Crombleholme, T.M., Adenoviral-mediated overexpression of platelet-derived growth factor-B corrects ischemic impaired wound healing, *J. Invest. Dermatol.,* 113, 375–383, 1999.

12. Liechty, K.W., Sablich, T.J., Adzick, N.S., and Crombleholme, T.M., Recombinant adenoviral mediated gene transfer in ischemic impaired wound healing, *Wound Repair Regen.,* 7, 148–153, 1999.

13. Crombleholme, T.M., Adenoviral-mediated gene transfer in wound healing, *Wound Repair Regen.,* 8, 460–472, 2000.

14. Galeano, M., Deodato, B., Altavilla, D., Cucinotta, D., Arsic, N., Marini, H., Torre, V., Giacca, M., and Squadrito, F., Adeno-associated viral vector-mediated human vascular endothelial growth factor gene transfer stimulates angiogenesis and wound healing in the genetically diabetic mouse, *Diabetologia,* 46, 546–555, 2003.

15. Deodato, B., Arsic, N., Zentilin, L., Galeano, M., Santoro, D., Torre, V., Altavilla, D., Valdembri, D., Bussolino, F., Squadrito, F., and Giacca, M., Recombinant AAV vector encoding human VEGF165 enhances wound healing, *Gene Ther.,* 9, 777–785, 2002.

16. Kennedy, P.G., Potential use of herpes simplex virus (HSV) vectors for gene therapy of neurological disorders, *Brain,* 120, 1245–1259, 1997.
17. Lu, B., Federoff, H.J., Wang, Y., Goldsmith, L.A., and Scott, G., Topical application of viral vectors for epidermal gene transfer, *J. Invest. Dermatol.,* 108, 803–808, 1997.
18. Eming, S.A., Snow, R.G., Yarmush, M.L., and Morgan, J.R., Targeted expression of insulin-like growth factor to human keratinocytes: modification of the autocrine control of keratinocyte proliferation, *J. Invest. Dermatol.,* 107, 113–120, 1996.
19. Eming, S.A., Lee, J., Snow, R.G., Tompkins, R.G., Yarmush, M.L., and Morgan, J.R., Genetically modified human epidermis overexpressing PDGF-A directs the development of a cellular and vascular connective tissue stroma when transplanted to athymic mice — implications for the use of genetically modified keratinocytes to modulate dermal regeneration, *J. Invest. Dermatol.,* 105, 756–763, 1995.
20. Reiser, J., Harmison, G., Kluepfel-Stahl, S., Brady, R.O., Karlsson, S., and Schubert, M., Transduction of nondividing cells using pseudotyped defective high-titer HIV type 1 particles, *Proc. Natl. Acad. Sci. U.S.A.,* 93, 15,266–15,271, 1996.
21. Cao, T., Wang, X.J., and Roop, D.R., Regulated cutaneous gene delivery: the skin as a bioreactor, *Hum. Gene Ther.,* 11, 2297–2300, 2000.
22. Slama, J., Davidson, J.M., and Eriksson, E., Gene transfer in cutaneous wound healing, in *Wound Healing and the Skin,* Falanga, V., Ed., Martin Dunitz Press, London, 2000.
23. Yao, F., Svensjo, T., Winkler, T., Lu, M., Eriksson, C., and Eriksson, E., Tetracycline repressor, tetR, rather than the tetR-mammalian cell transcription factor fusion derivatives, regulates inducible gene expression in mammalian cells, *Hum. Gene Ther.,* 9, 1939–1950, 1998.
24. Cupp, C.L. and Bloom, D.C., Gene therapy, electroporation, and the future of wound-healing therapies, *Facial Plast. Surg.,* 18, 53–57, 2002.
25. Eriksson, E., Yao, F., Svensjo, T., Winkler, T., Slama, J., Macklin, M.D., Andree, C., McGregor, M., Hinshaw, V., and Swain, W.F., *In vivo* gene transfer to skin and wound by microseeding, *J. Surg. Res.,* 78, 85–91, 1998.
26. Eriksson, E., Gene transfer in wound healing, *Adv. Skin Wound Care,* 13 (2 Suppl), 20–22, 2000.
27. Isner, J.M., Pieczek, A., Schainfeld, R., Blair, R., Haley, L., Asahara, T., Rosenfield, K., Razvi, S., Walsh, K., and Symes, J.F., Clinical evidence of angiogenesis after arterial gene transfer of phVEGF165 in patient with ischaemic limb [see comments], *Lancet,* 348, 370–374, 1996.
28. Romano Di Peppe, S., Mangoni, A., Zambruno, G., Spinetti, G., Melillo, G., Napolitano, M., and Capogrossi, M.C., Adenovirus-mediated VEGF(165) gene transfer enhances wound healing by promoting angiogenesis in CD1 diabetic mice, *Gene Ther.,* 9, 1271–1277, 2002.
29. Gelse, K., von der Mark, K., Aigner, T., Park, J., and Schneider, H., Articular cartilage repair by gene therapy using growth factor-producing mesenchymal cells, *Arthritis Rheum.,* 48, 430–441, 2003.
30. Jeschke, M.G., Richter, G., Herndon, D.N., Geissler, E.K., Hartl, M., Hofstatter, F., Jauch, K.W., and Perez-Polo, J.R., Therapeutic success and efficacy of nonviral liposomal cDNA gene transfer to the skin *in vivo* is dose dependent, *Gene Ther.,* 8, 1777–1784, 2001.
31. Nanney, L.B., Paulsen, S., Davidson, M.K., Cardwell, N.L., Whitsitt, J.S., and Davidson, J.M., Boosting epidermal growth factor receptor expression by gene gun transfection stimulates epidermal growth *in vivo, Wound Repair Regen.,* 8, 117–127, 2000.

32. Bryant, M., Drew, G.M., Houston, P., Hissey, P., Campbell, C.J., and Braddock, M., Tissue repair with a therapeutic transcription factor, *Hum. Gene Ther.,* 11, 2143–2158, 2000.
33. Bevan, S., Martin, R., and McKay, I.A., The production and applications of genetically modified skin cells, *Biotechnol. Genet. Eng. Rev.,* 16, 231–256, 1999.
34. Breitbart, A.S., Mason, J.M., Urmacher, C., Barcia, M., Grant, R.T., Pergolizzi, R.G., and Grande, D.A., Gene-enhanced tissue engineering: applications for wound healing using cultured dermal fibroblasts transduced retrovirally with the PDGF-B gene, *Ann. Plast. Surg.,* 43, 632–639, 1999.
35. Eming, S.A., Medalie, D.A., Tompkins, R.G., Yarmush, M.L., and Morgan, J.R., Genetically modified human keratinocytes overexpressing PDGF-A enhance the performance of a composite skin graft, *Hum. Gene Ther.,* 9, 529–539, 1998.
36. Garlick, J.A. and Fenjves, E.S., Keratinocyte gene transfer and gene therapy, *Crit. Rev. Oral Biol. Med.,* 7, 204–221, 1996.
37. Hunziker, E.B., Articular cartilage repair: basic science and clinical progress. A review of the current status and prospects, *Osteoarthritis Cartilage,* 10, 432–463, 2002.
38. Bell, E., Ehrlich, H.P., Buttle, D.J., and Nakatsuji, T., Living tissue formed *in vitro* and accepted as skin-equivalent tissue of full thickness, *Science,* 211, 1052–1054, 1981.
39. Cooper, M.L., Hansbrough, J.F., Spielvogel, R.L., Cohen, R., Bartel, R.L., and Naughton, G., *In vivo* optimization of a living dermal substitute employing cultured human fibroblasts on a biodegradable polyglycolic acid or polyglactin mesh, *Biomaterials,* 12, 243–248, 1991.
40. Badiavas, E., Mehta, P.P., and Falanga, V., Retrovirally mediated gene transfer in a skin equivalent model of chronic wounds, *J. Dermatol. Sci.,* 13, 56–62, 1996.

14 Wound Bed Preparation

Kevin Donohue, Holly Rausch, and Vincent Falanga

CONTENTS

14.1 BACKGROUND

Wound bed preparation has been defined as the global management of wounds to accelerate endogenous healing or to facilitate the effectiveness of advanced therapeutic products.[1] This formal approach in chronic wound treatment compartmentalizes the critical steps in optimizing the wound bed while considering the universal needs of the wound. For the most part, wound bed preparation is being used to address two key needs of wound care. First, chronic wounds are quite distinct from acute wounds, and a formal approach to wound bed preparation aids in understanding chronic wounds and how best to treat them. Second, wounds slated for treatment with advanced therapies such as bioengineered skin and growth factors need to be optimally prepared to maximize their benefit; wound bed preparation lends itself well to this need.

14.1.1 ACUTE VS. CHRONIC

For many years, the clinical study of wounds focused primarily on acute wounds, with chronic wounds for the most part considered an afterthought. The course of events that is classically used to describe the wound healing process, (i.e., three phases: inflammatory, proliferative, and remodeling) is based on acute injury, for

0-8493-1561-1/04/$0.00+$1.50

example by scalpel or trauma. With this as the primary model, it was inevitable that therapeutic interventions for facilitating optimal wound healing were originally geared toward acute wounds. In time these therapies were applied to chronic wounds, and for the most part were beneficial. This approach, however, came with an inherent flaw; it failed to address features unique to chronic wounds. Take debridement as an example. In an acute wound, debridement by any method is viewed as occurring early in treatment, having a defined time frame, and resulting in a sustained revitalization of the wound bed. In chronic wounds, though, debridement tends not to remove the underlying pathology and commonly results in a benefit that proves only temporary; the reaccumulation of a "necrotic burden" occurs, with the wound returning to stagnancy. However, the chronic wound can be reinvigorated with subsequent debridements. This leads us to now realize the need/benefit of a "maintenance debridement" phase that may continue throughout the life of the wound.[1]

14.1.2 ADVANCED THERAPIES

Advanced therapies such as bioengineered skin and growth factors are in great part the catalyst for elevating wound bed preparation from routine practice to an area of distinction requiring careful clinical consideration and further analysis and investigation to improve upon current practices. These therapies achieve their maximum benefit when the wound bed is adequately prepared.[2] As these products came into use, it was realized that for them to survive and advance the field of wound healing, wound bed preparation would need to become a widely recognized clinical concept. As it turns out, basic steps taken to ensure appropriate wound bed preparation help greatly in stimulating healing of all types of wounds. Wound bed preparation has encouraged improvements in old therapies and discovery of new ones, overall resulting in better wound care. This has created a revolution of sorts for the field of wound care. The potential for significant improvement in patient well-being based on new discoveries in wound bed preparation has made the science of chronic wounds one of the most exciting areas of research today.

14.2 INTRODUCTION

Wound bed preparation is not simply debridement of fibrinous and necrotic debris. In addition, we need to control exudate and bacterial burden. Also, we have started to consider the existence of a "cellular burden," comprised of phenotypically abnormal cells that undermine the ability of the wound to heal. Likewise, there is growing interest in the effectiveness and distribution of matrix metalloproteinases (MMPs).

Figure 14.1 provides a schematic overview of the features of chronic wounds that may impair healing, accompanied by corresponding therapeutic options.[3] It illustrates the complex interaction among multiple variables found in chronic wounds. On one side of the spectrum are basic abnormalities such as necrotic tissue, edema, infection, and hemodynamic instability. The corresponding therapeutic options to treat these abnormalities include debridement, antibiotics, and surgery. These basic characteristics and treatments are relevant to both acute and chronic wounds. On the other side of the spectrum, more complex abnormalities are being

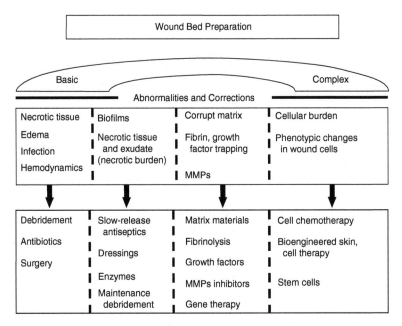

FIGURE 14.1 Wound bed preparation and the abnormalities present in chronic wounds and possible corrective measures. Arrows refer to corrective measures for the abnormalities in each compartment. Dashed lines indicate the overlapping among different compartments of abnormalities and corrective measures.

identified that are perhaps more specific to chronic wounds. For example, chronic wounds and their ability to heal are influenced by increased and often recurrent bacterial and necrotic tissue burdens. Additionally, a corrupt matrix containing fibrinous debris that traps growth factors may undermine their healing. Finally, the presence of phenotypically abnormal cells within chronic wounds may inhibit the normal healing process. As these more complex characteristics are identified in chronic wounds and further understood, appropriate treatment measures will be developed through both new technology and adaptation of existing therapies. Similar to how the major phases of the wound healing process often overlap, we find that wound therapies, from the basic to the advanced, often demonstrate benefit in more than one area of wound bed preparation.

We will now turn to examining individual components of wound bed preparation. First, we will address bacterial burden, debridement of necrotic tissue, and control of exudate. Afterward, we will investigate the increasingly important role of managing the molecular microenvironment of wounds. Finally, we will discuss systemic approaches to wound bed preparation.

14.3 CONTROL OF BACTERIAL BURDEN

The presence of bacteria within chronic wounds has significant influences on healing. While some have suggested that low levels of certain types of bacteria may have a positive influence on the healing process,[4,5] it is clear that bacterial presence in the form of overt tissue infection is detrimental to healing. Somewhere between these two extremes are bacterial colonization and increased bacterial burden, both of which have less well-defined impacts on the healing of chronic wounds. Unfortunately, it is often difficult to ascertain clinically whether one is dealing with colonization or infection.

Several factors influence the relationship between a wound and bacteria. These include the quantity of bacteria present in the wound as well as the particular bacterial strain. The host's resistance, however, may be the most important factor.[6] Host resistance, in turn, is impacted by a variety of local and systemic factors. Examples of local factors include wound size, depth, and duration. Systemic factors include, among others, the presence of underlying vascular disease, diabetes, peripheral edema, malnutrition, and immunosuppression.[7]

When an overt infection or even perhaps a high bacterial load exists, several mechanisms are believed to play a role in the inhibition of healing in chronic wounds. For example, the presence of bacteria may stimulate a persistent inflammatory reaction that ultimately leads to tissue necrosis. Furthermore, chronic infection has been hypothesized to result in down-regulation of the normal host immune response. Through these mechanisms, the chronic wound may experience impaired formation of granulation tissue and decreased tensile strength.[6]

A number of therapeutic options are available to correct the abnormalities that develop in chronic wounds as a result of bacterial imbalance. These include but are not limited to antibiotics, antiseptics, and debridement. We will specifically address slow-release antiseptics, which have proven very useful clinically.

Slow release antiseptics such as silver-impregnated dressings and cadexomer iodine are unique and innovative therapeutic measures. Evidence suggests that they aid the healing of wounds beyond their antimicrobial function through several different mechanisms, making them key examples of the previously mentioned overlapping benefits of many wound therapies.

In the past, much controversy has surrounded the use of iodine in chronic wounds. This is in part due to the fact that early iodine preparations were found to be cytotoxic and thus inhibitory to wound healing. However, more recently, low concentration slow-release formulations of iodine, such as cadexomer iodine, have been developed. They provide antibacterial action through a multitargeted effect on the bacterial cell membrane, organelles, and nucleic acid. The multiplicity of this effect, in theory, makes this treatment less susceptible to the development of bacterial resistance. Moreover, cadexomer iodine has been found to have broad antibacterial efficacy against organisms ranging from Gram-positive and Gram-negative bacteria to fungi.[8] Cadexomer iodine also provides a significant absorptive capacity, thereby decreasing the presence of exudate in the wound bed.[9] In addition, it provides effective debridement in chronic wounds.[10] Finally, it is thought that the iodine in these preparations may have a direct effect on the reepithelialization of the wound.[8]

Like iodine, silver has demonstrated antibacterial properties against most types of bacteria including vancomycin-resistant enterococci (VRE) and methicillin-resistant *Staphylococcus aureus* (MRSA), as well as antifungal properties. In the last decade, silver-impregnated dressings that provide a slow and sustained release of silver ions have been developed. Some can be kept on for up to 7 d and in our experience have been particularly helpful in heavily colonized and highly exudative wounds. The wound healing properties of silver beyond the antimicrobial will be covered later in this chapter.

14.4   DEBRIDEMENT OF NECROTIC TISSUE

A number of benefits are brought about by debridement. First, the necrotic tissue serves as a source for bacterial growth and infection and may impede the process of reepithelialization. Also, we are now recognizing the existence of a "cellular burden" comprised of phenotypically altered host cells that need to be corrected or removed. One example of phenotypically altered cells in chronic wounds is fibroblasts. Fibroblasts from chronic wounds have demonstrated altered responses to cytokines, decreased proliferation rates, and increased senescence.[3]

Although acute wounds may benefit from an isolated episode of debridement, it appears we should reconsider this simple approach when treating chronic wounds. Unique pathogenic processes occur in chronic wounds that may not be definitively corrected with a single episode of debridement. Because of this, a prolonged "maintenance debridement" phase may, in fact, be more appropriate for chronic wounds. The reaccumulation of a "necrotic burden" made up of fibrinous debris, nonviable tissue, exudate, etc. occurs. Therefore, we are now realizing the need for "maintenance debridement" in chronic wounds, defined as an ongoing process of periodic reassessment and elimination of this continuously accumulating necrotic burden. Enzymatic debridement is one therapeutic option available to facilitate this maintenance debridement phase.

Currently, two preparations for enzymatic debridement are commercially available. The first is a urea/papain product that acts through indiscriminant protein breakdown. The second, collagenase, has greater tissue specificity and acts by hydrolysis of native collagen. Enzymatic debridement is important in the context of wound bed preparation for several reasons. First, the topical preparations allow for a prolonged maintenance debridement phase, theoretically preventing the accumulation of the cellular burden we have discussed. Next, this treatment provides an excellent example of how the concept of wound preparation is allowing for new insight into old therapies. Beyond simple debridement, enzymatic methods may exert multiple additional effects on wound bed preparation and healing. Color Figure 14.2* suggests some proposed additional effects of collagenase on epithelialization and angiogenesis. Further, Figure 14.1[3] demonstrates the hypothetical overlap that may exist in the wound bed preparation properties of enzymatic debridement agents, including control of bacterial burden and exudate.

14.5   CONTROL OF EXUDATE

It has become increasingly evident that the presence of exudate has detrimental effects on the healing of chronic wounds. The exudate of chronic wounds has been

* Color figures follow page 110.

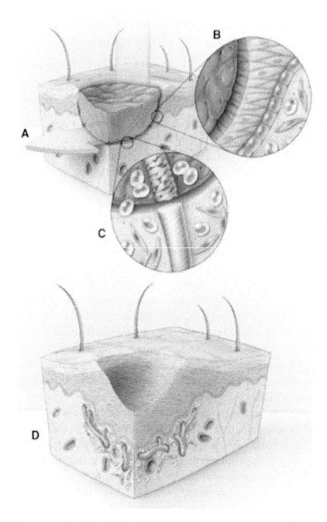

FIGURE 14.2 A proposed view of how a debriding agent (collagenase) might have beneficial effects on wound bed preparation and healing. A) The necrotic plug is being removed by enzymatic action. B) The collagen bundles are being cut at the necrotic–viable tissue interphase. C) Rapid epithelialization that might occur either indirectly (as necrotic tissue is removed) or through the direct effect of collagenase on keratinocyte migration. D) The wound, now free of necrotic tissue, has good granulation tissue and is mostly epithelialized. (See color figure following page 110.)

shown to decrease the proliferation of cells including keratinocytes, fibroblasts, and endothelial cells.[11,12] In particular, an imbalance of metalloproteinases within this fluid may play a role in the disruption of viable tissue matrix, leading to decreased reepitheliazation. Furthermore, there is evidence that substances within the exudate may bind essential growth factors, making wound healing less likely.[1,13]

Careful assessment of the wound will help in establishing the underlying causes of the exudate as well as the treatment approach that will be most beneficial. The treatment of exudate in chronic wounds essentially falls into one of two categories, indirect and direct. Indirect management involves the treatment of the underlying cause of exudate. For example, bacterial infection, hemodynamic imbalances, and chronic inflammatory conditions all may result in increased exudate that as previously described may hamper wound healing. Treatment of these causes is necessary to exudate management. Direct management of exudate involves the removal of the fluid itself. There are a number of therapeutic mechanisms to achieve this goal, including compression, appropriate dressing selection, irrigation, and negative pressure therapy.

Compression is the mainstay of venous ulcer treatment. One aspect is the control of exudate. For many years, the Unna boot was the standard. Other, less exudative wounds were often treated with a two-layer dressing of gauze and an elastic wrap. However, many patients with venous ulcers need a greater amount of compression than the Unna boot or two-layer dressing can supply. This has lead to the introduction of multilayer dressings that supply two elastic outer layers for greater compression, coupled with one or two nonelastic inner layers for stability and absorbency. These dressings are widely accepted in Europe and are slowly but steadily being adopted in the United States.

Negative pressure therapy is a dynamic, effective, and fast-growing tool for wound bed preparation. This treatment, first described in 1955, was developed in the 1980s into a device called vacuum-assisted closure (VAC). By applying suction evenly throughout the wound bed, VAC delivers a highly dependable therapy through actions on several areas of wound bed preparation. In addition to exudate removal, VAC has been found to increase granulation tissue by stimulating fibroblasts.[14] Further, it acts to disinfect the wound bed through continual removal and elimination of microorganisms.[14] VAC therapy has made its mark primarily in large and difficult surgical wounds that previously were some of the most frustrating to treat.

14.6 MANAGING THE BIOLOGICAL MICROENVIRONMENT

We are gradually acquiring an image of the biological microenvironment of the chronic wound. Dysfunctions at the cellular and molecular level are being discovered, helping us to understand the chronic wound and how to assist it.

Within chronic wounds, specific dysfunctions in the key cells involved in wound healing are being identified. These cells are thought to have undergone "phenotypic dysregulation" and make up what we have termed the "cellular burden" of chronic wounds. Venous ulcers, for example, have defective remodeling of the extracellular matrix, an inability to reepithelialize, and prolonged inflammation.[15-17] The epidermis in chronic wounds fails to migrate, particularly in venous ulcers, and there is acanthosis of the wound edge.[18] It has been suggested this process hinders epithelial migration and may be due to either increased proliferation or decreased apoptosis of keratinocytes.[18] Fibroblasts cultured from chronic wounds have demonstrated reduced response to growth factors, in particular PDGF-β and TGF-β1.[16,17] Some evidence indicates that this unresponsiveness is due to poorly expressed TGF-β type II receptors and may explain the failure of topical growth factors to heal some wounds, in that the cells are unable to respond to available growth factors.[18] Understanding the cellular physiology of wound healing is important and may assist in determining what areas of wound care to focus on for a particular wound.

In chronic wounds, particularly venous ulcers, fibrinogen leaks out into the dermis and polymerizes to fibrin. This and other molecules bind growth factors and other cytokines, possibly trapping and retaining them.[13,18] Even though considerable quantities of growth factors may be present in these wounds, they may be unavailable to the healing process.

Another set of molecules essential to wound repair are matrix metalloproteinases (MMPs). These are enzymes that basically serve as cutting tools. There are greater than ten known varieties that act by cleaving certain structural components such as collagen. Within chronic wounds, the concentration of MMPs is characteristically elevated. This would suggest the disruption of wound healing by way of a corrupted wound matrix. At first glance one might think too many MMPs means the wound matrix is being damaged by their enzymatic activation. Although this may be the case, some evidence suggests a greater complexity. In a comparison of fibroblasts from chronic leg wounds and from normal skin, an overabundance of tissue inhibitors of metalloproteinases-1 and -2 (TIMP-1, and TIMP-2) has been found.[15] Although MMPs from these chronic wound fibroblasts are also elevated, they have reduced function, with most seen to remain in the proenzyme form.[15] Fibroblasts' inability to properly organize the extracellular wound matrix was apparently due to these imbalances in MMPs and TIMPs.[15]

Interestingly, reduced levels of MMPs, as well as enhanced fibroplasia and increased cellular apoptosis have been seen to occur in a porcine model of contaminated wounds treated with a silver-impregnated dressing.[19] This silver dressing, designed for slow release of silver ions, demonstrated increased reepithelialization and faster healing than did a standard antimicrobial dressing. It was also hypothesized that silver enhanced angiogenesis. Furthermore, silver is thought to cause an earlier start of fibroplasia during the healing process based on the observation of fibroblasts in the silver-dressed wound beds 24 to 48 h sooner than expected.[19] When one considers the role of fibroplasia in angiogenesis, this finding supports the observation that silver dressings enhance the formation of well-vascularized granulation tissue.[20] In addition, more extensive apoptosis was observed in the silver-treated wounds.[19] It is believed that the inhibition of apoptosis within fibroblast and keratinocyte cell populations interferes with reepithelialization.[18] Therefore, the increase in apoptosis may be an instrumental finding. How the findings of decreased MMPs, enhanced fibroplasia, and increased apoptosis actually relate to the silver dressing is unclear. It is very exciting, however, and will undoubtedly encourage much further investigation into the molecular microenvironment of chronic wounds.

14.7 SYSTEMIC APPROACHES

Systemic approaches to wound bed preparation need to be considered as well. Disease states such as malnutrition, smoking, metabolic illnesses such as diabetes, and artherosclerotic vascular disease causing arterial insufficiency are well known to impair healing. Cigarette smoking, for example, undermines oxygen delivery to the wound by reduced hemoglobin carrying capacity due to carbon monoxide, as well as by constriction of arterioles from nicotine.[21] Deficiencies in vitamins A and C result in the compromise of numerous cellular activities essential to wound healing.[22] Therapies for systemic conditions, like these listed, range from patient education to surgery.

As of late, we are realizing the benefit of a number of oral medications that more directly act on the pathophysiology of wounds. In particular, stanozolol, isotretinoin, and pentoxifylline have been shown to accelerate wound healing. Pentoxifylline is a good example. In a number of studies, it has shown significant benefit in attaining complete closure in venous ulcers, and it has relatively little risk, making it a therapy we should consider using in all venous ulcer patients.[23] Doses of 800 mg three times daily (TID) have proven more effective and were equally well tolerated as the lesser, more common dose of 400 mg TID.[24] Pentoxifylline is known to reduce levels of tumor necrosis factor-α (TNF-α) and decreases leukocyte stimulation by TNF-α and interleukin-1.[25] These changes are thought to achieve benefit by reducing inflammation occurring in wounds.

14.8 CONCLUSION

We expect that an approach to chronic wound treatment through the concept of wound bed preparation will help to guide both the general practitioner and wound care specialist in their approach to care of chronic wounds. There is also a great potential for benefit from useful classification systems for wound bed preparation. Some attempts at this are underway.[2] Wound bed preparation is a dynamic model that will evolve as we continue to better understand wound pathophysiology, further facilitating the optimal implementation of present therapies and the investigation of as yet undiscovered ones.

REFERENCES

1. Falanga, V., *Wound Bed Preparation. Science of Wound Management,* Smith & Nephew Medical Limited, Hull, England, 2001.
2. Falanga, V., Classifications for wound bed preparation and stimulation of chronic wounds, *Wound Repair Regen.,* 8, 347–352, 2000.
3. Falanga, V., Wound bed preparation and the role of enzymes: a case for multiple actions of therapeutic actions, *Wounds,* 14, 47–57, 2002.
4. De Haan, B.B., Ellis, H., and Wilks, M., The role of infection on wound healing, *Surg. Gynecol. Obstet.,* 138, 693–700, 1974
5. Pollack, S.V., The wound healing process, *Clin. Dermatol.,* 2, 8–16, 1984.

6. Dow, G., Browne, A., and Sibbald, R.G., Infection in chronic wounds: controversies in diagnosis and treatment, *Ostomy Wound Manage.*, 45, 23–27, 29-40, quiz 41–42, 1999.

7. Sibbald, R.G., et al., Preparing the wound bed — debridement, bacterial balance, and moisture balance, *Ostomy Wound Manage.*, 46, 14–22, 24–28, 30–35, quiz 36–37, 2000.

8. Apelqvist, J. and Ragnarson Tennvall, G., Cavity foot ulcers in diabetic patients: a comparative study of cadexomer iodine ointment and standard treatment. An economic analysis alongside a clinical trial, *Acta Dermatol. Venereol.*, 76, 231–235, 1996.

9. Hanson, C.P.L.-M., Stenquist, B. et al., The effects of cadexomer iodine paste in the treatment of venous leg ulcers in comparison with hydrocolloid dressing and paraffin gauze dressing, *Int. J. Dermatol.*, 37, 390–396, 1998.

10. Skog, E. et al., A randomized trial comparing cadexomer iodine and standard treatment in the out-patient management of chronic venous ulcers, *Br. J. Dermatol.*, 109, 77–83, 1983.

11. Bucalo B.E.W. and Falanga V., Inhibition of cell proliferation by chronic wound fluid, *Wound Repair Regen.*, 1, 181–186, 1993.

12. Park, H.Y.S.K. and Phillips, T., The effect of heat on the inhibitory effects of chronic wound fluid on fibroblasts *in vitro*, *Wounds*, 10, 189–192, 1998.

13. Falanga, V. and Eaglstein, W.H., The "trap" hypothesis of venous ulceration, *Lancet*, 341, 1006–1008, 1993.

14. Teot, L., Negative pressure therapy in wound bed preparation, in *The Clinical Relevance of Wound Bed Preparation*, Harding, V.F.A.K., Ed., 2002, Springer-Verlag, Berlin, 2002, pp. 39–53.

15. Cook, H. et al., Defective extracellular matrix reorganization by chronic wound fibroblasts is associated with alterations in TIMP-1, TIMP-2, and MMP-2 activity, *J. Invest. Dermatol.*, 115, 225–233, 2000.

16. Agren, M.S. et al., Proliferation and mitogenic response to PDGF-BB of fibroblasts isolated from chronic venous leg ulcers is ulcer-age dependent, *J. Invest. Dermatol.*, 112, 463–469, 1999.

17. Hasan, A. et al., Dermal fibroblasts from venous ulcers are unresponsive to the action of transforming growth factor-beta 1, *J. Dermatol. Sci.*, 16, 59–66, 1997.

18. Falanga, V., Wound bed preparation, video presentation, 2000.

19. Wright, J.B. et al., Early healing events in a porcine model of contaminated wounds: effects of nanocrystalline silver on matrix metalloproteinases, cell apoptosis, and healing, *Wound Repair Regen.*, 10, 141–151, 2002.

20. Wright, J.B., Lam, K., and Burrell, R.E., Wound management in an era of increasing bacterial antibiotic resistance: a role for topical silver treatment, *Am. J. Infect. Control.*, 26, 572–577, 1998.

21. Silverstein, P., Smoking and wound healing., *Am. J. Med.*, 93, 22S–24S, 1992.

22. Mazzotta, M.Y., Nutrition and wound healing, *J. Am. Podiatr. Med. Assoc.*, 84, 456–462, 1994.

23. Jull, A.B., Waters, J., and Arroll, B., Pentoxifylline for treating venous leg ulcers, *Cochrane Database Syst. Rev.*, 1, 2002.

24. Falanga, V. et al., Systemic treatment of venous leg ulcers with high doses of pentoxifylline: efficacy in a randomized, placebo-controlled trial, *Wound Repair Regen.*, 7, 208–213, 1999.

25. Samlaska, C.P. and Winfield, E.A., Pentoxifylline, *J. Am. Acad. Dermatol.*, 30, 603–621, 1994.

15 Gene Transfer of Growth Factors for Wound Repair

Jan Jeroen Vranckx, Feng Yao, and Elof Eriksson

CONTENTS

15.1 INTRODUCTION

The healing wound is a site of intense metabolism and complex molecular interactions. Several classes of molecules, such as coagulation factors and products, kinins, cytokines, complement factors, vasoactive amines, proteases, and growth factors, are involved in the inflammatory response during wound healing. Growth factors are a diverse class of peptides that signal cells and guide growth, development, and reparative processes. They play key roles in regulating cell-to-cell interactions, cell migration, proliferation, differentiation, and extracellular matrix synthesis and breakdown during the process of wound repair. Growth factors can function in both autocrine and paracrine fashions.

Growth factors are produced by cells heavily involved in wound repair such as platelets, macrophages, fibroblasts, and epithelial and endothelial cells and are able to influence the growth rate of these cells when bound to specific receptors. Upon wounding, expression of growth factors and their corresponding receptors is elevated; it subsides once the wound has healed. Although they are present only in minute amounts, growth factors exert a powerful influence on the process of wound repair. Although growth factors are crucial in initiating, sustaining, and regulating post injury response, these same molecules have been implicated in impaired wound healing, scarring, and chronic cutaneous conditions.[1,2] Both the magnitude of this response and the temporal and spatial pattern of cytokine and growth factor expression are important during normal and impaired wound healing.

Over the past two decades, much research has been conducted to characterize the role and potential treatment applications of individual growth factors in impaired wound healing states. Topical administration of recombinant growth factors as proteins has major shortcomings, including short shelf life, low bioavailability, enzymatic inactivaton, and inefficient delivery to target cells. For example, with topical application of epidermal growth factor (EGF), only 1 to 9% of the applied dose reached a wound depth of 1 to 3 mm. Hence, to achieve its therapeutic effect, the costly use of repeated high doses is required.[3]

Gene therapy offers an attractive approach for direct delivery of growth factors to the healing wound; genetic material is introduced into the cells with the intent of altering protein synthesis to modify the healing response. Gene therapy can offer targeted local and persistent delivery of *de novo*-synthesized growth factor to the wound environment over many days.[4,5] Using gene therapy to selectively elevate or downregulate expression of a particular growth factor in the healing wound microenvironment has great promise in promoting tissue repair and regeneration, in particular if one considers that healing of a wound is a local event and requires high levels of transgene expression only for a limited period of time.

Skin is a good candidate for gene therapy not only because of its obvious accessibility but also for its capacity for regeneration and abundant vascularity.[6] Although many reasons have been proposed for why chronic open wounds fail to heal, no unifying theory exists, and the cause is most likely multifactorial. Altering local factors and meticulous care are paramount in preventing wound progression, but the local milieu of growth factors may also greatly influence wound healing. The major challenges facing wound repair are the problem of identifying an appropriate gene that is effective in tissue repair and then ensuring that the therapeutic gene is expressed reliably and at clinically beneficial levels. We also must find ways to control the timing and the level of gene expression.

15.2   GROWTH FACTORS AND WOUND HEALING

Upon injury, inflammatory cells are recruited to the site of injury by substances secreted by platelets, such as platelet-derived growth factors (PDGFs) and thrombin, and by substances generated by the coagulation cascade, such as fibrinopeptides. The fibrinopeptides, thrombin, and activated platelets attract macrophages into the

TABLE 15.1
Growth Factors Active in Wound Healing

	Growth Factor	Cell Source	Biological Activity in Skin Wounds
VEGF	Vasculoendothelial growth factor	Keratinocytes, fibroblasts, macrophages	Angiogenesis
EGF	Epidermal growth factor	Keratinocytes, macrophages Kidney, salivary, and lacrimal glands	Keratinocyte proliferation and migration and collagenase activity
FGF	Fibroblast growth factor	Fibroblasts, macrophages, endothelial cells, smooth muscle cells, chondrocytes	Keratinocyte proliferation and migration, angiogenesis, endothelial cell activation
KGF	Keratinocyte growth factor	Fibroblasts, endothelial cells	Keratinocyte proliferation and migration
PDGF	Platelet derived growth factor	Platelets, macrophages, keratinocytes, fibroblasts, endothelial cells	Activates fibroblasts, stimulates extracellular matrix formation
TGF-β	Transforming growth factor	Platelets, fibroblasts, macrophages, keratinocytes, hepatocytes	Fibroblast activation, extracellular matrix formation
IGF	Insulin growth factor	Fibroblasts, macrophages, liver, skeletal muscle, neutrophils	Keratinocyte and fibroblast proliferation, collagen synthesis, angiogenesis, endothelial cell activation

wound. Macrophages and then neutrophils are stimulated by fibrin, lactate, and hypoxia and start to release growth factors including PDGFs, insulin growth factors (IGFs), transforming growth factors (TGFs) and epidermal growth factors (EGFs), as well as cytokines and additional lactate, which will continue the process and stimulate fibroplasia, collagen deposition, and angiogenesis. Proliferation of fibroblasts leads to upregulation and release of fibroblast growth factors (FGFs), PDGFs, and IGFs and synthesis of collagen and proteoglycans of the connective tissue. It is shown that TGF-β and IGF-1 can lead to upregulating collagen gene transcription. Vasculoendothelial factors (VEGFs), PDGFs, and TGFs all have been shown to stimulate migration and/or proliferation of endothelial cells. Therefore, they are important factors in regulating angiogenesis. Epithelial cells respond to many of the same stimuli as fibroblasts and endothelial cells. EGFs, FGFs, and TGFs play a role in epithelialization. Finally the early tissue repair process is followed by tissue maturation, remodeling, and reorganization. The TGF-beta isoforms play an important role in these events.[1-5]

In Table 15.1, an overview is given of the growth factors that play a role in wound healing. Besides the cell source of growth factor production, the biological activities of these growth factors in the healing process of skin wounds are shown.

15.2.1 Vasculoendothelial Growth Factor

The VEGF group of molecules consists of VEGF-A and the VEGF-related factors VEGF-B and VEGF-C and placental growth factor (PIGF). VEGF-A is transcribed from a single gene, but as a result of alternative splicing, various isoforms exist ranging from 121 to 206 amino acid residues.[7–10]

VEGF121 does not contain exons 6 and 7 of the gene and is fully active as an inducer of angiogenesis with endothelial cell specific mitogenic and vascular permeability–enhancing activities.[11,12] VEGF is a highly conserved protein that has cross-species activity: among human, rat, and bovine VEGF, 84 to 94% sequence identity has been observed.[13] VEGF is released primarily by keratinocytes and also by fibroblasts and macrophages.[7–10] Numerous studies revealed that VEGF plays an elementary role in embryonic development.[8] Currently, transgenic mice models with tissue-specific or conditional VEGF-A expression are used to investigate the specific role of VEGF-A forms in neovascularization. Ferrara et al. demonstrated how VEGF-family antibodies inhibited angiogenesis in nude mice.[12] VEGF cDNA administered to experimental ischemic skin flaps led to an increased flap survival.[14,15] Takeshita et al. demonstrated in a rabbit model with hindlimb ischemia that the three isoforms VEGF121, VEGF165, and VEGF189 are biologically equivalent for *in vivo* angiogenesis.[16] Enhanced vascularity and bursting strength of a healing abdominal fascia was seen using adenovirus vector-mediated VEGF transfer in a mouse-model.[17] Supp and Boyce demonstrated the acceleration of early graft vascularization and improved healing of genetically modified cultured skin substitutes by overexpression of VEGF in athymic mice.[18] Yao et al. investigated age and growth factors in a study in porcine full thickness wound healing. The rate of reepithelialization decreased with increasing age, and the endogenous VEGF concentration in the older pigs peaked later and at one-fourth the level when compared to the younger age groups.[19]

There is huge interest in the role of VEGF in models of angiogenesis for tumor growth and treatment as well as in tissue engineering of three-dimensional constructs with intrinsic vascular networks.[4–18]

15.2.2 Epidermal Growth Factor

EGF is produced by platelets, keratinocytes, monocytes, and macrophages and is present in high quantities in the early phase of wound healing. It is a small molecule similar to TGF-α, with which it shares a receptor. EGF likely increases wound healing by stimulating the migration and proliferation not only of epithelial cells but also mesenchymal cells. EGF is also produced by the salivary glands, the kidney, and the lacrimal glands. EGF has been found to promote epidermal regeneration and to influence wound healing by stimulating the production of proteins and the migration of epithelial cells.[20] EGF might play a role in tensile strength and wound remodeling by stimulating fibroblast collagenase secretion. Reports suggest that aged dermal fibroblasts have a decreased EGF-receptor expression and may contribute to the impaired wound healing seen during aging.[21,22] EGF has been used in randomized clinical trials studying healing of skin graft donor sites and chronic wounds treated with silver sulfadiazine containing EGF. These preliminary data suggested that monotherapy of EGF might be of benefit in wound healing.

15.2.3 Fibroblast Growth Factor

FGF exists as an acidic aFGF (FGF-1) and a basic bFGF (FGF-2) isomer. There is a 50% amino acid homology between the two forms. They both bind to the same receptor, but bFGF is 10 times more potent. Both are released by macrophages, fibroblasts, smooth muscle cells, and endothelial cells, and they stimulate keratinocyte and fibroblast migration and proliferation.[23] bFGF also plays a role in angiogenesis by promoting endothelial cell growth and migration. In a recent study, recombinant bFGF accelerated wound healing significantly in burns, operative wounds, and chronic ulcers.[24,25] FGF-7 and FGF-10 are also known as keratinocyte growth factor (KGF)-1 and KGF-2 (see below).

15.2.4 Keratinocyte Growth Factor

KGF is a member of the FGF family. Two forms have been identified — KGF-1 and KGF-2 (= FGF-10). They interact with the same receptor. Both are secreted by fibroblasts and endothelial cells, whereas KGF receptors are only found on epithelial cells.[26,27] Both KGF isomers are important regulators of keratinocyte proliferation and maturation. The administration of recombinant KGF-1 and KGF-2 improved reepithelialization, collagen content, and wound breaking strength in murine models and in a porcine wound healing model.[28] Introduction of KGF expression was reduced and delayed during wound healing in genetically diabetic mice.[29] KGF is produced and secreted by mesenchymal cells but exerts its function on keratinocytes, which have ectodermal roots.

15.2.5 Transforming Growth Factor

TGF is composed of two polypeptide chains, α and β. TGF-α has a 30% homology with EGF. They both bind to the EGF receptor but with different actions. The initial identification of TGF-β was based on its ability to reversibly induce phenotypic transformation of select fibroblast cell lines.[30] TGF-β plays an important role in the control of the immune response and wound healing and in the development of various tissues and organs.[30–33] Three isoforms exist in mammalian cells (β1, β2, and β3), each encoded by its own gene; they have a sequence identity of 70 to 80%. Despite high homology at the sequence level, analysis of their *in vivo* function by gene knockouts has revealed striking differences, suggesting no significant functional redundancy among TGF-β1, 2, and 3. The TGF-β superfamily binds to type II and type I serine/threonine kinase receptors and transduces signals via Smad proteins.[32,33]

TGF-β induces a mitogenic or antiproliferative effect depending on the cell type.[32] It promotes cell proliferation in culture in several cell lines, predominantly of mesenchymal origin. In smooth muscle cells, fibroblasts, and chondrocytes, TGF-β induces a bimodal response in proliferative behavior. At lower concentrations, TGF-β induces PDGF-A expression, whereas higher concentrations inhibit the expression of the PDGF receptor α unit.[34]

Exogenous TGF-β administration *in vivo* has been shown to result in increased cell density, fibrosis, and angiogenesis.[35] TGF-β also is a potent inhibitor of cell proliferation of many cell types. Considerable evidence indicates that TGF-β plays an immunomodulatory role and functions as a potent differentiating, modulating, and immunosuppressive agent.[35-38] TGF-β appears in a latent form that is activated *in vivo* by many stimuli. Bauer et al. explored the influence of keratinocytes transfected with latent and active TGF-β on the modulation of extracellular matrix expression by dermal fibroblasts.[39]

Shah et al. demonstrated that the neutralization of TGF-β1 and TGF-β2 reduced scarring in cutaneous rat wounds. When exogenous TGF-β3 was added to the wounds, a similar reduction in scarring was noted.[40] Benn et al. evaluated overexpression of TGF-β1 by particle-mediated DNA transfer to rat skin and noted enhanced tensile strength in the treated wounds.[41] The role of TGF-β in the different physiologic and pathologic processes *in vivo* and the features of the Smads transcriptional activators of TGF-β responses are only now starting to be explored.[42,43]

15.2.6 INSULIN-LIKE GROWTH FACTOR

Insulin-like growth factors (IGFs) or somatomedins have a 50% amino acid homology with proinsulin and have insulin-like activity. IGF exists as the isomers IGF-1 and -2. IGF-1 is identical to somatedin-C, whereas IGF-2 is similar to sometidin. IGF-1 is produced by the liver, heart, lung, pancreas, and skeletal muscle and also by fibroblasts, neutrophils, and macrophages in the wound environment. IGF-2 appears to play a significant role in fetal growth. Target receptors are found on fibroblasts, keratinocytes, and endothelial cells. IGF-1 and IGF-2 have separate receptors.

IGF is bound to a carrier protein that plays a major role in regulating its effects.[44] IGF stimulates collagen synthesis and the proliferation of keratinocytes and fibroblasts. IGF influences endothelial cell turnover and might play a role in angiogenesis.[45] Exogenously administered IGF-1 improved wound healing in both diabetic and steroid-impaired subjects.[46]

15.2.7 PLATELET-DERIVED GROWTH FACTOR

PDGF is a disulfide-bonded cationic dimeric glycoprotein; it occurs as three isoforms — PDGF-AA, -BB, and -AB, named according to the arrangement of the two polypeptide chains A and B, which share 60% homology. These isomers exert their influence by binding to two receptors, α and β.

Human platelets contain all three forms of PDGF in the ratio 12% AA:65% AB:23% BB.[47] Platelets are the largest source of PDGF, but it is also produced by macrophages and fibroblasts. PDGF stimulates the production of fibronectin, hyaluronic acid, and collagenase. PDGF also acts with TGF-β and EGF to stimulate mesenchymal cells. The administration of exogenous PDGF-BB has improved wound closure in chronic and diabetic nonhealing ulcers in both humans and rodents.[48] A randomized prospective double-blind study of recombinant human PDGF-BB performed in patients with diabetic, neurotrophic foot ulcers demonstrated that PDGF could be applied topically and was effective and safe in promoting the healing of these ulcers in humans.[49–51] Gene transfer experiments with PDGF are currently under investigation. Eming et al. reported increased tensile strength by using particle-mediated gene transfer of PDGF isoforms in a rat model.[52]

15.3 PLASMID-DNA AND *DE NOVO*-SYNTHESIZED GROWTH FACTORS

Short shelf life and inefficient delivery to target cells are major concerns associated with topical administration of recombinant growth factors. Gene therapy offers an attractive approach for direct delivery of growth factors to the healing wound. It can offer targeted local and persistent delivery of *de novo*-synthesized growth factor to the wound environment over many days. Plasmid-DNA can be successfully delivered to and expressed in various tissues by viral and nonviral vector-mediated gene transfer. Plasmids are naturally occurring, self-replicating, double-stranded circular DNA molecules within bacteria, responsible for acquired bacterial traits such as antibiotic resistance. They behave as accessory genetic units that replicate and are inherited independently of the bacterial chromosome. Recombinant plasmid vectors typically contain a bacterial origin of replication, an antibiotic resistance gene, and a multiple cloning site. Gene transfer with plasmids to mammalian cells and tissues requires specific incorporation of at least two basic DNA elements into the plasmid: a mammalian cell enhancer/promoter element and a poly A signal sequence. Promoter sequences may be constitutive (always "on") or conditional (turned on or off only when exposed to specific environmental stimuli or transcriptional modulators). The poly A signal located downstream from the gene of interest provides a signal where transcription terminates. A typical mammalian cell messenger ribonucleic acid (mRNA) contains a poly A tail, which is required for stabilization of the mRNA and its efficient transport from the nucleus to the cytoplasm. Polyadenylatioin sequences downstream from the gene of interest are often used to stabilize the mRNA sequences after gene transcription has been initiated.[4–6]

15.4 STRATEGIES OF GENE DELIVERY

Numerous methods of gene delivery have been developed, modified, and improved; however, these technologies are still under intensive investigation, since no single gene transfer strategy is optimal for all medical applications: all have their specific attributes, each with advantages and disadvantages depending on the target tissues.

An important difference among gene transfer methods is whether the genetic modification induced is temporary or permanent. In temporary genetic modification, the delivered genes are normally not integrated into the genome of the target cells and do not feature the genetic elements required to be replicated as the cell divides. Over time, the genes will be lost and the expression will stop. In wound repair, this "temporary modification" might be ideal. When the delivered genes are integrated into the genome of the target cells, they will normally be replicated and expressed by each generation of daughter cells for the lifetime of the cell. However, gene transfer that mediates temporary genetic modification can produce permanent genetic modification of some cells (although the frequency is extremely low) and gene expression resulting from gene transfer that mediates permanent genetic modifications can be variable, especially *in vivo,* due to downregulation of the genetic expression or loss of the genetically modified cells (by apoptosis or immunologic reaction) resulting in "temporary modification."[4–6,53]

There are two major 'strategies' of gene delivery systems: non viral and viral. Both strategies may be carried out *in vivo* whereby genes are delivered directly to target cells or *ex vivo* in which cells are removed from the patient, genetically modified, and transplanted back into the tissues. Nonviral delivery systems involve physical or chemical transfer of genetic material ("transfection") and are dependent on cellular transport mechanisms for uptake and expression in the host cell.

Permanent genetic modification can be achieved by gene transfer with recombinant retroviruses, recombinant adeno-associated viruses, and recently by the recombinant lentiviruses. The other viral and nonviral strategies lead to temporary genetic modification.

15.4.1 VIRAL GENE TRANSFER STRATEGIES

Viral transfection strategies are based on the natural ability of viruses to infect cells. To ensure the safety of these strategies, sequences of the viral genome essential for viral replication are removed and replaced with the selected DNA sequence. This approach reduces the risk of inadvertent production of infective virus from the viral vector. Development of special "packaging cell" lines in which high titers of recombinant viruses can be produced has provided a means for generating adequate virus for transduction studies. Transduction is associated with higher transfection efficiency as compared to nonviral strategies. The viruses most often used in gene therapy are retroviruses, adenoviruses, adeno-associated viruses, and herpes simplex virus. The viral vectors differ in terms of integration into the host cells, packing abilities, and their capacities to infect dividing or nondividing (quiescent) cells.

Cytotoxicity and the risk for mutagenesis are essential factors in the selection of a viral vector for therapeutic means, as well as the host immune response (antigenicity) elicited. Some viral vectors are also dependent on helper viruses for replication (Table 15.2).

Retroviruses have genetic material composed of RNA, which is made into DNA by the specific enzyme reverse transcriptase when the virus enters the cell. Retroviruses are easy to modify. Classic retroviruses only infect dividing cells, and their genetic material integrates into the host genomes. Since few cells are actively proliferating *in vivo,* retroviruses are significantly limited for *in vivo* gene transfer. Another disadvantage is that integration into the host genome is at random and therefore a (small) risk exists that retroviruses could disrupt normal functioning of the host cells.[54] Recombinant retroviruses are the most widely used gene transfer vehicles in current clinical experience (40% of human gene therapy trials).[8]

Human lentiviruses are a new class of retroviruses analyzed as vectors for gene transfer. These viruses are stably integrated into the genome as well but both in

TABLE 15.2
Viral Gene Delivery Strategies

Viral Vector	Genome	Packing Ability (kb)	Expression in Host Cell	Infection to	Drawbacks
Retrovirus	Single-stranded RNA	8	Chromosomal integration in numerous cell types	Actively dividing cells only; 10^6 to 10^7 appm	Potential insertional mutagenesis; unstable viral particles; limited *in vivo* use
Adenovirus	Double-stranded DNA	7.5	Episomal	Both dividing and nondividing cells; 10^{10} to 10^{12} appm	Host immune response can be strong
Adeno-associated virus	Single-stranded DNA	4.6	Chromosomal integration	Both dividing and nondividing cells; 10^4 to 10^5 appm	Small packing ability; requires helper virus for replication that must be eliminated from the final stock
Lentivirus	Single-stranded RNA		Chromosomal integration in numerous cell types	Both dividing and nondividing cells; 10^4 to 10^5 appm	New vector system Low titers
Herpes simplex 1 virus	Double-stranded DNA	30 to 50	Episomal	To neurotropic cells only; 10^{11} to 10^{12} appm	Potential wild-type break-through; new HSV-1 amplicon vector has low antigenecity but low titers

Note: appm, active particles per milliliter in the produced purified viral stocks.

dividing and quiescent cells *in vivo*. This class of viruses includes human immunodeficiency virus and simian immunodeficiency virus.[55]

Recombinant adenoviral vectors account for 20% of human gene therapy trials. The E1, 2, and 3 genes regulate the replication of the adenoviral genome. After removal of these genes, 8 kb can be carried by this vector. The production of the adenoviral vector is efficient, and high titers can be obtained. The transferred DNA does not become integrated within the genome and limits the potential of this vector for long-term transfection, such as in chronic diseases. The proteins of the virus particles of the adenoviral vector can elicit an inflammatory response *in vivo* and evoke significant lasting immune reactivity. In order to reduce vector immunogenicity and to prolong transgene expression, a new generation of helper-dependent or "gutless" adenoviral (Ad)-vectors were developed in which all viral coding sequences were deleted.[56,57] This vector remains particularly useful for transient transfection such as in wound healing or cancer treatment.[58]

Adeno-associated virus (AAV) is a parvovirus that has never shown pathogenicity or toxicity in humans. Six serotypes exist, of which serotype 2 is the most commonly used in gene therapy protocols. Recombinant adeno-associated viral vectors are stably integrated into the genome of quiescent and dividing cells and thus useful for permanent *in vivo* genetic modification. Genomic integration of the wild type AAV occurs 70% of the time in chromosome 19, and it has been shown to persist in a latent phase throughout more than 100 passages of the cell culture.[59] However, recombinant vectors have lost this specificity and are integrated at random. AAV vector requires a helper virus in order to replicate. This helper virus (such as adenovirus) must be eliminated from the final stock. Also, the AAV vector can only harbor 4.6 kb of foreign DNA. Recently, adenovirus-free AAV vectors were produced and high titer vector stocks obtained.[60] This vector represents the most promising current vector for chronic diseases.

15.4.2 NONVIRAL GENE TRANSFER STRATEGIES

Nonviral gene transfer strategies have lower transfection efficiencies in comparison to viral gene transfer, varying greatly from 5 to 20% for nonpermissive cells up to 90% for certain cell lines.

Examples of nonviral gene delivery are direct injection of plasmid DNA (mostly in a direct *in vivo* gene transfer protocol)[67] or delivery of plasmid DNA into cells by electroporation,[68] particle bombardment,[61,62], microseeding,[63] and cationic liposomes.[65,66] (See Table 15.3.)

Particle-mediated gene transfer (particle bombardment, gene gun technology) is applicable to a wide variety of mammalian tissues.[20,61,62] Microprojectiles (1 to 5 μm) consisting of DNA coated with microscopic gold (or tungsten) particles are loaded into a "macroprojectile" inside the gene gun. The macroprojectile is accelerated at high velocity by a helium burst or a voltage discharge through a vacuum chamber, and the microprojectiles are shot into the target tissue, overcoming the mutually repelling electrostatic forces. The resulting spray penetrates the target tissue, and the bombarded cells express the encoded genes.

We successfully delivered human (hEGF) plasmid DNA directly into the cells of partial-thickness wounds by particle bombardment. This resulted in hEGF expression for several days in the targeted tissue.[8] *In vivo* gene transfer of TGF-β by the gene gun accelerated healing of murine incisional wounds and moreover, with the use of the same animal model, it was demonstrated that transfection of PDGF-expressing plasmid into wounds could lead to increased wound tensile strength compared with untransfected control wounds.[52,62] Particle-mediated gene transfer

TABLE 15.3
Nonviral Gene Delivery Strategies

Method	Advantages	Disadvantages	Efficiency
Injection of naked DNA/plasmids	Simple	Nonspecific, dissipates	Low transfection efficiency
Electroporation	Nontoxic; large amounts can be delivered	Complex equipment; feasibility *in vivo*?	Low transfection efficiency
Cationic liposomes	Low immunogenecity; simple, local; large amounts of DNA can be delivered	Toxic to cells: must be titrated, short-term transfection	Efficiency 5 to 90%
Gene gun: particle bombardment	Simple with gun; large amounts of DNA can be delivered	Nonspecific, superficial; foreign bodies, mechanical damage?	Relatively low transfection efficiency
Microseeding	Large amounts can be delivered; deep penetration	Inflammatory reaction by punctures?	High transfection efficiency
Epigenetic approaches; antisense nucleotides	Simple, nontoxic	Nonspecific, hit or miss sequences, Short-term effect	To be investigated

carries minimal intrinsic toxicity, although the high pressure might kill cells biomechanically. Large DNA constructs can be included, and multiple genes can be delivered simultaneously.

For the *in vivo* gene transfer experiments in our animal wound model we use the *microseeding technique*.[63] A linear set of six solid microneedles surrounded by a guiding steel cylinder is attached to a piston driven by an electric motor. The plasmid DNA or vector solution is delivered to the oscillating needles via fine silicone tubing connected to a $30^{1}/_{2}$ G. needle and a 1 cc syringe controlled by an infusion pump. The depth of the penetration can be varied depending on needle design and the purpose of the experiment. Varying the DNA concentration and the amount of solution delivered to the needles may regulate the magnitude of gene expression. The yield of hEGF in microseeded partial thickness wounds was about threefold higher than that of wounds bombarded by the Accell gene gun and sevenfold higher than gene transfer by single injection. Since no special preparation is required, recombinant viral vectors such as adenoviral vectors can also be efficiently delivered to skin wounds by microseeding. After microseeding 1×10^9 particles per wound of Ad-VEGF121 to full thickness skin wounds in an aged porcine model, high titers of VEGF were measured in wound fluid during 6 d.[64]

Liposomes are self-assembling particles formed from phospholipids, which are able to encapsulate substances within their layers. Cationic liposomes are synthetically prepared vesicles consisting of a positively charged lipid and a co-lipid. Cationic liposomes can efficiently form a noncovalent complex with negatively charged

DNA molecules through electrostatic interaction. The resulting liposome-DNA complexes interact with the cell membrane of transfected cells.[65] The DNA molecules are introduced into the cells presumably through endocytosis. Transfection with liposomes is achieved either by direct application or by injection into a defined arterial or venous system. Initial transfection rates were very low, but newer specialized techniques are being developed to increase transfection efficiency.[66] The efficiency of cationic liposome-mediated gene transfer *in vitro* can range from 5 to 20% for nonpermissive cells and up to 90% for certain cell lines.

Liposomes can package relatively large amounts of genetic material. They lack immunogenicity and the technique is simple: *in vitro* gene delivery to cells in culture is achieved simply by mixing the liposome/DNA complex with cells; soon after treatment, cells *in vitro* take up and express the genes. With this method, genes can be delivered to both dividing and nondividing (quiescent) cells. In our laboratory, we intensively use this strategy for the *ex vivo* gene transfer of growth factor recombinant DNA to cell suspension cultures of fibroblasts and keratinocytes. These transfected cell cultures are transplanted into standard full thickness wounds in a porcine wound model. On a daily basis, we retrieve wound fluid, and the overexpression of the growth factors by the transplanted cells and their impact on wound repair are analyzed (cf. Section 15.5).

Human artificial chromosomes (HAC) are currently still under development but are heralded as the most promising nonviral vectors of the future. They represent "mini-chromosomes" containing specific DNA fragments that will enter the cell and permanently reside there without being incorporated into the native genome, avoiding insertional mutagenesis while keeping the ability to transfer the inserted gene into daughter cells during cell division.[53]

15.5   GENE TRANSFER OF GROWTH FACTORS TO FULL THICKNESS WOUNDS IN A PORCINE EXPERIMENTAL MODEL

Pig skin is very comparable to human skin.[69,70] The dermal–epidermal thickness ratio is similar.[71] The epidermis shows a similar staining pattern for a number of antigens, such as keratins 10 and 16, fillagrin, collagen IV, fibronectin, and vimentin.[72] The body hair of pigs is sparse and progresses through a hair cycle independently of neighboring follicles, just as in human skin. Functionally, pig and human skin are similar in terms of epidermal cell turnover time, type of keratinous proteins, and lipid composition of the stratum corneum. The papillary dermis displays rete ridges, and the porcine dermal collagen is similar to human collagen biochemically.[73] The number and distribution of blood vessels also are similar, although there are differences such as the less developed subepidermal plexus in pigs. Pig skin has apocrine glands along with hair follicles, similar to human skin, but there are no eccrine sweat glands. These structural similarities to human skin make porcine skin very useful to investigate the roles of cell engineering and gene transfer of growth factors in the repair of skin wounds. Based on the omnipresence of growth factors in each phase of the wound healing process, it is hypothesized that wound repair can be accelerated by the overexpression of highly targeted delivery of exogenous growth factor genes into the wound microenvironment.

We developed a standardized full thickness skin (FTW) wound model in young and old pigs (Yorkshire and Yucatan pigs) to analyze the impact of *in vivo* and *ex vivo* gene transfer of growth factors such as EGF, KGF, PDGF, VEGF, and TGF-β_1 on wound repair. For the *in vivo* gene transfer experiments, DNA-solution is "microseeded" at a depth of 2 to 3 mm into the wound base and borders at a rate of 7500 r/min with the needles of the motor device set at a 60 degree angle to the wound surface. The infusion pump speed is set at 60 μl/min, and the total amount of virus solution administered is 60 to 100 μl per wound. We used the microseeding technique for *in vivo* experiments of gene transfer of hEGF, Ad-VEGF, PDGF-AA and BB, and KGF-2 to investigate the role of *in vivo* gene transfer of growth factors to partial- and full-thickness skin wounds in a porcine model.

For *ex vivo* gene transfer, we process a fresh split skin graft, and keratinocytes and fibroblasts are grown as single cell suspensions. The keratinocytes are seeded on collagen I-coated culture dishes. After first passage, highly proliferative cells attach to the dish. These cells have high clonogenic potential in the applied growth medium, which favors proliferation and migration instead of differentiation. After 24 h, these cells are transfected with plasmid DNA using cationic liposomes. This procedure results in a 10 to 20% transfection efficiency, based on the quality and age of the cultured cells. Stable cell lines can be created by selection during the culturing process, resulting in high and long-term gene expression by the transplanted cells. After another incubation period of 48 to 72 h, the transfected cells are released from the culture dishes, carefully mixed, and counted using the hemocytometer. Separate syringes with a predetermined number of transfected cells (per protocol) are meticulously prepared, constantly mixing the cell solutions, and shortly stored on ice for transfer to the operating room where simultaneously the standard wounds are made on the dorsum of the pig by other team members. The cell suspensions are injected into transparent wound chambers that are attached over each of the full-thickness wounds. These wound chambers place the wounds in a wet environment that promotes wound healing.[76] We allow the cells to settle into the wounds for 2 h before waking the pig. On a daily basis, we place the animal in a custom-made sling under light mask anesthesia to retrieve wound fluid from the transparent wound chambers. This wound fluid is transferred on ice and stored in a −80°C freezer. The cell supernatant and the wound fluid are analyzed by ELISA assays.

15.6 REGULATION OF THE GENE PRODUCT

Successful implementation of gene therapy relies not only on delivering a therapeutic gene into target cells efficiently, but ultimately on developing a genetic device in which expression of a therapeutic gene could be regulated in a predictable and effective way. New strategies involve the inclusion of promoter regions that are only active in specific tissues or at specific stages of cell differentiation or that can be regulated by exogenously supplied drugs. To date there are four such major systems.[74,75] The common feature lies in their employment of a minimal mammalian cell promoter, which by itself exhibits little basal activity, fused to its cis-corresponding DNA binding elements and a hybrid transactivator whose transactivating activity is regulated by a pharmacological molecule, such as tetracycline in the tetracycline-inducible system. Our laboratory developed a new tetracycline-inducible system, not relying on the human cytomegalovirus (hCMV) minimal promotor and tetracylin-controlled tramactivator (tTA), which is a fusion protein between the transactivating domain of herpes simplex virus (HSV)-1 VP16 and tetracycline repressor (tetR), but relying on the wild-type hCMV major immediate–early promotor and tetR itself. It was shown that gene expression from the tetracycline operator-bearing hCMV major immediate–early enhancer promotor could be regulated by tetR over three orders of magnitude in response to tetracycline when the reporter was cotransfected with the tetR-expressing plasmid in transient expression assays switch.[74,75] We recently performed an *ex vivo* gene transfer experiment in a porcine full-thickness wound model with the use of a double stable cell line R11/OEGF, in which the expression of hEGF stands under the control of a tet-operator can be regulated by the presence and absence of tetracycline. By transplanting these cells to porcine full-thickness wounds in the presence and absence of locally delivered tetracycline, over 1000-fold regulation in hEGF expression was detected. The levels reached 80 ng/ml. Furthermore, the levels of hEGF expression in R11/OEGF transplanted wounds could be controlled by tetracycline at different concentrations.

15.7 FUTURE APPLICATIONS AND PITFALLS

The healing response is complex and, given the redundant and synergistic effects of the mediators involved, gene therapy directed at one growth factor may not attenuate pathological wound healing responses. It is plausible that combinations of various growth factors given at meticulously timed intervals may promote wound healing.

Timing and bioavailability of these growth factors are essential features of gene therapy strategies. Coupling tissue-specific promoting genes with growth factor genes may further direct gene therapy to particular cell lines in order to simultaneously improve the therapeutic effect and diminish therapeutic toxicity.

Gene therapy is not limited to the expression of active proteins. *In vivo* and *ex vivo* gene transfer of a dominant-negative mutant polypeptide or a single-chain antibody specific to a particular growth factor or cytokine in the localized wound microenvironment might be an effective therapy in controlling overhealing. The functional knockout of a specific growth factor can also be achieved by gene transfer of soluble growth factor receptors.

Epigenetic approaches do not involve introduction of a DNA sequence that will be used to translate a protein. Rather, one introduces DNA sequences that modify the cell's ability to express its own endogenous genes. An "antisense" cDNA to a growth factor would block the cell from translating that protein. There has been a resurgence of interest in antisense technology through oligonucleotides with the completion of the human genome project. New delivery techniques should make oligonucleotide therapy more efficient. Another new approach is the use of ribozomes, which are specifically designed segments of RNA that have catalytic activity preventing the production of proteins. Moreover, the newly emerged siRNA technology could be also used as potential wound therapy.

15.8 CONCLUSION

Using gene therapy to selectively elevate or downregulate expression of a particular growth factor in the healing wound microenvironment has great promise in promoting tissue repair and regeneration, in particular if one considers that healing of a wound is a local event and requires high levels of transgene expression only for a limited period of time. Skin is a good candidate for gene therapy not only because of its obvious accessibility but also for its capacity for regeneration and abundant vascularity. Although many reasons have been proposed for why chronic open wounds fail to heal, no unifying theory exists, and the cause is most likely multifactorial. Altering local factors and meticulous care are paramount in preventing wound progression, but the local milieu of growth factors may also greatly influence wound healing. The major challenges facing wound repair are the problem of identifying an appropriate gene that is effective in tissue repair and then ensuring that the therapeutic gene is expressed reliably and at clinically beneficial levels. Ultimately, a genetic device must be developed with which expression of a therapeutic gene could be regulated in a predictable and effective way.

REFERENCES

1. Rumalla, V.K. and Borah, G.L., Cytokines, growth factors and plastic surgery, *Plast. Reconstr. Surg.,* 108, 719, 2001.
2. Singer, A. and Clark, R.A., Mechanisms of disease: cutaneous wound healing, *N. Engl. J. Med.,* 341, 738–746, 1999.
3. Steed, D.L., Modifying the wound healing response with exogenous growth factors, *Clin. Plast. Surg.,* 25, 397–405, 1998.
4. Morgan, J. and Yarmush, M., Gene therapy in tissue engineering, in *Frontiers in Tissue Engineering,* Patrick, C., Mikos, A., and McIntire, L., Eds., Pergamon, Oxford, 1998, p. 283–289.
5. Cutroneo, K. and Chiu, J.F., Comparison and evaluation of gene therapy and epigenetic approaches for wound healing, *Wound Repair Regen.,* 8, 494–502, 2000.
6. Yao, F. and Eriksson, E., Gene therapy in wound repair and regeneration, *Wound Repair Regen.,* 8, 443–451, 2000.
7. De Vries C., Escobedo, J.A., Ueno, H., Houck, K., Ferrara, N., and Williams, L.T., The fms-like tyrosine kinase, a receptor for vascular endothelial growth factor, *Science,* 255, 989, 1992.
8. Carmeliet, P., Ferreira, V., Breier, G., Pollefeyt, S., Kieckens, M., Gertsenstein, M., and Fahrig, M., Abnormal blood vessel development and lethality in embryos lacking a single VEGF allele, *Nature,* 380, 435–439, 1996.
9. Carmeliet, P. and Collen, D., Molecular analysis of blood vessel formation and disease, invited review, *Am. Physiol. Soc.,* H2091–H2104, 1997.
10. Houck, K.A., Ferrara, N., Winer, J., Cachianes, G., Li, B., and Leung, D.W., The vascular endothelial growth factor family: identification of four molecular species and characterization of alternative splicing of RNA, *Mol. Endocrinol.,* 5, 1806, 1991.

11. Maglione, D., Guerriero, V., Viglietto, G., Delli-Bovi, P., and Persico, H., Isolation of human placenta cDNA coding for a protein related to the vascular permeability factor, *Proc. Natl. Acad. Sci. U.S.A.,* 88, 9267–9271, 1991.

12. Ferrara, N., Vascular endothelial growth factor, *Eur. J. Cancer,* 32A, 2413–2422, 1996.

13. Neufeld, G., Tessler, S., Gitay-Goren, H., Cohen, T., and Levi, B.Z., Vascular endothelial growth factor and its receptors, *Prog. Growth Factor Res.,* 5, 89, 1994.

14. Taub, P.J., Marmur, J.D., Zhang, W.X., Senderoff, D., Nhatt, P.D., Phelps, R., Urken, M., Silver, L., and Weinberg, H., Locally administered vascular endothelial growth factor cDNA increases survival of ischaemic experimental skin flaps, *Plast. Reconstr. Surg.,* 102, 2033–2039, 1998.

15. Lubiatowski, P., Gurunluoglu R., Carnevale K., and Siemionow, M., Enhancement of epigastric skin flap survival by adenovirus-mediated VEGF gene therapy, *Plast. Reconstr. Surg.,* 109, 1986–1993, 2002.

16. Takeshita, S., Tsurumi, Y., Couffinahl, T., Asahara, T., and Isner, J., Gene transfer of naked DNA encoding for three isoforms of VEGF stimulates collateral development *in vivo, J. Lab. Invest.,* 75, 487–501, 1996.

17. Ailawadi, M., Lee, J.M., Lee, S., Hackett, N., Crystal, R.G., and Korst, R.J., Adenovirus vector-mediated transfer of the VEGF cDNA to healing abdominal fascia enhances vascularity and bursting strength in mice with normal and impaired wound healing, *Surgery,* 131, 219–227, 2002.

18. Supp, D.M. and Boyce, S.T., Overexpression of VEGF accelerates early vascularization and improves healing of genetically modified cultured skin substitutes, *J. Burn Care Rehabil.,* 23, 10–20, 2002.

19. Yao, F., Visovatti, S., Johnson, S., Chen, M., Slama, J., Wenger, A., and Eriksson, E., Age and growth factors in porcine full thickness wound healing, *Wound Repair Regen.,* 9, 371–377, 2001.

20. Andree, C., Swain, W.F., Page, C.P., Macklin, M.D., Slama, J., Hatzis, D., and Eriksson, E., *In vivo* gene transfer and expression of human epidermal growth factor accelerates wound repair, *Proc. Natl. Acad. Sci. U.S.A.,* 91, 12,188–12,192, 1994.

21. Brown G.L. and Nanney, L.B., Enhancement of wound healing by topical treatment with epidermal growth factor, *N. Engl. J. Med.,* 321, 76–80, 1989.

22. Shiraha, H., Gupta, K., Drabik, K., and Wells, A., Aging fibroblasts present reduced epidermal growth factor responsiveness due to preferential loss of EGF receptors, *J. Biol. Chem.,* 275, 19,343, 2000.

23. Hebda, P.A., Klingbeil, C.K., Abraham, J.A., and Fiddes, J.C., Basic fibroblast growth factor stimulation of epidermal wound healing in pigs, *J. Invest. Dermatol.,* 95, 626, 1990.

24. Fu, X., Shen, Z., and Chen, Y., Basic fibroblast growth factor and wound healing: a multicenter clinical trial in 1024 cases, *Chung Kuo Hsiu Fu Chung Chien Wai Ko Tsa Chih,* 12, 209, 1998.

25. Robson, M.C., Mustoe, T.A., and Hunt, T.K., The future of recombinant growth factors in wound healing, *Am. J. Surg.,* 176, 80S–82S, 1998.

26. Xia, Y.P., Zhao, Y., and Marcus, J., Effects of keratinocyte growth factor-2 on wound healing in an ischaemia impaired rabbit ear model and on scar formation, *J. Pathol.,* 188, 431, 1999.

27. Werner, S., Smola, H., and Liao, X., The function of KGF in morphogenesis of epithelium and reepithelialization of wounds, *Science,* 266, 819, 1994.

28. Werner, S., Breeden, M., Hubner, G., Greenhalgh, D.G., and Longaker, M.T., Introduction of keratinocyte growth factor expression is reduced and delayed during wound healing in the genetically diabetic mouse, *J. Invest. Dermatol.,* 103, 469, 1994.

29. Staiano-Coico, L., Krueger, J.G., Rubin, J.S., D'limi, S., Vallat, V.P., Valentino, L., Fahey, T., Hawe, A., Kingston, G., and Madden, M.R., Human keratinocyte growth factor effects in a porcine model of epidermal wound healing, *J. Exp. Med.,* 178, 865–878, 1993.

30. Derynck, R., Jarrett, J.A., Chen, E.Y., Eaton, D.H., Bell, J.R., Assoian, R.K., Roberts A.B., Sporn, M.B., and Goeddel, D.V., Human transforming growth factor-beta complementary DNA sequence and expression in normal and transformed cells, *Nature,* 316, 701, 1985.

31. Moses, H.L.,Yang, E.Y., and Pietenpol, J.A., TGF-beta stimulation and inhibition of cell proliferation: new mechanistic insights, *Cell,* 635, 245–247, 1990.

32. Massague, J., The transforming growth factor beta family, *Annu. Rev. Cell Biol.,* 6, 597–641, 1990.

33. Niesler, C.U. and Ferguson, M.W., TGF-beta superfamily cytokines in wound healing, in *TGF-beta and Related Cytokines in Inflammation,* Breit, S.N., and Wahl, S.M., Eds. Birkhauser Verlag, Basel, 2001, pp. 173–198.

34. Battegay, E., Rupp, J., Iruela-Arispe, L., Sage, E., and Pech, M., PDGF-BB modulates endothelial proliferation and angiogenesis *in vitro* via PDGF-beta receptors, *J. Cell Biol.,* 125, 917–928, 1994.

35. Roberts, A.B. and Sporn, M.B., Physiologic actions and clinical applications of transforming growth factor betas and wound healing, *Int. J. Biochem. Cell. Biol.,* 29, 63, 1997.

36. Boyd, F.T., Cheifetz, S., Andres, J., Laiho, M., and Massague, J., TGF-beta receptors and binding proteoglycans, *J. Cell. Sci. Suppl.,* 13, 131–138, 1990.

37. Geng, Y. and Weinberg, R.A., TGF-beta effects on expression of G1 cyclins and cyclin-dependent protein kinases, *Proc. Natl. Acad. Sci. U.S.A.,* 90, 10, 315–319, 1993.

38. Vinals, F. and Poussegur, J., Transforming growth factor beta-1 promotes endothelial cell survival during *in vitro* angiogenesis via an autocrine mechanism implicating TGF-a signaling, *Mol. Cell. Biol.,* 21, 7218–7230, 2001.

39. Bauer, B.S., Tredget, E.E., Marcoux, Y., Scott, P.G., and Ghahary, A., Latent and active transforming growth factor beta 1 released from genetically modified keratinocytes modulates extracellular matrix expression by dermal fibroblasts in a coculture system., *J. Invest. Dermatol.,* 119, 456–463, 2002.

40. Shah, M., Foreman, D.M., and Ferguson, M.W., Neutralization of TGF-beta 1 and TGF-beta 2 or exogenous addition of TGF-beta 3 to cutaneous rat wounds reduces scarring, *J. Cell. Sci.,* 108, 985, 1995.

41. Benn, S.I., Whitsitt, J.S., Broadley, K.N., Nanney, L.B., Perkins, D., He, L., Patel, M., Morgan, J.R., Swain, W.F., and Davidson, J.M., Particle-mediated gene transfer with transforming growth factor beta 1 cDNAs enhances wound repair in rat skin, *J. Clin. Invest.,* 98, 2894–2902, 1996.

42. Derynck, R., Zhang, Y., and Feng, X.H., Smads: transcriptional activators of TGF-beta responses, *Cell.,* 95, 737, 1998.

43. Roberts, A.B. and Derynck, R., Signaling schemes for TGF-beta, *Sci STKE* 18: PE 43, 2001.

44. Kratz, G., Lake M., and Gidlund, M., Insulin-like growth factor-I and II and their role in the reepithelialization of wounds: interaction with insulin-like growth factor binding protein type 1, *Scand. J. Plast. Reconstr. Surg. Hand Surg.,* 28, 107, 1994.

45. Taylor, W.R. and Alexander, R.W., Autocrine control of wound repair by insulin-like growth factor-I in cultured endothelial cells, *Am. J. Physiol.,* 265, C801, 1993.

46. Bitar, M.S., Insulin-like growth factor-1 reverses diabetes-induced wound healing impairment in rats, *Horm. Metab. Res.,* 29, 383, 1997.

47. Bennett, N. and Schultz, P., Growth factors and wound healing: biochemical properties of growth factors and their receptors, *Am. J. Surg.,* 165, 728–737, 1993.

48. Pierce, G.F., Tarply, J.E., Yanagihara, D., Mustoe, T.A., Fox, G.M., and Thomasson, A., Platelet derived growth factor (BB-homodimer), transforming growth factor-beta 1, and basis fibroblast growth factor in dermal wound healing: neovessel and matrix formation and cessation of repair, *Am. J. Pathol.,* 140, 1375, 1992.

49. Steed, D.L., Diabetic ulcer study group: clinical evaluation of recombinant human platelet derived growth factor for the treatment of lower extremity diabetic ulcers, *J. Vasc. Surg.,* 21, 71–81, 1995.

50. Falanga, V., Eaglestein, W.H., Bucalo, B., Katz, M.H., Harris, B., and Carson, P., Topical use of human recombinant epidermal growth factor in venous ulcers. *J. Dermatol. Surg. Oncol.,* 18, 604–606, 1992.

51. Robson, M.C., Phillips, L.G., Thomason, A., Robson, L.E., and Pierce, G.F., Platelet-derived growth factor BB for the treatment of chronic pressure ulcers, *Lancet,* 339, 23–25, 1992.

52. Eming, S.A., Whitsitt, J.S., He, L., Krieg, T., Morgan J.R., and Davidson, J.M., Particle mediated gene transfer of PDGF isoforms promotes wound repair, *J. Invest. Dermatol.,* 112, 297–302, 1999.

53. *Culver, K.W.,* Methods for gene transfer and repair, in *Gene Therapy: A Primer for Physicians,* Culver, K.W., Ed., Marie-An Liebert Inc., Larchmont, N.Y., 1996, pp. 19–21.

54. Morgan, J.R. and Eden, C.A., Retroviral-mediated gene transfer into transplantable human epidermal cells, *Prog. Clin. Biolog. Res.,* 365, 417–428, 1991.

55. Naldini, L., Blomer, U., Gallay, P., Ory, D., Mulligan, R., Gage, F., Verma, I., and Trono, D., *In vivo* gene delivery and stable transduction of non dividing cells by a lentiviral vector, *Science,* 272, 263–267, 1996.

56. Mitani, K., Graham, H., Caskey, C.T., and Kochanek, S., Rescue, propagation and potential purification of a helper-virus dependent adenovirus vector, *Proc. Natl. Acad. Sci. U.S.A.,* 92, 3854–3858, 1995.

57. Fisher, K.J., Chojl H., Burda, J., Chen, S.J., and Wilson, J.M., Recombinant adenovirus deleted of all viral genes for gene therapy of cystic fibrosis, *Virology,* 217, 11–22, 1996.

58. Liechty, K.W., Sablick, T.J., Adzick, N.S., and Cromblestone, T.M., Recombinant adenoviral mediated gene transfer in ischaemic impaired wound healing, *Wound Repair Regen.,* 7, 148–153, 1999.

59. Cheung, A.K., Hoggan, M.D., and Hauswirth, W.W., Integration of the adeno-associated virus genome into cellular DNA in latently infected human Detroit 6 cells, *J. Virol.,* 33, 739–748, 1980

60. Xiao, W., Chirmule, N., Berta, S.C., McCullough, B., Gao, G., and Wilson, J., Gene therapy vectors based on adeno-associated virus type 1, *J. Virol.,* 73, 3994–4003, 1999.

61. Yang, N.S., Burkholder, J., Roberts, B., Martinell, B., and McCabe, D., *In vivo* and *in vitro* gene transfer to mammalian somatic cells by particle bombardment, *Proc. Natl. Acad. Sci. U.S.A.,* 87, 9568–9572, 1990.

62. Benn, S.I., Whitsitt, J., Broadley, K., Nanney, L., Perkins, D., He, L., Patel, M., Morgan, J., Swain, W., and Davidson, J.M., Particle mediated gene transfer with transforming growth factor beta1 cDNAs enhances wound repair in rat skin, *J. Clin. Invest.,* 98, 2894–2902, 1996.

63. Eriksson, E., Yao, F., Svensjo, T., Winkler, T., Slama, J., Macklin, M., Andree, C., McGregor, M., Hinshaw, V., and Swain, W., *In vivo* gene transfer to skin by micro-seeding, *J. Surg. Res.*, 78, 85–91, 1998.
64. Vranckx, J.J., Yao, F., Petrie, N., Augustinova, H., Hoeller, D., Visovatti, S., Chen, M., and Eriksson, E., *In-vivo* gene delivery of Ad-VEGF$_{121}$ to full-thickness wounds in aged pigs results in a high VEGF-expression but not in accelerated healing, Submitted. Proc. PSRC 2003. p. 256.
65. Felgner, P.L., Gadek, T.R., and Holm, M., Lipofection: a highly efficient, lipid mediated DNA transfection procedure, *Proc. Natl. Acad. Sci. U.S.A.*, 84, 7413–7417, 1987.
66. Wheeler, C.J., Felgner, P.L., Tsai, Y., Marshall, J., Sukhu, L., Doh, G., Hartikka, J., Manthorpe, M., Nichols, M., Plewe, M., Liang, X., Norman, J., Smith, A., and Cheng, S., A novel cationic lipid greatly enhances plasmid DNA delivery and expression in mouse lung, *Proc. Natl. Acad. Sci. U.S.A.*, 93, 11,454–11,459, 1996.
67. Hengge, U.R., Walker, P.S., and Vogel, J.C., Expression of naked DNA in human, pig and mouse skin, *J. Clin. Invest.*, 97, 2911–2916, 1996.
68. Titomorov, A.V., Sukharev, S., and Kistanova, E., *In vivo* electroporation and stable transformation of skin cells of newborn mice by plasmid DNA, *Biochem. Biophys. Res. Commun.*, 220, 633–636, 1996.
69. Kangesu, T., Navsaria, H., Manak, S., Shurey, C., Jones, C., Fryer, P., Leigh, I., and Green, C., A porcine model using skin graft chambers for studies on cultured keratinocytes, *Br. J. Plast. Surg.*, 46, 393–400, 1993.
70. Sullivan, T.P., Eaglstein, W., Davis, S.C., and Mertz, P., The pig as a model for human wound healing, *Wound Repair Regen.*, 9, 66, 2001.
71. Vardaxis, N.J., Brans, T.A., Boon, M.E., Kreis, R., and Marres, L., Confocal laser scanning microscopy of porcine skin: implications for human wound healing studies, *J. Anatomy*, 190, 601–611, 1997.
72. Wollina, U., Berger, U., and Mahrle, G., Immunohistochemistry of porcine skin, *Acta Histochem.*, 90, 87–91, 1991.
73. Heinrich, W., Lange, P.M., Stirz, T., and Lancu, C., Isolation and characterization of large cyanogen bromide peptides from the a1 and a2-chains in pig skin collagen, *FEBS Lett.*, 16, 63–67, 1971.
74. Yao, F., Svensjo, T., Winker, T., Lu, M., and Eriksson, E., Tetracycline repressor, tetR, rather than tetR-mamalian cell transcription fusion derivative, regulates inducible gene expression in mammalian cells, *Hum. Gene Ther.*, 9, 1939–1950, 1998.
75. Yao, F. and Eriksson, E., A novel tetracycline-inducible viral replication switch, *Hum. Gene Ther.*, 10, 419–427, 1999.
76. Vranckx, J.J., Slama, J., Preuss, S., Perez, N., Svensjo, T., Breuiing, K., Bartlett, R., Pribaz, J., Weiss, D., and Eriksson E., Wet wound healing, *Plast. Reconstr. Surg.*, 110, 1680, 2002.

16 Autologous Skin Transplantation

Tor Svensjö and Elof Eriksson

CONTENTS

16.1 INTRODUCTION

Restoration of an intact barrier is of critical importance following wounding and may be achieved by normal wound healing, by direct wound closure, or by skin transplantation. Skin transplantation is defined as the transposition of skin from one part of the body (donor site) to another location (recipient site). It most commonly refers to skin grafting. Skin grafts lack their own blood supply and therefore rely on revascularization from the recipient site. It is believed that skin grafting was performed by the natives of India more than 2000 years ago,[1,2] but widespread interest did not develop until the nineteenth century.[1,3] Skin may also be transferred without disruption of its main vascular supply (or sometimes microsurgically, by reanastomosis with vessels at the recipient site) by use of skin flaps. Flap surgery requires greater anatomical knowledge and planning and is generally performed by physicians with training in plastic and reconstructive surgery. The earliest skin flap procedure described is probably that of Sushruta, the father of Hindu surgery, who described nasal reconstruction using a cheek flap sometime between 800 and 750 B.C.[3] Other techniques of skin transplantation include the use of minced skin and pinch grafts. These are essentially variants of skin grafts and will also be discussed in that section.

During the past three decades, tissue culture techniques have gone through tremendous development. This has allowed the production of various cultured skin components. Epidermal cells may be cultured and expanded *in vitro,* and when sufficient numbers of cells have been generated, they are transplanted to the skin defect.[4,5] The technique is particularly useful when donor sites are limited due to extensive skin loss, as in severely burned patients. More recently, the possibility of transplanting gene-modified cultured skin has been demonstrated.[6,7] In the future it may be possible to transplant genetically modified skin with the dual purpose of resurfacing skin defects as well as augmenting skin wound healing.[8] The various clinical methods for skin transplantation that are discussed in this chapter are summarized in Table 16.1.

16.2 SKIN FLAPS AND SKIN EXPANSION

Numerous skin flaps have been described. A brief overview is presented here, but for more in-depth reading several other sources are recommended.[9–14] Skin flaps may be indicated for wound coverage for several reasons. Among the most important is impaired healing of the recipient site that renders normal skin grafting difficult, e.g., arterial insufficiency, irradiated skin, or diabetes. Skin flaps are also employed when there is a requirement for good functional and cosmetic outcome, for example on the face. Specialized flaps are also used to cover gliding tendons, to reconstruct bony defects, and for specialized sensory function.

In principle, a flap is a unit of tissue that is transferred from one site (the donor site) to another (the recipient site) while maintaining its own blood supply. The various types of flaps that exist may be categorized according to:

1. Type of blood supply
2. Type of tissue that is transferred
3. Location of donor site

Type of blood supply — A flap can maintain its blood supply in two ways. If the blood supply is not derived from a recognized artery but rather comes from many small unnamed vessels, the flap is referred to as a random flap. If the blood supply comes from a recognized artery or group of arteries, it is referred to as an axial flap.

Type of tissue that is transferred — In general, flaps may comprise in part or in whole almost any component of the human body as long as an adequate blood supply to the flap is ensured after tissue transfer. Skin flaps may consist of skin only (cutaneous flaps) or of several different types of tissue (skin and fascia — fascio-cutaneous; or skin, fascia, and muscle — musculo-cutaneous).

Location of donor site — Skin flaps may be transferred from an area adjacent to the defect. This is known as a "local" flap. Tissue transferred from a remote anatomic site is referred to as a "distant" flap. Distant flaps are either "pedicled" (transferred while still attached to their original blood supply) or "free." Free flaps have been physically detached from their native blood supply and then reattached to vessels at the recipient site. As stated above, skin flaps generally result in a good cosmetic and functional outcome. Extensive use of flaps is limited, however, since the donor site also must be closed. When the skin is transferred from regions that display excessive skin/tissue, such as the abdomen, donor site closure may be performed by direct suture. In other cases, it is often closed with a skin graft. The donor site may also undergo tissue expansion beforehand (see below), and in such cases there is usually enough remaining skin to immediately close the skin defect.

The phenomenon of tissue expansion of the skin and underlying soft tissues has long been observed in pregnancy, slow-growing tumors, and fluid collections, where the local tissue expands and enlarges in response to the tension generated by the increased volume of the mass. Skin expansion usually refers to the surgical introduction of subcutaneous silicone chambers that are subsequently filled with saline in a stepwise fashion to slowly expand the overlying tissue(s). The expanded skin is usually transferred to the recipient site as a local skin flap. Common indications include treatment of alopecia (e.g., traumatic or male pattern baldness), breast reconstruction, and reconstructive surgery of the head, neck, and face regions.[15] The gain in surface area appears to result from increased mitotic activity and represents new tissue. Tissue expansion offers a reliable method to obtain local donor skin of fine texture and color match with minimal donor site morbidity and scarring. It has also been used at various locations in the body to provide tissue with specialized sensory function, as with skin flaps in breast reconstruction. Disadvantages include temporary cosmetic deformity during the expansion phase, the requirement of multiple operations, and a prolonged outpatient course. The expansion involves the dermal and epidermal components; however, skin appendages such as sweat glands and hair follicles do not change in number. In addition, the adipose tissue undergoes permanent atrophy of 30 to 50% with loss of fat cells.

16.3 SKIN GRAFTS

A skin graft differs from a skin flap in that its survival depends entirely on the blood supply from the recipient site. Skin grafts consist of the entire epidermis and a dermal component of variable thickness. If the entire thickness of the dermis is included, the appropriate term is full-thickness skin graft (FTSG).[16] If less than the entire thickness of the dermis is included, appropriate terms are partial or split-thickness skin graft (STSG). The choice between full- and split-thickness skin grafting depends on wound condition, location, and size as well as aesthetic concerns. In general, wounds covered with full-thickness grafts contract less than those covered with split-thickness grafts, and those covered with thick STSGs contract less than those treated with thin split-thickness grafts.[17] Furthermore, wounds covered with thin STSGs contract less than open wounds do.[18]

The most critical component of successful skin grafting is preparation of the recipient site. Physiologic conditions must be optimized to accept and nourish the graft. Skin grafts will not survive on tissue without a blood supply, such as bone devascularized by removal of the periosteum, cartilage without the perichondrium, tendon without parathenon, or nerve without perineurium. Skin grafts will survive

TABLE 16.1
Overview of Clinical Methods for Autologous Skin Transplantation

	Advantages	Disadvantages	Primary use
Skin flaps	Cosmetic outcome Functionality Mechanical durability Skin appendages (hair follicles, sweat glands, apocrine glands) are maintained Higher survival rate in recipient sites with compromised healing as compared to skin grafts Inhibit contraction to a high extent	Require special knowledge, handling and planning Distant flaps require microsurgical vessel anastomosis Donor site defect is equivalent to recipient site defect and must be closed primarily or resurfaced with a split-thickness graft from another site No expansion allowed	Compromised healing at the recipient site (post trauma radiation therapy, diabetes, vascular disease) High demands on cosmetic and functional outcome (e.g., face, sensory function, mechanical durability)
Skin expansion	Essentially as above	Temporary cosmetic deformity during the expansion phase The time period needed for expansion Need for multiple procedures Complications associated with the implant and placement Atrophy of adipose tissue Skin appendages (hair follicles and sweat glands) are not multiplied during expansion	Alopecia Breast reconstruction Reconstructive surgery in head, neck, and facial areas
Full-thickness skin grafts	Cosmetic outcome, functionality and mechanical durability usually equal or somewhere between skin flaps and STSG Simplicity of method Skin appendages (hair follicles, sweat glands, apocrine glands) are maintained fully or partially Inhibit contraction to a moderate to high extent	Donor site defect is equivalent to recipient site defect and must be closed by approximation or resurfaced with a split-thickness graft from another site Increased thickness of the graft lead to increased risk of graft failure FTSG require a healthy and sufficiently vascularized recipient site No expansion allowed	Wound closure in the face or hand and over joints

TABLE 16.1 (CONTINUED)
Overview of Clinical Methods for Autologous Skin Transplantation

	Advantages	Disadvantages	Primary use
Split-thickness skin grafts	Donor sites heal completely (thin grafts without scarring) and may be reharvested Fairly simple method STSG may be meshed to allow grafting of large skin defects (graft expansion) Inhibit contraction (but correlates to graft thickness and depends on the anatomical location of the recipient site) Meshing allows expansion	Significant pain at the donor site Worse cosmetic and functional outcome, as well as mechanical durability, when compared to FTSG and flaps Skin appendages are usually not preserved, leading to hairless, dry, and sometimes itching skin Require a harvest instrument, e.g., a dermatome Unattractive honeycomb appearance of healed recipient site when grafting meshed STSG	Resurface donor sites (skin flap, FTSG) Leg ulcers Burn wounds Post traumatic and post surgical reconstruction Leg ulcers (venous, vasculitic and mixed etiology)
Pinch grafts	Simplicity Cost Feasibility in primary care facilities	Poor cosmetic outcome at both donor and recipient sites Time required to harvest and graft	Leg ulcers (venous, vasculitic, and mixed etiology)
Minced skin	High expansion factor	Time required to harvest and graft usually longer than procedures using meshed STSG Still at an experimental stage	Extensive burns
Cultured epidermis	Expansion (enough skin to cover the entire body can be generated from a small skin biopsy) Minimal donor site morbidity	Expensive Time needed to culture skin typically 3-4 weeks Poor cosmetic outcome Poor mechanical durability Lack of skin appendages Necessity to coordinate culture lab and operating theater Dermis or a dermal substitute is necessary to increase graft take and function Do not prevent wound contraction	Extensive burns

on periosteum, perichondrium, parathenon, perineurium, dermis, fascia, muscle, and granulation tissue. Wounds secondary to irradiation have a poor blood supply and are unlikely to support a graft. Patients with wounds resulting from venous stasis or arterial insufficiency need to have the underlying condition treated prior to grafting to increase the likelihood of graft survival.

16.3.1 FULL-THICKNESS SKIN GRAFTS

Full-thickness skin grafts are ideal for visible areas of the face that are inaccessible to local flaps or when local flaps are not indicated. Full-thickness grafts retain more of the characteristics of normal skin including color, texture, and thickness in comparison to split-thickness grafts. Full-thickness grafts also undergo less contraction while healing. This is important on the face, as well as on the hands and over mobile joint surfaces. Full-thickness grafts in children are also more likely to grow with the individual. However, full-thickness skin grafts are limited to relatively small, uncontaminated, well-vascularized wounds and thus do not have as wide a range of application as split-thickness grafts do. Donor sites must be closed primarily or, sometimes, resurfaced with a STSG from another site.

Full-thickness skin grafts may be harvested with a scalpel. The graft is dissected from underlying subcutaneous fat. Residual adipose tissue may be trimmed from the underside of the graft with a scissors because the fat reduces revascularization from the wound bed.

16.3.2 SPLIT-THICKNESS SKIN GRAFTS

Split-thickness skin grafts can tolerate less-ideal conditions for survival and have a much broader range of application. They are harvested with a dermatome, a specialized instrument, equipped with an oscillating knife, which cuts STSG of adjustable depth and wideness. Split-thickness skin grafts are categorized as thin (0.005 to 0.012 in.), intermediate (0.012 to 0.018 in.), or thick (0.018 to 0.030 in.), based on the thickness of the graft harvested[14,19,20] (Figure 16.1). They are used to resurface large wounds, line cavities, resurface mucosal defects, close donor sites of flaps, and resurface muscle flaps.

Split-thickness skin graft donor sites heal spontaneously with cells supplied by the remaining epidermal appendages, and these donor sites may be reharvested once healing is complete. Thin STSG donor sites heal faster and with less scarring than thicker skin graft sites do. This should be considered when donor sites are limited, with the resulting necessity of harvesting skin from previous donor sites.

Split-thickness skin grafts also have significant disadvantages that must be considered. They are more fragile, especially when placed over areas with little underlying soft-tissue bulk for support, and usually cannot withstand subsequent radiation therapy. They contract more during healing, do not grow with the individual, and tend to be smoother and shinier than normal skin because of the absence of skin appendages.[20] They also tend to be abnormally pigmented, either pale or white, or alternatively hyperpigmented, particularly in darker-skinned individuals.[20] Because of their disadvantages, STSGs are less than ideal, particularly in exposed areas.

Once harvested, an STSG may be meshed by placing the graft on a carrier and passing it through a mechanical meshing instrument.[21] The mesher cuts multiple parallel slits in the graft, allowing it to be pulled out to several times its width, giving it a chicken-wire or honeycomb appearance. This allows expansion of the graft to up to nine times the donor site surface area. This is indicated when insufficient donor skin is available for large wounds, as in major burns, or when the recipient site is

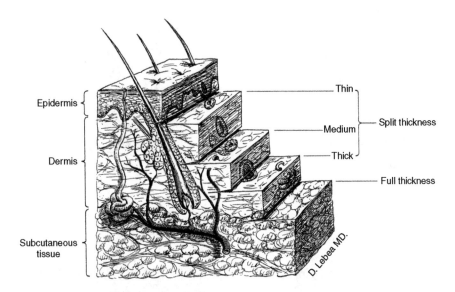

Epidermis

Dermis

Subcutaneous
tissue

Thin

Medium

Thick

Split thickness

Full thickness

D. Lebea MD.

FIGURE 16.1 Drawing illustrating the difference between a split thickness and a full thickness skin graft. Split thickness skin grafts are also further categorized as thin (0.005–0.012 in), intermediate (0.012–0.018), or thick (0.018–0.030). Reproduced from Wood, R.J. and Jurkiewicz, M.J., in *Principles of Surgery*, 7th ed., Schwartz, S.I., Shires, G.T., Spencer, F.C., Daly, J.M., Fischer, J.E., and Galloway, A.C., Eds., McGraw-Hill Professional Publishing, New York, 1998. With permission from McGraw-Hill Professional Publishing.

irregularly contoured, and adherence is a concern. Expansion slits also allow wound fluid to escape through the graft rather than accumulating beneath the graft and preventing adherence. Expansion slits must heal by reepithelialization and may contract significantly. In addition, mesh-grafted wounds have a characteristic honeycomb appearance. Meshed grafts are therefore usually avoided in the face, hands, and other highly visible areas.

16.3.3 PINCH GRAFTS

Reverdin is usually credited with providing, in 1869, the first detailed description of pinch grafting.[1,2] The method refers to transplantation of small fragments of skin, typically 3 to 5 mm in diameter, which contain portions of both dermis and epidermis.[22] The grafts are most commonly harvested by horizontal excision of skin that has been raised with a small needle (Figure 16.2).[23,24] The procedure was at one time performed by pinching up the superficial skin with a forceps and cutting or pinching it off with scissors; for this reason, the grafts were called "pinch grafts."[24] Similar grafts may also be obtained utilizing a punch biopsy instrument (i.e., a punch graft)[25] or a specialized instrument, the trigger-fired pinch graft harvester.[26] Pinch grafting may be employed on any kind of wound, but it has been found to be particularly useful and efficient as a complement to conservative therapy of leg ulcers.[22,27] A fine granulation surface on the ulcer and absence of clinical signs of infection are considered prerequisites before attempts are made to graft the wound.[22] The grafts are evenly administered over the wound surface with typically 0.5 to 1

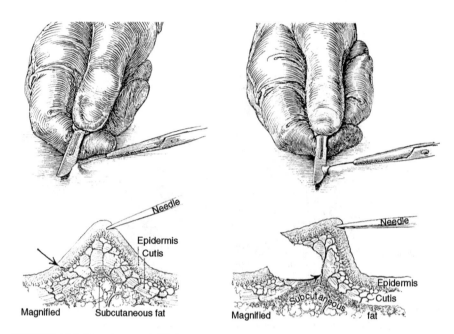

FIGURE 16.2 Drawing exemplifying the common method of harvesting a pinch graft. Reproduced from Davis, J.S., *Ann. Surg.*, 91, 633–635, 1930.

cm free space between the grafts. Moist dressings are then used to cover the wound, and in venous leg ulcers, compression bandages are overlaid. The advantages of pinch grafting are its simplicity, the fact that it requires no special equipment to perform, and its feasibility in primary care facilities, the location where it also is the least expensive to perform.[22] Disadvantages include poor cosmetic outcome, at both the recipient and donor sites, and the long time required to graft large ulcers.[19]

16.3.4 MINCED SKIN GRAFTS

Minced skin is not a defined term; however, it generally refers to skin that has been cut or sliced into small pieces less than or equal to approximately one millimeter in diameter. It is often referred to as microskin; however, we have chosen to use the more descriptive term "minced skin." The rationale for mincing skin is that it may allow for greater expansion of grafts than can be achieved with traditional skin meshers (i.e., donor-to-recipient site ratio greater than approximately 1:9). This would be of particular use when donor sites are limited, such as in patients with massive burns. The basic principle is that each small graft will support reepithelialization once grafted to the wound. In theory, the smallest graft possible would be one that contains one epidermal cell with the ability to replicate.

The concept of creating small skin grafts for transplantation dates back to at least 1895, at which time von Mangoldt described his method. He held a razor blade oriented perpendicular to the skin and scraped the surface of it to yield small skin particles. The resulting mixture of epidermal and possibly dermal cells as well as blood was then applied to the granulating surface of wounds with reported success in terms of healing.[28] The method was successfully adopted by some clinicians,[1] but it never seemed to gain any widespread use.

Najarian and others described utilization of a kitchen blender to mince rabbit STSGs to yield particles of epidermal cells, dermal elements, hair shafts, and hair follicles.[29] The epidermal particles consisted of approximately 10 to 100 epidermal cells. They were successfully grafted to rabbit full-thickness skin wounds in a ratio of 1:10 (relation between donor and recipient site areas). The rate of epithelialization was essentially the same whether they were applied to granulation tissue or directly on fascia of freshly excised wounds.[29] Comparable results were also reported by Cox and Nichol utilizing a similar method;[30] however, to date, no clinical study has reported on their methods.

A different procedure was designed by Nyström,[31] who constructed an apparatus for mincing STSGs. His cutting apparatus had several stainless steel lamellas run in parallel at a 1-mm distance from one another. The STSG was laid onto the lamella, fixed, and then cut into strips with a scalpel blade. The processed STSG was then lifted, turned 90°, and repositioned over the lamella again, allowing it to be cut into small grafts with a size of 1 × 1 mm. Unlike Najarian and Cox, Nyström used the minced skin to graft burns and leg ulcers in a limited number of humans with seemingly fair results in terms of reepithelialization. Nyström's method did not gain widespread use, however, perhaps because of the introduction of the faster and more practical skin meshing technique by Vandeput and colleagues in 1963.[21] This allowed fast expansion of STSG up to approximately 1:9. However, meshed grafts are typically not expanded beyond 1:4 to 6 because of practical difficulties in the handling of such grafts.[32,33]

In 1994, Lin and Horng described a method to produce small skin grafts, 1.2 × 1.2 mm, by processing the STSG through a skin mesher twice. This technique is essentially a refinement of Nyström's method, as it produces grafts of comparable architecture and size; however, it is faster and simpler.[34] Clinical results with this method were reported to be equivalent to those obtained with an older mincing method (cutting with scissors) in terms of healing.[34,35] The authors preferred an expansion rate of 1:10, as it ensured reepithelialization in a reasonable time. The healed skin displayed only mild hypertrophy and good pliability; however, a cobblestone appearance gave grafted sites a poor cosmetic result. The latter should, however, be compared to the honeycomb appearance of wounds grafted with meshed STSGs. One disadvantage with the mincing process is that dermal and epidermal cells of the small grafts are exposed to air in inverse proportion to the size of the skin graft. The smaller the grafts, the more vulnerable they become to desiccation, and special handling techniques may be required. Biobrane®[34,35] and skin allografts[31,35,36] have been used in humans to cover the grafts.

In a recent experimental study, minced skin was transplanted to porcine wounds enclosed in a liquid environment.[37] The skin particles were created with modified scalpel blades that were used to mince skin *in situ* and yielded particles in the range of 50 to 600 μm. The grafted minced skin particles and the wounds were maintained in a liquid environment, and the rate of reepithelialization increased and contraction decreased in proportion to the amount of minced skin transplanted. The histological appearance of the neo-epidermis was similar, whether the wounds had been grafted with minced skin, cultured keratinocytes, or noncultured keratinocytes.

In summary, minced skin transplantation is still at an experimental stage. There is a need for future studies that directly compare minced skin to meshed STSGs and/or cultured epidermis, to determine if the technique may replace or be a complement to the already-established treatment options.

16.4 CELLULAR GRAFTS

This heterogeneous group encompasses transplantation of skin cells, either cultured or noncultured. The latter are obtained by enzymatic digestion of skin samples. Research has mainly focused on transplantation of keratinocytes and/or fibroblasts, but reports have also appeared on the grafting of endothelial cells,[38,39] melanocytes,[40–47] and preadipocytes.[48] Of these cells, only keratinocytes may resurface the wound and reestablish the protective barrier function of the epidermis. Other cell types have been transplanted with the purpose of enhancing keratinocyte grafting, to augment skin regeneration, and/or for cosmetic reasons.

16.4.1 KERATINOCYTES

Billingham and Reynolds[49] were the first to exclusively study transplantation of epidermal cells. They digested STSGs with trypsin and further processed the STSGs in sodium citrate solution to yield either sheets of epidermis or epidermal cell suspensions. Both types of grafts were shown to reepithelialize rabbit full-thickness skin wounds, and no apparent difference in the histological appearance of neo-epidermis from sheet grafts or suspensions was found.

Twenty-two years later, Rheinwald and Green presented their landmark study on the serial cultivation of human keratinocytes in a defined medium and with a culture feeder layer consisting of irradiated 3T3 mouse fibroblasts.[50] These cells could be used to generate coherent stratifying sheets a thousand-fold larger than the original epidermal specimen, and may be released from the culture dishes by treatment with the protease dispase.[4] It was further shown that such human sheet grafts could resurface full-thickness skin defects in immunodeficient mice.[51]

The first clinical pilot, published in 1981, demonstrated that autologous sheet grafts, or cultured epithelial autografts (CEAs), as they are usually referred to, could be used in the treatment of patients with third-degree burn wounds and that permanent wound coverage with CEAs was possible.[5] In 1984, it was shown that CEA grafting could be lifesaving in pediatric patients with massive burn wounds.[52] Since then, several clinical studies have reported on the use of cultured autologous keratinocyte grafts to resurface burn wounds,[52–56] in the treatment of certain skin diseases,[57–59] and for the treatment of skin ulcers.[60] In 1988, CEAs prepared by the method of Rheinwald and Green became commercially available (e.g., Genzyme Tissue Repair Corporation, Cambridge, Mass., U.S.A.), thereby expanding the scope of application of this therapy.

The grafts are mounted onto a backing material of Vaseline-impregnated gauze to provide enough structural support to be handled surgically, but they are fragile and great care must be taken to minimize manipulation and trauma of the CEA. As with other grafting procedures, successful take of the CEAs relies on adequate hemostasis and debridement of the recipient site as well as the absence of infection of the wound bed. Grossly, the CEA appears translucent and has a mucoid consistency, The graft stays invisible on the recipient site until a stratum corneum has developed, which normally takes about 8 d.[5] Microscopically, CEAs appear as stratified sheets of keratinocytes with basal and suprabasal layers that are polarized towards the attachment surface of the culture flask.[61] The sheets are typically 3 to 9 cell layers thick and display a relatively undifferentiated morphology. After transplantation, the CEAs rapidly differentiate and appear as normally stratified epidermis (but initially hypertrophic) with granular and cornified layers.[61] Rete ridges develop after about 2 to 12 months.[56]

One of the most significant problems in the clinical use of CEAs has been the variable take rates reported. When grafted to wound bed granulation tissue, the average take-rate of CEAs is 55 to 60%.[61] The introduction of a two-step grafting procedure by Cuono and coworkers[62] has improved take rates significantly. In this procedure, CEA is transplanted to the dermal remnants of engrafted, partially excised skin allografts. New clinical data from seven burn centers in the United States, using commercially produced CEAs with the two-step procedure, have shown that the rate of successful engraftment averages 85%, a take rate comparable to that of meshed STSGs.[61] This approach is also practical since skin allograft, so far, is the best known temporary wound cover available for large skin defects. One drawback with the use of skin allograft is the potential risk of transmitting viruses to the recipient. Careful screening of prospective donors reduces the risk of transmission of infective agents, but the risk is not completely eliminated.

Some investigators have also described the phenomenon of late graft loss, which appears to be independent of mechanical and infectious causes.[63] Clinically already healed wounds may undergo blistering and ulceration, sometimes resulting in total autograft destruction.[63,64] It has been speculated that this destruction is immunologically mediated and initiated by the foreign fibroblasts used as a feeder layer to optimize keratinocyte growth during culture.[63,65]

Human keratinocytes can be cultured and serially passaged without a fibroblast feeder layer using a defined low-calcium environment,[66] but this approach has not gained widespread clinical use, possibly because these keratinocytes lack desmosomal interconnections, preventing them from forming the stratified coherent sheets[67] that are practical to handle.

Several systems have been designed to grow keratinocytes on membranes that are transferred upside-down onto the wound bed.[68] This provides a temporary mechanical support for the noncoherent keratinocytes, and the feasibility of such systems has been demonstrated, but their possible advantage still remains to be proven in a clinical setting. Another alternative is to transplant the keratinocytes in the form of suspensions. This principle allows the use of feeder-free culture protocols as well as the possibility of grafting preconfluent cultures. The latter may shorten the preparation time of grafts, typically 3 to 5 weeks, since there would be no need to await confluence and stratification of the keratinocyte culture.

Some success has been achieved by applying suspended keratinocytes with fibrin glue.[69–71] Cultured keratinocytes suspended in fibrin or growth medium have also been applied to the wound surface in a spray by utilizing an aerosolization apparatus.[72,73] Another system employs liquid-tight chambers that are sealed around the skin defects. The suspended keratinocytes are directly injected into the chamber and allowed to settle on the wound surface.[8] The advantages of this method are faster healing in a liquid environment[74,75] and prevention of graft desiccation, as well as the opportunity to noninvasively monitor healing of keratinocyte-grafted wounds.[8,76]

Transplantation of suspensions also raises the possibility of completely eliminating the culture process by transplanting freshly harvested keratinocytes directly onto the wound. This principle has been tested in human ulcers with reported success;[77] however, the advantage of this method remains to be proven clinically. Experimental studies suggest that the lower colony-forming capacity of noncultured keratinocytes, in relation to cultured ones, significantly decreases the efficacy of grafting,[37,76,78] thereby limiting expansion rates.

It has also been suggested that the proteolytic enzyme dispase, used to release the sheet grafts from the culture discs, may affect the early take rate of CEA. This is based on studies that show internalization of integrin $\alpha 64$, as well as other hemidesmosomal components, in epidermal sheets released by the action of dispase.[79,80] Integrins are members of a large family of surface receptors involved in cell–cell interaction as well as in cell adhesion to the extracellular matrix.[81] Interestingly, insufficient attachment of transplanted epidermis seems to have been observed already by Billingham and Reynolds in 1953.[49] They found that the neo-epidermis initially displayed rete ridge-like formations, but at a later stage the dermo-epidermal junction turned essentially flat. Despite a robust, heavily keratinized appearance, the epithelium was weakly attached to the underlying stroma, so that it could be easily peeled off as a coherent sheet of hyperplastic epidermis, which also proved viable on transplantation. A moderate degree of union was not attained until about 30 to 40 days post grafting, when the underlying stroma had become differentiated into characteristic dense fibrous tissue. Billingham and Reynolds used another proteolytic enzyme, trypsin, to produce epidermal sheets and suspensions. Interestingly, this has also been shown to induce structural changes in keratinocyte suspensions, including invagination, vacuolation, and redistribution of desmosome tonofibril complexes.[82] The use of composite grafts that contain a dermal portion onto which the keratinocytes are seeded and allowed to mature prior to grafting has been described.[83,84] This might overcome possible effects induced by proteases, but even so, it remains to be shown in an experimental or clinical study that this is more than just a theoretical concern. However, the fact that the anchoring fibril regeneration of the interstices of reepithelialized meshed STSG grafts appears similar to that of CEA-grafted wounds[61] indicates that the observed weak attachment may be intrinsic to the healing wound rather than a result of the methods of handling the transplanted keratinocytes. The weak attachment of the neo-epidermis after transplantation with CEA and keratinocyte suspensions is likely a reflection of the immaturity of the anchoring fibrils of the basement membrane, [56,85] which has been observed to last up to 3 years post grafting.[61]

Despite many drawbacks of keratinocyte grafting, cultured grafts are used in the treatment of extensive skin loss in the absence of sufficient autologous donor skin. Advances in methods that reduce the time to generate sufficient graftable cultured skin, lessen their initial weak attachment, and improve the cosmetic and functional outcome of the grafted skin would significantly enhance the use of cultured keratinocytes in treatment of skin wounds.

16.4.2 FIBROBLASTS

Granulation tissue typically starts to build up in the skin wound about 3 or 4 days post injury. This neodermal tissue consists of a framework of fibroblasts transpierced with a capillary network that nourishes the healing wound. Wound fibroblasts participate in the healing process by secreting various growth factors and synthesizing a collagen-rich extracellular matrix necessary for cell ingrowth.[86] The fibroblasts, unlike the keratinocytes, can be generated from any tissues that have been wounded, such as dermis, subdermal fat, fascia, muscle, and periosteum. There is, however, a typical lag phase of 3 to 4 days before fibroblast proliferation reaches significant proportions.[86–88] The general hypotheses of many transplantation studies have been that transplanted fibroblasts may shorten the lag phase, augment the outcome of dermal repair, and/or improve the outcome of cotransplanted keratinocytes.

Since fibroblasts normally do not form coherent sheets as keratinocytes do, several other methods of transplanting the cells have been tested. The cells have most commonly been grafted onto the wound with aid of a supporting vehicle containing collagen and elastin[89–91] or just collagen,[92–95] and both vehicles are often referred to as "skin equivalents." Other techniques employed for transplantation of fibroblasts include attachment of the graft suspension onto the wound bed with fibrin glue,[87] application with the aid of a spraying gun,[96] utilizing fibrin derived microbeads as carriers,[97] introduction of small volumes of concentrated fibroblast suspensions into moist experimental wound chambers,[98] and allowing the fibroblasts to settle by gravitational force after injection of the cell suspension into liquid-containing chambers overlying the wounds.[99]

Studies in rats utilizing radiographic or fluorescence techniques indicate that transplanted fibroblasts proliferate[90] and survive at least up to 5 weeks[94] after grafting. Other studies utilizing genetically engineered fibroblasts have demonstrated survival up to at least 3 and 8.5 months, respectively, as determined by analysis of the transgene product[100] and detection of the transferred vector sequence[101] in skin areas grafted with modified fibroblasts. It is not entirely clear what the relations between transplanted and native fibroblasts are in the healed wound, but one study indicates that the proportion of grafted fibroblasts is relatively high, although it seems to decrease with time. This was revealed by identifying female fibroblasts, through a karyotyping procedure, in cell cultures established from male isogenic rats that had been grafted with the female fibroblasts.[92] The proportion of grafted fibroblasts was 82% at 9 d, 64% at 1 month, and 42% at 13 months after transplantation, indicating long-time survival but gradual displacement by or ingrowth of native fibroblasts.

It has been known for almost three decades that the presence of a fibroblast feeder layer facilitates the *in vitro* growth and cultivation of human keratinocytes.[50] The first *in vivo* studies on keratinocyte and fibroblast cotransplantation published in the early eighties were carried out in mice and demonstrated a greater percentage of successful keratinocyte grafts when fibroblasts were included,[98,102] Comparable results were also observed in a pig study of full-thickness wounds grafted with suspensions of fibroblasts and keratinocytes.[99] In this study, cotransplanted wounds exhibited about twice as many keratinocyte colonies in wound histologies as compared to wounds grafted with keratinocytes only (Color Figure 16.3).* This indicates increased proliferation and/or take of the keratinocytes, but the exact mechanisms by which the fibroblasts exert their effect on keratinocytes in the wound still remains unclear. Based on *in vitro* observations of keratinocytes supported by a fibroblast feeder layer, it is believed that the synthesis of extracellular matrix elements and soluble factors is important.[67] It has also been speculated that part of the stimulus is related to fibroblast absorption or inactivation of transforming growth factor β (TGF-β) introduced into the culture medium as a constituent of the added fetal calf serum[103] and present in wound fluid collected from healing skin wounds.[104,105] Another theory emphasizes cell–cell interaction and is based on the observation that *in vitro,* cocultured keratinocytes induce in the fibroblast feeder layer the expression of growth factors known to exert stimulatory effects on keratinocyte proliferation in a paracrine fashion, such as keratinocyte growth factor (KGF) and interleukin 6.[106]

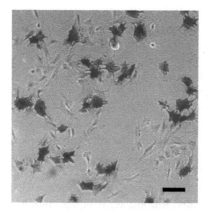

FIGURE 16.3A Transplantation of cultured fibroblasts to porcine full thickness skin wounds. A. Cultured fibroblasts were transfected *in vitro* with β-galactosidase (a marker gene) prior to transplantation. Transfected cells are stained blue. Scale bar: 50 μm. (See color figure following page 110.) (Figures 16.3A, B, C, and D reproduced from Svensjo, T., Yao, F., Pomahac, B., Winkler, T., and Eriksson, E., *Transplantation,* 73, (7) 1033–1041, 2002. With permission from *Journal of Surgical Research,* Lipincott, Williams & Wilkins.)

---

* Color figures follow page 110.

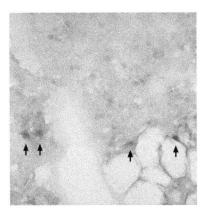

FIGURE 16.3B Transplanted transfected fibroblasts stained blue in a histological section in a wound 4 d post grafting demonstrating integration of the grafted cells into the neodermis (granulation tissue). Scale bar: 50 μm. (See color figure following page 110.)

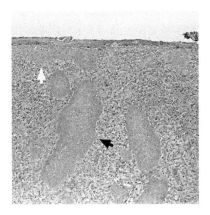

FIGURE 16.3C Histological section from a wound transplanted with cultured keratinocytes only (8 d post transplantation). The white arrow indicates the neodermal and neoepidermal border. The black arrow indicates one of the several keratinocyte colonies observed in the granulation tissue. Scale bar: 100 μm.

In the porcine study of fibroblasts and keratinocyte cotransplantation,[37] it was also observed that wounds grafted with only fibroblasts exhibited faster reepithelialization as compared to nongrafted control wounds. Studies on radiation-impaired wound healing in rodent models have shown that injection of irradiated wounds with cultured fibroblasts also improves healing by increasing the mechanical strength of injected wounds.[107,108] Furthermore, a clinical study utilizing allogenic fibroblasts and keratinocytes in a synthetic skin substitute to treat leg ulcers has also shown faster healing in approximately 20% of grafted wounds.[109] None of these techniques has yet become a routine clinical procedure, however. The exact mechanisms by

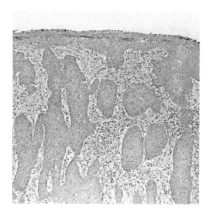

FIGURE 16.3D Histological section from a wound transplanted with both keratinocytes and fibroblasts. These wounds displayed increased numbers of keratinocyte colonies, greater reepithelialization and thicker neoepidermis as compared to wounds seeded with keratinocytes only. Scale bar: 100 μm.

which fibroblasts augment skin wound repair are not known, but it is likely that secretion of growth factors and synthesis of extracellular matrix early during wound repair are important. When transplanting actively proliferating fibroblasts, it is also possible that the initial lag phase of typically 3 to 4 days (i.e., before any granulation tissue is evident) is decreased.[87]

Interestingly, some studies have also reported regeneration of hair follicles in wounded skin of mice after cotransplantation with keratinocytes and fibroblasts, but not with keratinocytes alone.[98,102] The hair-inductive capabilities of fibroblasts have so far been restricted to the dermal papilla cells of the hair follicle.[110] The inductive capacity is also lost after repeated subculture of dermal papilla cells.[111-113] These results have been restricted to rodent models, and to date, no similar data has been published regarding the regeneration of hair follicles in pigs or humans.

16.4.3 Melanocytes

Melanocytes are present in cultures of keratinocytes prepared according to the method of Rheinwald and Green and hence are also present at the time of CEA transplantation. Functional epidermal melanin units, however, are not seen in groin- or axilla-derived grafts for 6 to 8 weeks or in sole-derived epidermis until a year or more post transplantation.[56] This possibility of transplanting melanocytes has been used for the treatment of vitiligo, a hypopigmentation skin disorder. Vitiligo is caused by the disappearance of pigment cells from the epidermis, resulting in well-defined white patches, which are cosmetically disfiguring and more sensitive to sunburn[114] Patients who have areas of vitiligo with stable activity are candidates for transplantation with grafts taken from nonaffected skin areas. Methods utilized for this purpose include punch grafting, insertion of mini skin grafts into small incisions of the depigmentated skin, ultrathin split thickness skin grafting, and engraftment with the epidermal roof obtained from suction-induced blisters of healthy skin.[115] More refined methods that have been tested in patients employ cultured[41,43,44] or noncultured[42,47] melanocytes applied to hypopigmented recipient sites made graftable by either dermabrasion[43,44,47] or blister induction with liquid nitrogen.[41,42] In the latter case, suspended keratinocytes and melanocytes were injected into intact blisters[42] or, alternatively, grafted as sheets onto denuded skin after blister removal.[41] All of the refined methods have resulted in repigmentation. The best long-term results were obtained in patients with stable vitiligo that did not exceed 30% of the body area.[44,45] Already established treatment options such as engraftment with ultrathin STSGs, however, still remain the treatments of choice for reasons of cost and practicality,[115] as well as long term results.[45]

16.5 GENE THERAPY AND SKIN TRANSPLANTATION

Clinical wound healing trials with growth factors, such as platelet-derived growth factor-BB (PDGF-BB)[116,117] and epidermal growth factor (EGF),[118] have reported significant improvements in wound healing; however, the results have been rather modest. It has also been necessary to use large repetitive doses along with a long duration of therapy to obtain these results. Possible factors responsible for the limited effect of exogenous growth factors include binding of the growth factor to macro-molecules at the base of the wound, rendering them biologically unavailable,[119] rapid degradation of applied growth factor as a result of elevated matrix metalloproteinases in chronic wounds,[120] or insufficient penetration into wound granulation tissue of topically applied growth factor.[121] Somatic gene therapy offers a potentially useful strategy for the delivery of growth factors to enhance tissue repair as well as for the correction of specific genetic skin diseases. It may potentially offer targeted local and persistent delivery of *de novo* synthesized growth factor to the skin and wound environment over many days.

The skin is particularly attractive as a target for gene transfer for several reasons:

1. Skin cells, such as fibroblasts[122,123] and keratinocytes,[50,66] can be easily obtained and serially cultivated *in vitro*, thereby permitting use of autol-ogous cells and *ex vivo* genetic modification and testing.
2. Systems have been established for transplanting both keratinocytes[5,8] and fibroblasts.[92,94,99]
3. If unwanted effects occur in the genetically modified skin, for example a tumor, they can be readily detected and removed.
4. Since genetically modified keratinocytes have been shown to reconstitute epidermis of grafted wounds,[8] they may be transplanted with the dual purpose of resurfacing the wound as well as supplying growth factors that augment tissue repair.
5. Although long-term sustained gene expression remains a major obstacle in gene therapy applications for many diseases, short-term expression may be sufficient or even desirable to accelerate and augment a time-limited process such as skin repair.

Several experimental studies have demonstrated the feasibility and augmentation of skin wound repair by gene therapy. Gene transfer protocols that have resulted in augmented skin wound repair include:

1. Acceleration of reepithelialization with EGF after particle-mediated gene transfer[124]
2. Reversal of impaired wound repair in inducible nitric oxide synthase (iNOS)–deficient mice by topical adenoviral-mediated iNOS gene transfer[125]
3. Adenoviral-mediated overexpression of PDGF-B to correct ischemic impaired wound healing[126]
4. Adeno-associated viral vector-mediated vascular endothelial growth factor (VEGF) gene transfer to improve angiogenesis and wound healing in diabetic mice[127]
5. Improvement of dermal and epidermal regeneration after nonviral liposome-mediated KGF gene transfer[128]
6. Accelerated wound repair in diabetic mice by expression of an oxygen-regulated protein after adenoviral gene transfer[129]

Similar gene transfer procedures may potentially be applied in skin transplantation by *ex vivo* gene transfer to autologous keratinocytes and/or fibroblasts and subsequent transplantation to skin wounds with the dual purpose of resurfacing the wound and accelerating wound repair. The feasibility of such gene transfer protocols has been demonstrated in pigs,[8,76,99,130] which are particularly suitable for preclinical testing due to their skin's close resemblances to human skin in architecture and function.[131–134] Although the feasibility of gene therapy has been successfully demonstrated in animal models, there have so far been no successful clinical trials published regarding gene therapy to skin with the aim of treating a genetic skin disease or skin wounds. The principle of corrective gene therapy for a specific human genetic skin disorder has been proven, however. Jonkman and colleagues demonstrated a form of natural gene therapy in a patient suffering from one of the forms of epidermolysis bullosa, a skin disease that is characterized by continuous blistering of the skin since birth. The disorder is an inherited autosomal recessive pattern and is caused by a defective gene for type XVII collagen, a transmembrane cell–matrix adhesion molecule. The study showed that reversion of the mutation had occurred naturally (by means of mitotic gene conversion) in some of the keratinocytes of the affected patient, thus leading to several patches of normal skin.[135] This raises the possibility of treating this particular patient by transplanting self-corrected keratinocytes to recipient sites carrying the defective gene.

An experimental study utilizing gene therapy to directly enhance the outcome of skin transplantation has been published. Human keratinocytes were genetically modified to overexpress platelet-derived growth factor A (PDGF-A)[136] and subsequently seeded into composite grafts of modified keratinocytes and acellular dermis. The genetically modified grafts were transplanted to full-thickness skin wounds of immuno-incompetent nude mice, resulting in significantly greater cell densities in the neodermis as well as an increase in staining for collagen types I and IV. The latter two collagens are basement membrane proteins that are involved in the attachment of epidermis to the underlying dermis and thus may be important for adequate mechanical durability after epidermal transplantation. Wound contraction was also found to be significantly inhibited. It was concluded that gene transfer with PDGF-A enhances the performance of this particular composite graft.

During the past decade, information has been gathered about the various peptides that function as natural antibiotics, particularly in the skin.[137] The introduction of such genes into graftable skin could hypothetically be used to control deleterious infections which otherwise may lead to graft failure. Another hypothetical gene therapy application may be aimed at modulating or down-regulating genes that express immunogenic proteins. This would allow for a living transplantable allogenic skin that is immediately available and hopefully tolerated by any recipient. Finally, the introduction of gene therapy in skin transplantation also requires a system to efficiently regulate transgene expression *in vivo*. Recently, a tetracycline-inducible switch that allows for tight control of gene expression was developed.[138] The system allows regulation of transgene expression in wounds by local or systemic delivery of tetracycline.[138] The regulated delivery of growth factors in the wound and graft microenvironment would maximize their biological effect and decrease the potential toxicity resulting from overexpression. Ultimately, gene therapy with multiple growth factors might be more effective than single growth factor therapy alone. Different genes can be delivered at the same time, while expression of one or more genes can be delayed in a controlled fashion with the regulatory switch. This sequential delivery of transgenes will make it possible to deliver enhancing growth factors early and retarding (scar reducing) factors late in wound repair.

ABBREVIATIONS

CEA	Cultured epithelial autograft
EGF	Epidermal growth factor
FTSG	Full-thickness skin graft
iNOS	Inducible nitric oxide synthase
KGF	Keratinocyte growth factor
PDGF-A	Platelet-derived growth factor A
PDGF-B	Platelet-derived growth factor B
STSG	Split-thickness skin graft
TGF-β	Transforming growth factor β
VEGF	Vascular endothelial growth factor

REFERENCES

1. Ehrenfried, A., Reverdin and other methods of skin grafting, *Boston Med. Surg. J.,* 161, 911–917, 1909.
2. Hauben, D.J., Baruchin, A., and Mahler, A., On the histroy of the free skin graft, *Ann. Plast. Surg.,* 9, 242–245, 1982.
3. Davis, J.S., The story of plastic surgery, *Ann. Surg.,* 113, 641–56, 1941.

4. Green, H., Kehinde, O., and Thomas, J., Growth of cultured human epidermal cells into multiple epithelia suitable for grafting, *Proc. Natl. Acad. Sci. U.S.A.*, 76, 5665–5668, 1979.

5. O'Connor, N.E., Mulliken, J.B., Banks-Schlegel, S., Kehinde, O., and Green, H., Grafting of burns with cultured epithelium prepared from autologous epidermal cells, *Lancet*, 2, 75–78, 1981.

6. Morgan, J.R., Barrandon, Y., Green, H., and Mulligan, R.C., Expression of an exogenous growth hormone gene by transplantable human epidermal cells, *Science*, 237, 1476–1479, 1987.

7. Garver, R.I., Chytil, A., Courtney, M., and Crystal, R.G., Clonal gene therapy: transplanted mouse fibroblast clones express human alpha1-antitrypsin gene *in vivo*, *Science*, 237, 762–764, 1987.

8. Vogt, P.M., Thompson, S., Andree, C., Liu, P., Breuing, K., Hatzis, D., Mulligan, R.C., and Eriksson, E., Genetically modified keratinocytes transplanted to wounds reconstitute the epidermis, *Proc. Natl. Acad. Sci. U.S.A,*. 91, 9307–9311, 1994.

9. Chrysopoulo, M.T. and Desvigne, L.D., Flaps, Classification, www.emedicine.com, 2002.

10. Woodberry, K.M. and Robertson, K., Flaps, Fasciocutaneous Flaps, www.emedicine.com, 2001.

11. Nahabedian, M.Y., Flaps, Free Tissue Transfer, www.emedicine.com, 2002.

12. Jansen, D., McGee, J., and Newsome, R.E., Flaps, Muscle and Musculocutaneous Flaps, www.emedicine.com, 2002.

13. Woodberry, K.M., Flaps, Random Skin Flaps, www.emedicine.com, 2002.

14. Wood, R.J. and Jurkiewicz, M.J., Plastic and reconstructive surgery, in *Principles of Surgery*, 7th ed., Schwartz, S.I., Shires, G.T., Spencer, F.C., Daly, J.M., Fischer, J.E., and Galloway, A.C., Eds., McGraw-Hill Professional Publishing, New York, 1998, pp. 2091–2143.

15. Chia, C. and Stadelmann, W., Skin, Tissue Expansion, www.emedicine.com, 2002.

16. Revis, D.R. and Seagel, M.B., Skin Grafts, Full-thickness, www.emedicine.com, 2002.

17. Revis, D.R. and Seagel, M.B., Skin, Grafts, www.emedicine.com, 2001.

18. Livesey, S.A., Herndon, D.N., Hollyoak, M.A., Atkinson, Y.H., and Nag, A., Transplanted acellular allograft dermal matrix, *Transplantation*, 60 (1), 1–9, 1995.

19. Kirsner, R.S. and Falanga, V., Techniques of split-thickness skin grafting for lower extremity ulcerations, *J. Dermatol. Surg. Oncol.*, 19, 779–783, 1993.

20. Revis, D.R. and Seagel, M.B., Skin Grafts, Split-thickness, www.emedicine.com, 2001.

21. Vandeput, J., Nelissen, M., Tanner, J.C., and Boswick, J., A review of skin meshers, *Burns*, 12, 364–370, 1995.

22. Öien, R.F., Leg Ulcer Management in Primary Care with Special Reference to Pinch Grafting, thesis, Lund University, Malmö, Sweden, 2002.

23. Davis, J.S., The small deep graft, *Ann. Surg.*, 91, 633–635, 1930.

24. Davis, J.S., The small deep graft. Relationship to the true Reverdin graft, *Ann. Surg.*, 89, 902–916, 1929.

25. Robinson, J.K., Surgical gem. An alternate method of obtaining a pinch graft, *J. Dermatol. Surg. Oncol.*, 8, 162, 1982.

26. Greenwood, J.E., Parry, A.D., Williams, R.M., and McCollum, C.N., Trigger-fired pinch-graft harvester for use in chronic venous ulcers, *Br. J. Surg.*, 84, 397–398, 1997.

27. Christiansen, J., Ek, L., and Tegner, E., Pinch grafting of leg ulcers. A retrospective study of 412 treated ulcers in 146 patients, *Acta Dermatol. Venereol.*, 77, 471–473, 1997.

28. Von Mangoldt, F., V. Die ueberhäutung von Wundflächen und Wundhöhlen durch Epithelaussaat, eine neue Methode der Transplantation, *Deutsch. Med. Wochenschr.*, 48, 798–799, 1895.

29. Najarian, J.S., Crane, J.T., and McCorkle, H.J., An experimental study of the grafting of a suspension of skin particles, *Surgery*, 42, 218–227, 1957.

30. Cox, W.A. and Nichol, W.W., Evaluation of the fine-particle skin autograft technique, *Arch. Surg.*, 77, 870–874, 1958.

31. Nyström, G., Sowing of small skin graft particles as a method for epithelialization especially of extensive wound surfaces, *Plast. Reconstr. Surg.*, 23, 226–239, 1959.

32. Lari, A.R. and Gang, R.K., Expansion technique for skin grafts (Meek technique) in the treatment of severely burned patients, *Burns*, 27, 61–66, 2001.

33. Chang, L.Y. and Yang, J.Y., Clinical experience of postage stamp autograft with porcine skin onlay dressing in extensive burns, *Burns*, 24, 264–269, 1998.

34. Lin, T.-W. and Horng, S.-Y., A new method of microskin mincing, *Burns*, 20, 526–528, 1994.

35. Lin, T.-W., An alternative method of skin grafting: the scalp microdermis graft, *Burns*, 21, 374–378, 1995.

36. Zhang, M.L., Chang, Z.D., Wang, C.Y., and Fang, C.H., Microskin grafting in the treatment of extensive burns: a preliminary report, *J. Trauma*, 28, 804–807, 1988.

37. Svensjö, T., Pomahac, B., Yao, F., Slama, J., Wasif, N., and Eriksson, E., Autologous skin transplantation: comparison of minced skin to other techniques, *J. Surg. Res.*, 103, 19–29, 2002.

38. Soejima, K., Negishi, N., Nozaki, M., and Sasaki, K., Effect of cultured endothelial cells on angiogenesis *in vivo*, *Plast. Reconstr. Surg.*, 101, 1552–1560, 1998.

39. Supp, D.M., Wilson-Landy, K., and Boyce, S.T., Human dermal microvascular endothelial cells form vascular analogs in cultured skin substitutes after grafting to athymic mice, *FASEB J.*, 16, 797–804, 2002.

40. Boyce, S.T., Medrano, E.E., Abdel-Malek, Z., Supp, A.P., Dodick, J.M., Nordlund, J.J., and Warden, G. D., Pigmentation and inhibition of wound contraction by cultured skin substitutes with adult melanocytes after transplantation to athymic mice, *J. Invest. Dermatol.*, 100, 360–365, 1993.

41. Falabella, R., Escobar, C., and Borrero, I., Transplantation of *in vitro*-cultured epidermis bearing melanocytes for repigmenting vitiligo, *J. Am. Acad. Dermatol.*, 21, 257–264, 1989.

42. Gauthier, Y. and Surleve-Bazeille, J.E., Autologous grafting with noncultured melanocytes: a simplified method for treatment of depigmented lesions, *J. Am. Acad. Dermatol.*, 26, 191–194, 1992.

43. Lontz, W., Olsson, M.J., Moellmann, G., and Lerner, A.B., Pigment cell transplantation for treatment of vitiligo: a progress report, *J. Am. Acad. Dermatol.*, 30, 591–597, 1994.

44. Olsson, M.J. and Juhlin, L., Transplantation of melanocytes in vitiligo, *Br. J. Dermatol.*, 132, 587–591, 1995.

45. Olsson, M.J. and Juhlin, L., Long-term follow-up of leucoderma patients treated with transplants of autologous cultured melanocytes, ultrathin epidermal sheets and basal cell layer suspension, *Br. J. Dermatol.*, 147, 893–904, 2002.

46. Swope, V.B., Supp, A.P., and Boyce, S.T., Regulation of cutaneous pigmentation by titration of human melanocytes in cultured skin substitutes grafted to athymic mice, *Wound Repair Regen.*, 10, 378–386, 2002.

47. van Geel, N., Ongenae, K., De Mil, M., and Naeyaert, J.M., Modified technique of autologous noncultured epidermal cell transplantation for repigmenting vitiligo: a pilot study, *Dermatol. Surg.*, 27, 873–876, 2001.

48. von Heimburg, D., Zachariah, S., Heschel, I., Kuhling, H., Schoof, H., Hafemann, B., and Pallua, N., Human preadipocytes seeded on freeze-dried collagen scaffolds investigated *in vitro* and *in vivo*, *Biomaterials*, 22, 429–438, 2001.

49. Billingham, R.E. and Reynolds, J., Transplantation studies on sheets of pure epidermal epithelium and on epidermal cell suspensions, *Br. J. Plast. Surg.*, 5, 25–36, 1953.

50. Rheinwald, J.G. and Green, H., Serial cultivation of strains of human epidermal keratinocytes: the formation of keratinizing colonies from single cells, *Cell*, 6, 331–343, 1975.

51. Banks-Schlegel, S. and Green, H., Formation of epidermis by serially cultivated human epidermal cells transplanted as an epithelium to athymic mice, *Transplantation*, 29, 308–313, 1980.

52. Gallico, G.G., O'Connor, N.E., Compton, C.C., Kehinde, O., and Green, H., Permanent coverage of large burn wounds with autologous cultured human epithelium, *N. Engl. J. Med.*, 311, 448–451, 1984.

53. Teepe, R.G.C., Kreis, R.W., Koebrugge, E.J., Kempenaar, J.A., Vloemans, A.F.P.M., Hermans, R.P., Boxma, H., Doktor, J., Hermans, J., Ponec, M., and Vermeer, B.J., The use of cultured autologous epidermis in the treatment of extensive burn wounds, *J. Trauma*, 30, 269–275, 1990.

54. Munster, A.M., Weiner, S.H., and Spence, R.J., Cultured epidermis for the coverage of massive burn wounds, *Ann. Surg.*, 211, 676–680, 1990.

55. Herzog, S.R., Meyer, A., Woodley, D., and Peterson, H.D., Wound coverage with cultured autologous keratinocytes: use after burn wound excision, including biopsy follow up, *J. Trauma*, 28, 195–198, 1988.

56. Compton, C.C., Gill, J.M., Bradford, D.A., Regauer, S., Gallico, G.G., and O'Connor, N.E., Skin regenerated from cultured epithelial autografts on full-thickness burn wounds from 6 days to 5 years after grafting. A light, electron microscopic and immunohistochemical study, *Lab. Invest.*, 60, 600–612, 1989.

57. Green, H., Cultured cells for the treatment of disease, *Scientific American* (November), 96–102, 1991.

58. Myers, S., Navsaria, H., Sanders, R., Green, C., and Leigh, I., Transplantation of keratinocytes in the treatment of wounds, *Am. J. Surg.*, 170, 75–83, 1995.

59. Rennekampff, H.O., Kiessig, V., and Hansbrough, J.F., Current concepts in the development of cultured skin replacements, *J. Surg. Res.*, 62, 288–295, 1996.

60. Limat, A., Mauri, D., and Hunziker, T., Successful treatment of chronic leg ulcers with epidermal equivalents generated from cultured autologous outer root sheath cells, *J. Invest. Dermatol.*, 107, 128–135, 1996.

61. Compton, C.C., Cultured epithelial autografts for burn wound resurfacing: review of observations from an 11-year biopsy study, *Wounds*, 8, 125–133, 1996.

62. Cuono, C., Langdon, R., and McGuire, J., Use of cultured epidermal autografts and dermal allografts as skin replacement after burn injury, *Lancet*, 1, 1123–1124, 1986.

63. Hultman, S.C., Brinson, G.M., Siltharm, S., deSerres, S., Cairnes, B.A., Peterson, H.D., and Meyer, A.A., Allograft fibroblasts used to grow cultured epidermal autografts persist *in vivo* and sensitize the graft recipient for accelerated second-set rejection, *J. Trauma*, 41, 51–58, 1996.

64. Rue, L.W., Cioffi, W.G., McManus, W.F., and Pruitt, B.A., Wound closure and outcome in extensively burned patients treated with cultured autologous keratinocytes, *J. Trauma,* 34, 662–668, 1993.

65. Cairnes, B.A., deSerres, S., Brady, L.A., Hultman, C.S., and Meyer, A.A., Xenogeneic mouse fibroblasts persist in human cultured epidermal grafts: a possible mechanism of graft loss, *J. Trauma,* 39, 75–79, 1995.

66. Boyce, S.T. and Ham, R.G., Calcium-regulated differentiation of normal human epidermal keratinocytes in chemically defined clonal culture and serum-free serial culture, *J. Invest. Dermatol.,* 81, S33–S40, 1983.

67. Navsaria, H.A., Myers, S.R., Leigh, I.M., and McKay, I.A., Culturing skin *in vitro* for wound therapy, *Trends Biotechnol.,* 13, 91–100, 1995.

68. Jones, I., Currie, L., and Martin, R., A guide to biological skin substitutes, *Br. J. Plast. Surg.,* 55, 185–193, 2002.

69. Hafemann, B., Hettich, R., Ensslen, S., Kowol, B., Zühlke, A., Ebert, R., Königs, M., and Kirkpatrick, C.J., Treatment of skin defects using suspension of *in vitro* cultured keratinocytes, *Burns,* 20, 168–172, 1994.

70. Lam, P.K., Chan, E.S., Liew, C.T., Yen, R.S., Lau, H.C., and King, W.W., Dermal fibroblasts do not enhance the graft take rate of autologous, cultured keratinocyte suspension on full-thickness wounds in rats, *Ann. Plast. Surg.,* 46, 146–149, 2001.

71. Stark, G.B. and Kaiser, H.W., Cologne Burn Centre experience with glycerol-preserved allogenic skin: part II: Combination with autologous cultured keratinocytes, *Burns,* 20 suppl, S34–S38, 1994.

72. Fraulin, F.O., Bahoric, A., Harrop, A.R., Hiruki, T., and Clarke, H.M., Autotransplantation of epithelial cells in the pig via an aerosol vehicle, *J. Burn Care Rehabil.,* 19, 337–345, 1998.

73. Grant, I., Warwick, K., Marshall, J., Green, C., and Martin, R., The co-application of sprayed cultured autologous keratinocytes and autologous fibrin sealant in a porcine wound model, *Br. J. Plast. Surg.,* 55, 219–227, 2002.

74. Vogt, P.M., Andree, C., Breuing, K., Liu, P.Y., Slama, J., Helo, G., and Eriksson, E., Dry, moist and wet skin repair, *Ann. Plast. Surg.,* 34, 493–500, 1995.

75. Svensjö, T., Pomahac, B., Yao, F., Slama, J., and Eriksson, E., Accelerated healing of full-thickness skin wounds in a wet environment, *Plast. Reconstr. Surg.,* 106, 602–612, 2000.

76. Svensjö, T., Yao, F., Pomahac, B., and Eriksson, E., Autologous keratinocyte suspensions accelerate epidermal wound healing in pigs, *J. Surg. Res.,* 99, 211–221, 2001.

77. Hunyadi, J., Farkas, B., Bertenyi, C., Olah, J., and Dobozy, A., Keratinocyte grafting: a new means of transplantation to full thickness wounds, *J. Dermatol. Surg. Oncol.,* 14, 75–78, 1988.

78. Butler, C.E., Yannas, I.V., Compton, C.C., Correia, C.A., and Orgill, D.P., Comparison of cultured and uncultured keratinocytes seeded into a collagen-GAG matrix for skin replacements, *Br. J. Plast. Surg.,* 52, 127–132, 1999.

79. Poumay, Y., Roland, I.H., Leclercq-Smekens, M., and Leloup, R., Basal detachment of the epidermis using dispase: tissue spatial organization and fate of integrin alpha6ß4 and hemidesmosomes, *J. Invest. Dermatol.,* 102, 111–117, 1994.

80. Poumay, Y., Leclercq-Smekens, M., Grailly, S., Degen, A., and Leloup, R., Specific internalization of basal membrane domains containing the integrin alpha6ß4 in dispase-detached cultured human keratinocytes, *Eur. J. Cell Biol.,* 60, 12–20, 1993.

81. Jones, P.H. and Watt, F.M., Separation of human epidermal stem cells from transit amplifying cells on the basis of differences in integrin function and expression, *Cell,* 73, 713–724, 1993.

82. Barton, S.P. and Marks, R., Changes in suspensions of human keratinocytes due to trypsin, *Arch. Dermatol. Res.*, 271, 245–257, 1981.

83. Cooper, M.L., Andree, C., Hansbrough, J.F., Zapata-Sirvent, R.L., and Spielvogel, R.L., Direct comparison of a cultured composite skin substitute containing human keratinocytes and fibroblasts to an epidermal sheet graft containing human keratinocytes on athymic mice, *J. Invest. Dermatol.*, 101, 811–819, 1993.

84. Medalie, D.A., Eming, S.A., Tompkins, R.G., Yarmush, M.L., Krueger, G.G., and Morgan, J.R., Evaluation of human skin reconstituted from composite grafts of cultured keratinocytes and human acellular dermis transplanted to athymic mice, *J. Invest. Dermatol.*, 107, 121–127, 1996.

85. Woodley, D.T., Peterson, H.D., Herzog, S.R., Stricklin, G.P., Burgeson, R.E., Briggaman, R.A., Cronce, D.J., and O'Keefe, E.J., Burn wounds resurfaced by cultured epidermal autografts show abnormal reconstitution of anchoring fibrils, *JAMA*, 259, 2566–2571, 1988.

86. Martin, P., Wound healing — aiming for perfect skin regeneration, *Science,* 276, 75–81, 1997.

87. McClain, S.A., Simon, M., Jones, E., Nandi, A., Gailit, J.O., Tonnesen, M.G., Newman, D., and Clark, R.A.F., Mesenchymal cell activation is the rate-limiting step of granulation tissue induction, *Am. J. Pathol.*, 149, 1257–1270, 1996.

88. Hadfield, G., The tissue origin of the fibroblasts of the granulation tissue, *Br. J. Surg.*, 50, 870–881, 1963.

89. Lamme, E.N., van Leeuwen, R.T., Brandsma, K., van Marle, J., and Middelkoop, E., Higher numbers of autologous fibroblasts in an artificial dermal substitute improve tissue regeneration and modulate scar tissue formation, *J. Pathol.*, 190, 595–603, 2000.

90. Lamme, E., van Leeuwen, R., Jonker, A., van Marle, J., and Middelkoop, E., Living skin substitutes: survival and function of fibroblasts seeded in a dermal substitute in experimental wounds, *J. Invest. Dermatol.*, 111, 989–995, 1998.

91. de Vries, H.J., Middelkoop, E., van Heemstra-Hoen, M., Wildevuur, C.H., and Westerhof, W., Stromal cells from subcutaneous adipose tissue seeded in a native collagen/elastin dermal substitute reduce wound contraction in full thickness skin defects, *Lab. Invest.*, 73, 532–540, 1995.

92. Hull, B.E., Sher, S.E., Rosen, S., Church, D., and Bell, E., Fibroblasts in isogeneic skin equivalents persist for long periods after grafting, *J. Invest. Dermatol.*, 81, 436–438, 1983.

93. Hull, B.E., Sher, S.E., Rosen, S., Church, D., and Bell, E., Structural integration of skin equivalents grafted to Lewis and Sprague-Dawley rats, *J. Invest. Dermatol.*, 81, 429–436, 1983.

94. Bell, E., Ehrlich, H.P., Buttle, D.J., and Nakatsuji, T., Living tissue formed *in vitro* and accepted as skin-equivalent tissue of full thickness, *Science,* 211, 1052–1054, 1981.

95. Coulomb, B., Friteau, L., Baruch, J., Guilbaud, J., Chretien-Marquet, B., Glicenstein, J., Lebreton-Decoster, C., Bell, E., and Dubertret, L., Advantage of the presence of living dermal fibroblasts within *in vitro* reconstructed skin for grafting in humans, *Plast. Reconstr. Surg.*, 101, 1891–1903, 1998.

96. Wisser, D. and Steffes, J., Skin replacement with a collagen based dermal substitute, autologous keratinocytes and fibroblasts in burn trauma, *Burns,* 29, 375–380, 2003.

97. Gorodetsky, R., Clark, R.A., An, J., Gailit, J., Levdansky, L., Vexler, A., Berman, E., and Marx, G., Fibrin microbeads (FMB) as biodegradable carriers for culturing cells and for accelerating wound healing, *J. Invest. Dermatol.*, 112, 866–872, 1999.

98. Worst, P.K.M., Mackenzie, I.C., and Fusenig, N.E., Reformation of organized epidermal structure by transplantation of suspensions and cultures of epidermal and dermal cells, *Cell Tissue Res.,* 225, 65–77, 1982.

99. Svensjo, T., Yao, F., Pomahac, B., Winkler, T., and Eriksson, E., Cultured autologous fibroblasts augment epidermal repair, *Transplantation,* 73, 1033–1041, 2002.

100. Scharfmann, R., Axelrod, J.H., and Verma, I.M., Long-term *in vivo* expression of retrovirus-mediated gene transfer in mouse fibroblasts implants, *Proc. Natl. Acad. Sci. U.S.A.,* 88, 4626–4630, 1991.

101. Palmer, T.D., Rosman, G.J., Osborne, W.R., and Miller, A.D., Genetically modified skin fibroblasts persist long after transplantation but gradually inactivate introduced genes, *Proc. Natl. Acad. Sci. U.S.A.,* 88, 1330–1334, 1991.

102. Mackenzie, I.A. and Fusenig, N.E., Regeneration of organized epithelial structure, *J. Invest. Dermatol.,* 81, S184–S194, 1983.

103. Rollins, B.J., O'Connell, T M., Bennett, G., Burton, L.E., Stiles, C.D., and Rheinwald, J.G., Environment-dependent growth inhibition of human epidermal keratinocytes by recombinant human transforming growth factor-beta, *J. Cell Physiol.,* 139, 455–462, 1989.

104. Breuing, K., Andree, C., Helo, G., Slama, J., Liu, P.Y., and Eriksson, E., Growth factors in the repair of partial thickness porcine skin wounds, *Plast. Reconstr. Surg.,* 100, 657–664, 1997.

105. Vogt, P.M., Lehnhardt, M., Wagner, D., Jansen, V., Krieg, M., and Steinau, H.U., Determination of endogenous growth factors in human wound fluid: temporal presence and profiles of secretion, *Plast. Reconstr. Surg.,* 102, 117–123, 1998.

106. Smola, H., Thiekotter, G., and Fusenig, N.E., Mutual induction of growth factor gene expression by epidermal-dermal cell interaction, *J. Cell Biol.,* 122, 417–429, 1993.

107. Krueger, W.W., Goepfert, H., Romsdahl, M., Herson, J., Withers, R.H., and Jesse, R.H., Fibroblast implantation enhances wound healing as indicated by breaking strength determinations, *Otolaryngology,* 86, ORL–804–11, 1978.

108. Ferguson, P.C., Boynton, E.L., Wunder, J.S., Hill, R.P., O'Sullivan, B., Sandhu, J.S., and Bell, R.S., Intradermal injection of autologous dermal fibroblasts improves wound healing in irradiated skin, *J. Surg. Res.,* 85, 331–338, 1999.

109. Jones, J.E. and Nelson, E.A., Skin grafting for venous leg ulcers, *Cochrane Database Syst. Rev.,* 2, 2000.

110. Jahoda, C.A.B., Horne, K.A., and Oliver, R.F., Induction of hair growth by implantation of cultured dermal papilla cells, *Nature,* 311, 560–562, 1984.

111. Reynolds, A.J. and Jahoda, C.A., Cultured dermal papilla cells induce follicle formation and hair growth by transdifferentiation of an adult epidermis, *Development,* 115, 587–93, 1992.

112. Jahoda, C.A., Reynolds, A.J., and Oliver, R.F., Induction of hair growth in ear wounds by cultured dermal papilla cells, *J. Invest. Dermatol.,* 101, 584–590, 1993.

113. Jahoda, C.A.B. and Reynolds, A.J., Dermal-epidermal interaction. Adult follicle-derived cell populations and hair growth, *Dermatol. Clin.,* 14, 573–583, 1996.

114. Njoo, M.D. and Westerhof, W., Vitiligo. Pathogenesis and treatment, *Am. J. Clin. Dermatol.,* 2, 167–181, 2001.

115. Hann, S.-K., Vitiligo, www.emedicine.com, 2001.

116. Mustoe, T.A., Cutler, N.R., Allman, R.M., Goode, P.S., Deuel, T.F., Prause, J.A., Bear, M., Serdar, C.M., and Pierce, G.F., A phase II study to evaluate recombinant platelet-derived growth factor-BB in the treatment of stage 3 and 4 pressure ulcers, *Arch. Surg.,* 129, 213–219, 1994.

117. Wieman, T.J., Smiell, J.M., and Su, Y., Efficacy and safety of a topical gel formulation of recombinant human platelet-derived growth factor-BB (becaplermin) in patients with chronic neuropathic diabetic ulcers. A phase III randomized placebo-controlled double-blind study, *Diabetes Care,* 21, 822–827, 1998.

118. Brown, G.L., Nanney, L.B., Griffen, J., Cramer, A.B., Yancey, J.M., Curtsinger, L.J.D., Holtzin, L., Schultz, G.S., Jurkiewicz, M.J., and Lynch, J.B., Enhancement of wound healing by topical treatment with epidermal growth factor, *N. Engl. J. Med.,* 321, 76–79, 1989.

119. Falanga, V. and Eaglstein, W.H., The "trap" hypothesis of venous ulceration, *Lancet,* 341, 1006–1008, 1993.

120. Grinnell, F., Ho, C.H., and Wysocki, A., Degradation of fibronectin and vitronectin in chronic wound fluid: analysis by cell blotting, immunoblotting, and cell adhesion assays, *J. Invest. Dermatol.,* 98, 410–416, 1992.

121. Cross, S.E. and Roberts, M.S., Defining a model to predict the distribution of topically applied growth factors and other solutes in excisional full-thickness wounds, *J. Invest. Dermatol.,* 112, 36–41, 1999.

122. Martin, G.M., Sprague, C.A., and Epstein, C.J., Replicative life-span of cultivated human cells. Effects of donor's age, tissue, and genotype, *Lab. Invest.,* 23, 86–92, 1970.

123. Hayflick, L. and Moorhead, P.S., The serial cultivation of human diploid cell strains, *Exp. Cell Res.,* 25, 585–621, 1961.

124. Andree, C., Swain, W.F., Page, C., Macklin, M.D., Slama, J., Hatzis, D., and Eriksson, E., *In vivo* transfer and expression of a human epidermal growth factor gene accelerates wound repair, *Proc. Natl. Acad. Sci. U.S.A.,* 91, 12,188–12,192, 1994.

125. Yamasaki, K., Edington, H.D., McClosky, C., Tzeng, E., Lizonova, A., Kovesdi, I., Steed, D.L., and Billiar, T.R., Reversal of impaired wound repair in iNOS-deficient mice by topical adenoviral-mediated iNOS gene transfer, *J. Clin. Invest.,* 101, 967–971, 1998.

126. Liechty, K.W., Nesbit, M., Herlyn, M., Radu, A., Adzick, N.S., and Crombleholme, T.M., Adenoviral-mediated overexpression of platelet-derived growth factor-B corrects ischemic impaired wound healing, *J. Invest. Dermatol.,* 113, 375–383, 1999.

127. Galeano, M., Deodato, B., Altavilla, D., Cucinotta, D., Arsic, N., Marini, H., Torre, V., Giacca, M., and Squadrito, F., Adeno-associated viral vector-mediated human vascular endothelial growth factor gene transfer stimulates angiogenesis and wound healing in the genetically diabetic mouse, *Diabetologia,* 46, 546–555, 2003.

128. Jeschke, M.G., Richter, G., Hofstadter, F., Herndon, D.N., Perez-Polo, J.R., and Jauch, K.W., Non-viral liposomal keratinocyte growth factor (KGF) cDNA gene transfer improves dermal and epidermal regeneration through stimulation of epithelial and mesenchymal factors, *Gene Ther.,* 9, 1065–1074, 2002.

129. Ozawa, K., Kondo, T., Hori, O., Kitao, Y., Stern, D.M., Eisenmenger, W., Ogawa, S., and Ohshima, T., Expression of the oxygen-regulated protein ORP150 accelerates wound healing by modulating intracellular VEGF transport, *J. Clin. Invest.,* 108, 41–50, 2001.

130. Bevan, S., Woodward, B., Ng, R.L., Green, C., and Martin, R., Retroviral gene transfer into porcine keratinocytes following improved methods of cultivation, *Burns,* 23, 525–532, 1997.

131. Winter, D.D., Epidermal regeneration studied in the domestic pig, in *Epidermal Wound Healing,* Maibach, H.I. and Rovee, D.T., Eds., Year Book Medical Publishers, Inc., Chicago, 1972, pp. 71–111.

132. Weinstein, G.D., Autoradiographic studies of turnover time and protein synthesis in pig epidermis, *J. Invest. Dermatol.*, 44, 413–419, 1965.
133. Kangesu, T., Navsaria, H.A., Manek, S., Shurey, C.B., Jones, C.R., Fryer, P.R., Leigh, I. M., and Green, C.J., A porcine model using skin graft chambers for studies on cultured keratinocytes, *Br. J. Plast. Surg.*, 46, 393–400, 1993.
134. Sullivan, T.P., Eaglstein, W.H., Davis, S.C., and Mertz, P., The pig as a model for human wound healing, *Wound Repair Regen.*, 9, 66–76, 2001.
135. Jonkman, M.F., Sceffer, H., Stulp, R., Pas, H.H., Nijenhuis, M., Heeres, K., Owaribe, K., Pulkkinen, L., and Uitto, J., Revertant mosaicism in epidermolysis bullosa caused by mitotic gene conversion, *Cell*, 88, 543–551, 1997.
136. Eming, S., Medalie, D., Tompkins, R., Yarmush, M., and Morgan, J., Genetically modified human keratinocytes overexpressing PDGF-A enhance the performance of a composite skin graft, *Hum. Gene Ther.*, 9, 529–539, 1998.
137. Gallo, R.L. and Huttner, K.M., Antimicrobial peptides: an emerging concept in cutaneous biology, *J. Invest. Dermatol.*, 111, 739–743, 1998.
138. Yao, F., Svensjö, T., Winkler, T., Lu, M., Eriksson, C., and Eriksson, E., Tetracycline repressor, tetR, rather than the tetR-mammalian cell transcription factor fusion derivatives, regulates inducible gene expression in mammalian cells, *Hum. Gene Ther.*, 9, 1939–1950, 1998.

17 Retinoids and the Epidermis

Stephen Mandy, Leslie Baumann, and Monica Halem

CONTENTS

17.1 INTRODUCTION

The field of dermatology was dramatically changed over 70 years ago when retinol, vitamin A alcohol, was first formulated. In 1937, the Nobel Chemistry Prize was won by Karrer et al.[1] for determining the chemical structure of retinol. Then, a decade later, retinol was first synthesized, and it became commercially available. In the 1960s, a dermatologist in Berlin by the name of Stuttgen and a researcher with Hoffman-LaRoche laboratories in Switzerland began to study both oral and topical retinoids as treatment for dermatologic disease.[2] Initially, their research focused on the treatment of hyperproliferative and hyperkeratotic dermatologic disorders. They found profound efficacy with the use of oral retinoids; however, the therapeutic affect was seen only at toxic levels.[3]

Due to this toxic effect, emphasis in the research community at the time began to switch to a topical formulation of vitamin A that could be used to treat dermatologic diseases. Vitamin A acid, also known as retinoic acid or tretinoin, was studied. Tretinoin, the physiologically active metabolic product of vitamin A, was known to be beneficial in hyperkeratotic disorders. During the late 1960s, Kligman studied the effect of tretinoin on acne vulgaris and found topical tretinoin to be therapeutic in the treatment of this condition.[4] This was a landmark paper, and it launched the study of topical tretinoin's use in the treatment of various dermatologic diseases such as acne, psoriasis, photoaging, and skin cancer.

Since that time, the retinoid field has proliferated with new compounds now numbering over 2500 new products.[3] Initially, the definition of a retinoid was a compound the structure and action of which resembled those of the parent compound, vitamin A. Through the last several decades, chemists have made extensive modifications to the naturally occurring molecule that have resulted in the development of three generations of retinoids (Figure 17.1). Currently, a variety of first-, second-, and third-generation retinoids are available. The latest retinoids bear little structural resemblance to retinol and qualify as retinoids solely because they share one or more functions with the parent compound. Each new compound has had the challenge of having to demonstrate advantages over tretinoin. Some of these include greater specificity for particular diseases as well as more tolerability and less irritancy to the patients.

Currently, there has been an explosion of interest in the therapeutic uses of both oral and topical retinoids not only in dermatology, but in all areas of medicine. Some of these include the areas of oncology, rheumatology and connective tissue diseases, periodontal diseases, and immunodeficiencies. Researchers are focusing on the numerous mechanisms of action of retinoids to be able to apply them to both dermatologic and nondermatologic disease states. The advancement of new retinoid compounds and new applications continues to progress.

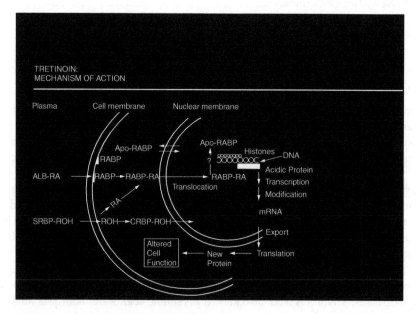

FIGURE 17.1 The mechanism of action for tretinoin.

This chapter will focus on the structure and mechanism of action of retinoids and their uses in dermatology. We will then discuss the evolving role of retinoids in the epidermis as it relates to epidermal wound healing as well as some new approaches to the future use of retinoids.

17.2 MECHANISM OF ACTION

17.2.1 DEFINITION AND STRUCTURE

In order to understand how retinoids affect the epidermis, a thorough understanding of the structure and pharmacologic properties of retinoids is necessary. Retinoids are currently defined as compounds that mimic the pharmacologic and biologic properties of retinol (Vitamin A). Retinoic acid, a naturally occurring derivative of vitamin A, is a lipid-soluble molecule known to affect cell growth, differentiation, homeostasis, apoptosis, and embryonic development. In fact, retinoids are essential for the growth, differentiation, and maintenance of epithelial tissues. Retinoids elicit their effects at the molecular level by regulating gene transcription and affecting activities such as cellular differentiation and proliferation (Figure 17.1). These agents can act directly by inducing transcription from genes with promoter regions that contain retinoid response elements or indirectly by inhibiting the transcription of certain other genes.[5] Three domains within the retinoic acid molecule govern its biological activity: an acidic function at one extremity and a lipophilic domain at the other, linked by a group that determines their relative spatial orientation.[6] The third-generation retinoids have resulted from remodification of the retinoic acid skeleton with addition of aromatic rings in place of the vulnerable double bonds found in retinoic acid. This makes the third-generation retinoids less irritating and more photostable when compared to the first- and second-generation compounds.[7]

17.2.2 RETINOID RECEPTORS

Retinoid-binding proteins were first discovered in the 1970s.[8] In 1987, the discovery of retinoic acid receptors led to the realization that tretinoin is a hormone.[9,10] Since that time, much research has been performed to determine the exact roles of these binding proteins and receptors. The biologic effects of retinoic acid are now known to be mediated by several receptors including cellular retinoic acid binding proteins I and III (CRABP I and II), cellular retinol binding protein (CRBP),[11] and nuclear receptors that are divided into two categories — the retinoic acid receptors (RARs) and the retinoid X receptors (RXRs).[12] All of these receptors are members of a large superfamily called *nuclear hormone superfamily receptors,* which includes the receptors for vitamin D, estradiol, glucocorticoids, and thyroid hormone.[13]

The retinoic acid receptor family is composed of two types of receptors, the RARs and the RXRs. The RARs and the RXRs are divided into α, β, and γ subtypes. The RARα, RARβ, and RARγ genes have been localized to chromosomes 17q21, 3p24, and 12q13, respectively, and the RXRα, RXRβ, and RXRγ genes have been mapped to chromosomes 9q34.3, 6p21.3, and 1q22–23, respectively.[14] These receptors are able to regulate gene expression in two ways:

1. They induce gene expression by binding to specific deoxyribonucleic acid (DNA) sequences known as retinoic acid responsive elements (RAREs).
2. They inhibit gene expression by downregulating the actions of other transcription factors (such as activator protein 1 [AP-1] and nuclear factor [NF]-IL6).

All of the α, β, and γ subtypes exhibit distinct affinities for retinoic acid and show a characteristic tissue distribution. For example, RARγ and RXRα are found in the epidermis whereas RARα is ubiquitous. RARβ is primarily found in the dermis, although it is found in other body tissues.[6] Ninety percent of the RARs in the epidermis and cultured keratinocytes are RARγ, which is the receptor associated with terminal differentiation; therefore, this receptor is the target of the retinoids used in dermatology.[15]

The interactions of the retinoid receptors among themselves and with other receptors of the nuclear hormone superfamily are complex. RARs are known to heterodimerize with RXR and mediate classic retinoid activity and toxicity. RXRs, however, are more promiscuous, heterodimerizing with several other members of the steroid receptor superfamily including peroxisome proliferator-activated receptors (PPAR), vitamin D receptors, thyroid hormone receptors, and a number of orphan receptors, such as liver x receptor (LXR), pregnane x receptor (PXR), and farnesoid x receptor (FXR).[16] The interactions of these receptors are being studied intensively; however, more research is necessary to fully delineate the mechanisms of action of retinoid agents. The main goal is to synthesize retinoids that are even more selective for individual receptor subtypes so that they will affect only specific pathways of a targeted disease. In addition to studying receptor-selective retinoids, current retinoid research is leading to the development of novel types of function-selective retinoids such as RAR inverse agonists and RAR antagonists. These retinoids are expected to be of clinical benefit not only in dermatology but also in oncology, diabetes, and diseases associated with human papilloma virus.[17]

17.2.3 Effects and Mechanism of Action

Retinoids have diverse biologic effects. They affect cell growth and differentiation, angiogenesis, morphogenesis, inhibition of tumor promotion and malignant cell growth, immunomodulatory actions, and alterations in cellular cohesiveness.[18] Most of these biologic effects are due to the effects retinoids have on the RAR and RXR nuclear receptors, which activate specific gene transcription as described above. Some of the genes regulated are DNA-binding proteins or other regulatory proteins. Retinoids can increase or suppress the expression of these genes. They have been shown to alter the expression of growth factors, oncogenes, keratins, and transglutaminases.[19] In addition, retinoids are known to speed up the cell cycle, increasing cellular turnover and regularizing keratinization.

Several studies have been published showing that retinoids increase heparin-binding (HB) epidermal growth factor (EGF)-like growth factor (HB-EGF). Induction of mRNA expression of HB-EGF-like growth factor in human keratinocytes and skin is seen in the setting of topical retinoid treatment.[20] HB-EGF is known to stimulate basal cell growth via intracellular signaling. These events may underlie retinoid action in epidermal regeneration during wound healing. Retinoids have also been shown to increase keratinocyte growth factor (KGF).[21] KGF plays an important role in the development and maintenance of epithelial structures and in epithelial wound healing. The effects of retinoids on KGF expression provide a mechanism by which retinoids can regulate the growth and diffentiation of epithelia.

Recently, researchers have been focusing on the effects retinoids have on matrix metalloproteinases (MMPs). MMPs were originally thought to be facilitators of clearing debris from the skin and allowing new tissue to form. Today they are known to be a specific class of proteolytic enzymes. These enzymes are known as collagenase, gelatinase, and stromelysin and are responsible for the breakdown of many dermal components. Increasing evidence indicates that retinoids decrease MMP secretion and activity, thus decreasing collagenase levels in the skin.[22] Most of the evidence of how MMPs affect the skin comes from studies looking at the affects of retinoids in photoaging (cf. section on reversal of photoaging). However, newer research is looking at MMP suppression in other tissues. A recent study showed that oral administration of retinoic acid after vein graft implantation decreased MMP secretion and activity and decreased vein graft intimal hyperplasia leading to an increased graft patency rate.[23] By suppressing the expression of MMPs, retinoids can affect multiple tissues in the body including both skin and smooth muscle.

17.3   USE OF RETINOIDS IN DERMATOLOGY

The therapeutic utilization of retinoids for the treatment of acne, photoaging, hyper-keratotic disorders, and malignancies has been clinically described and further sup-ported through an understanding of their pharmacologic parameters.[18] In fact, there are over 125 distinct dermatologic disorders for which there is credible evidence of retinoid efficacy.[3] A few important therapeutic applications of retinoids in the man-agement of acne, actinic keratosis, and the reversal of photoaging are described here.

17.3.1   ACNE

For many years, retinoids have been used topically and systemically for the treatment of dermatologic diseases, particularly acne. Acne is an inflammatory disease of the pilosebaceous units in the skin. The pathogenesis of the formation of acne is mul-tifactorial. Research suggests that the development of acne is influenced by andro-gen-induced sebum production; abnormal desquamation of sebaceous-follicle epi-thelium, or comedogenesis; proliferation of the anaerobic diphtheroid *Propioni-bacterium acnes*; and the resulting inflammation.[24] Acne is classified as comedonal, papulopustular, or cystic. Currently, three topical retinoid agents (tretinoin, ada-palene, and tazarotene) and one systemic agent (isotretinoin) are approved by the U.S. Food and Drug Administration (FDA) for the treatment of acne.

Tretinoin acts by normalizing the desquamation of the follicular epithelium, by promoting drainage of existing comedones, and by inhibiting the formation of new comedones.[25] In addition, the follicles become more accessible to antimicrobial penetration, decreasing the number of bacteria. Adapalene is a synthetic retinoid that possesses some of the biologic activities of tretinoin. In comparison, adapalene has increased chemical and light stability, rigidity, and high lipophilicity.[26] In addition, studies on adapalene have shown that it affects the cellular differentiation, keratinization, and inflammatory processes associated with acne.[26] It is believed that cutaneous irritation may be reduced without losing retinoid efficacy. New formulations of existing agents, such as tretinoin in a slow release microsphere gel, are now under investigation for acne. In addition, current research is focused on enhancing receptor selectivity with the belief that increased receptor selectivity would lead to improved benefits and an increased safety profile.

Tazarotene is an example of a retinoid that is selective for the RAR gamma receptor. A multicenter, double-blind, randomized, parallel-group study compared the efficacy and tolerability of tazarotene 0.1% gel and tretinoin 0.025% gel in the treatment of acne vulgaris.[27] A total of 143 patients with mild-to-moderate facial acne vulgaris were randomized to receive tazarotene 0.1% gel or tretinoin 0.025% gel once daily for 12 weeks. Tazarotene 0.1% gel was more effective than tretinoin 0.025% gel in reducing the open comedo count, the total noninflammatory lesion count, and the total inflammatory lesion count. These investigators concluded that tazarotene 0.1% gel is more effective than tretinoin 0.025% gel in reducing noninflammatory lesions and similarly effective in reducing inflammatory lesions. Of course, it is important to note that the concentration of tazarotene used in this trial was greater than that of tretinoin.

Another study assessed acne improvement and tolerability during 12 weeks of short-contact treatment with 0.1% tazarotene gel vs. a nonmedicated gel control.[28] This was a randomized, vehicle-controlled trial. Ninety-nine volunteers with facial acne were enrolled. Thirty-three patients were randomly assigned to each of three groups: one group applied 0.1% tazarotene gel twice daily, another applied 0.1% tazarotene gel once daily and vehicle gel once daily, and the third group applied vehicle gel twice daily. By week 12 the tazarotene group achieved significantly greater improvement in acne than vehicle based on mean percentage reduction in noninflammatory lesions and inflammatory lesions, percentage of treatment successes, and reduction in overall disease severity. Local adverse effects such as peeling, burning, and itching did not differ significantly among the three groups after week 4. The authors concluded that short-contact 0.1% tazarotene gel therapy is a safe and effective method of acne treatment.

More recently, the efficacy and tolerability of tazarotene 0.1% gel and adapalene 0.1% gel were compared in a multicenter, double-blind, randomized, parallel-group study in which 145 patients with mild-to-moderate facial acne vulgaris were enrolled.[29] Both treatments were applied once daily in the evenings for up to 12 weeks. Compared with adapalene, treatment with tazarotene was associated with a significantly greater incidence of treatment success (78 vs. 52%; $P = 0.002$) and significantly greater reductions in overall disease severity ($P < .0001$), noninflammatory lesion count ($P < 0.0001$), and inflammatory lesion count ($P = 0.0002$). In addition, mean usage of study medication was 0.32 g per application of tazarotene and 0.42 g per application of adapalene, which resulted in cost-effectiveness ratios of $79.95 per treatment success for tazarotene and $107.88 per treatment success for adapalene. These researchers concluded that tazarotene 0.1% gel was more effective than adapalene 0.1% gel in the treatment of acne vulgaris and was also a more cost-effective treatment option.

Another recent study evaluated the efficacy and tolerability of tazarotene 0.1% gel vs. tretinoin 0.1% microsponge gel in a multicenter, double-blind, randomized, parallel-group study in patients with mild-to-moderate inflammatory facial acne vulgaris.[30] Both agents were associated with significant reductions from baseline in the noninflammatory and inflammatory lesion counts. Tazarotene treatment was associated with a significantly greater reduction in overall disease severity than tretinoin microsponge treatment. Both drugs were well tolerated, with minimal side effects. In conclusion, topical retinoids offer a superb treatment option for acne with minimal side effects.

Finally, oral retinoids such as isotretinoin are indicated for the treatment of cystic acne or for patients who have failed topical therapy. Isotretinoin affects all four pathogenic factors of acne. It suppresses sebum production, reduces the size of sebaceous glands, inhibits sebaceous gland differentiation, and decreases bacterial load.[31] Isotretinoin is strictly contraindicated in pregnancy due to its teratogenic effects.

17.3.2 ACTINIC KERATOSIS AND SKIN CANCERS

Excessive exposure to the sun can lead to the development of solar or actinic keratoses (AKs). These are characterized as epidermal cutaneous neoplasms that are erythematous, scaled, and tan or darkly pigmented. They are usually found in areas of chronic sun exposure, such as the face, neck, arms, or dorsal surface of the hands. These are premalignant lesions and can lead to squamous cell cancer. Histologically, AKs consist of altered keratinocytes with a variation in cell size, nuclear heterogeneity, and loss of polarity.[32] The evidence on the positive effect retinoids have on AKs comes from studies on the use of topical retinoids for photodamage. Retinoids may reduce the risk of photocarcinogenesis through the same mechanism by which they prevent photodamage. By inhibiting the action of AP-1, they also decrease the formation of cyclooxygenase, an enzyme thought to be important in the production of skin cancer.[33] In a large multicenter study, 0.05% topical tretinoin applied once or twice daily was found to significantly decrease the number and size of facial AKs by 50% after 15 months of treatment.[34] Another multicenter double-blind study included 1265 patients who were treated for AK with either 0.05% tretinoin, 0.1% tretinoin, or vehicle for 15 months.[35]

In addition to AKs, retinoids are being studied for their therapeutic effect for skin cancers. A randomized, double-blind, vehicle-controlled Phase III study was conducted to evaluate the efficacy and safety of alitretinoin gel 0.1% for the topical treatment of the cutaneous lesions of acquired immune deficiency syndrome (AIDS)-related Kaposi's sarcoma (KS).[36] Treatment of patients with alitretinoin gel resulted in a significant antitumor effect. The overall patient response rate (complete plus partial response) was 37% (23 of 62) for the alitretinoin-treated patients and 7% (5 of 72) for the vehicle-treated patients ($P = 0.00003$). The difference in response rates for the two treatment groups remained significant even after taking into consideration numerous variables. The results of this study provided convincing evidence of the superiority of alitretinoin gel over vehicle gel for the treatment of the cutaneous lesions of AIDS-related KS.

Other studies have shown that retinoids inhibit the growth of squamous cell carcinoma and other malignancies.[37] One study treated squamous cell carcinoma (SCC-13) cells with all-*trans* retinoic acid (tRA) and 13-*cis* retinoic acid (cRA). The growth rate was inhibited for SCC cells treated with tRA and cRA vs. vehicle control. These researchers concluded that retinoic acids inhibit cell growth in SCC-13 cells. In another study, patients with advanced SCC were successfully treated with oral isotretinoin. In the cases described in this study, tumor regression lasted from 2 to 23 months.[38]

Recently, awareness of the usefulness of retinoids in the chemoprevention of skin cancers has increased. Isotretinoin (13-*cis*-retinoic acid) significantly decreases the incidence of second primary skin tumors in patients with head-and-neck cancer and reduces appearance of nonmelanoma skin cancer in patients with xeroderma pigmentosum.[39] Several clinical trials have further concluded that isotretinoin is the most effective retinoid for the prevention of nonmelanoma skin cancers in high-risk patients.[40] The use of retinoids as a chemopreventative agent for those at risk for other types of malignancies is very promising as well.

Transplant recipients have an increased risk of developing actinic keratoses and nonmelanotic skin cancers when compared with the general population. Systemic retinoids have been shown to be beneficial in the treatment of such lesions in recipients of renal or heart transplants.[41] In one recent study, five heart transplant recipients with multiple new skin cancer presentations were treated with acitretin at doses of either 10 or 25 mg/day. The researchers concluded that low-dose acitretin proved to be a valuable addition in the long-term strategy of reduction and treatment of nonmelanotic skin cancers in heart transplant recipients with multiple skin cancers and actinic keratoses. Ongoing studies in chemoprevention are focusing on efficacy/toxicity ratios that can result in highly effective chemopreventative therapy for both skin and nonskin cancer.[42]

17.3.3 REVERSAL OF PHOTOAGING

The potential benefits of retinoids for the treatment and prevention of photoaging have been explored over the last two decades. This research has led to a greater understanding of the etiology of skin aging. Concurrent but unrelated research has also recently demonstrated that doses of ultraviolet (UV) light too low to cause visible skin reddening are nevertheless capable of activating the enzymatic machinery that leads to photoaging.[43] Examination of the ways retinoids affect photoaged skin has helped to increase understanding of how retinoids affect the epidermis and epidermal wound healing.

The first anecdotal evidence that retinoids could improve aged skin was seen in female patients treated for acne. These patients reported that their skin felt smoother and less wrinkled after treatment.[11] This observation was followed by a clinical trial showing that patients treated with tretinoin demonstrated improvement of sunlight-induced epidermal atrophy, dysplasia, keratosis, and dispigmentation.[44] A plethora of clinical trials have confirmed such early observations. Although many different topical retinoids on the market today are useful against photodamage, Renova™ and Avage™ are the only topical agents approved specifically for this purpose. It should be noted, though, that oral retinoids are also being used to treat photodamage.

Multiple studies have examined the use of retinoids for the prevention and treatment of photoaging. The first of these clinical trials to demonstrate clinical improvement of photoaged skin were published in 1986 and 1988; both used tretinoin[44,45] Since then, many other studies and much clinical experience have shown similar results. In one randomized single-center study, 100 subjects were divided into three treatment groups.[46] One group was treated with 0.1% tretinoin, another with 0.025% tretinoin, and the last group with vehicle\cream. Treatment with either 0.1% or 0.025% tretinoin resulted in statistically significant improvement of photoaged skin compared with vehicle treatment. The histologically observed changes with the use of retinoids include abolition of cellular atypia, increased compacting of the stratum corneum, less clumping of melanin in basal cells, and a correction of polarity of keratinocytes, with more orderly differentiation as cells move upward. The ultrastructural changes seen with retinoid use include evidence of hyperproliferation of keratinocytes (larger nuclei, increased ribosomes, etc.) and a reduction in the size of melanosomes.

Although tretinoin and tazarotene have been approved for the *treatment* of photoaging, recent evidence suggests that they also play a role in the *prevention* of photoaging. This occurs in part because of inhibitory effects on damaging metalloproteinases. Ultraviolet exposure dramatically upregulates the production of several collagen-degrading enzymes known as matrix metalloproteinases (MMPs). As described above, activation of the MMP genes results in production of collagenase, gelatinase, and stromelysin, which have been shown to fully degrade skin collagen.[47] Fisher et al. demonstrated that application of tretinoin inhibits the induction of all three of these harmful MMPs.[43]

In addition to increasing levels of destructive enzymes such as collagenase, UV exposure has also been shown to decrease collagen production. Fisher et al.[48] demonstrated that expression of Type I and III collagen is substantially reduced within 24 h after a single UV exposure. Pretreatment of the skin with all-*trans* retinoic acid was shown to inhibit this loss of procollagen synthesis. Therefore, pretreatment of the skin with topical retinoids, when used consistently, is likely to be beneficial in preventing as well as treating photodamage.[49]

The effect of retinoids on the production of MMPs has been well characterized. Two transcription factors, c-jun and c-fos, must combine to produce AP-1. AP-1 is able to activate the MMP genes, resulting in production of collagenase, gelatinase, and stromelysin. All-*trans* retinoic acid blocks the UV-induced increase in c-jun protein. Although high levels of c-jun mRNA are still present, signifying that the c-jun gene has been activated, the levels of c-jun protein are decreased. Topical retinoic acid likely acts to reduce UV induction of c-jun protein by stimulating its breakdown through the ubiquitin–proteasome pathway.[49]

Changes in collagen and the ratio of collagen I to collagen III have been found to be important in the photoaging process. Retinoids have been shown to increase collagen synthesis in photoaged humans.[50] In addition to preventing the breakdown of collagen as described above, topical application of tretinoin 0.1% to photodamaged skin partially restores levels of collagen type I. An increase in anchoring fibrils (collagen VII) is also seen after application of tretinoin 0.1%.[50] Understanding these same mechanisms of how retinoids are used to treat and prevent photoaging has led researchers to understand the many roles retinoids play in wound healing.

17.3.4 EPIDERMAL WOUND HEALING

All cutaneous wounds undergo a highly organized programmed repair process. This process includes inflammation, removal of devitalized tissue, fibroplasia, matrix accumulation, angiogenesis, epithelial proliferation and reepithelialization, and tissue remodeling.[51] There are classically three principal phases: inflammatory, proliferative, and remodeling. The proliferative phase traditionally includes cell migration and proliferation. The remodeling phase encompasses the tertiary binding of collagen molecules.[52] The influence of retinoids on epithelialization, fibroplasia, angiogenesis, and collagen synthesis led scientists to study the effects of retinoids on epidermal wound healing.

Researchers have been aware of the beneficial effects of Vitamin A on cutaneous lesions since the 1930s.[53] Vitamin A deficiency resulted in a retardation of epithelialization, wound closure, collagen synthesis, and crosslinking of newly formed collagen.[64] Vitamin A further increases the rate of reepithelialization of wounded skin and normalizes the epithelial tissue.[55] It is well known that corticosteroids suppress collagen synthesis and inhibit wound healing. As early as 1968, scientists understood that vitamin A may reverse these potentially serious side effects that corticosteroids have on impaired wound healing.[56] Since that time, there have been numerous studies published in different fields of medicine supporting this original data on vitamin A.

Retinoids have been shown in well-documented studies to have a positive effect on wound healing as well by influencing epithelialization, fibroplasia, collagen synthesis, and angiogenesis.[57,58] Early wound healing studies began looking at the healing effects of oral retinoic acid on full-thickness skin wounds and epithelial corneal abrasions in experimental animals. These studies found that there was an enhancement of the thickness of the skin wounds and an increased healing of corneal epithelial wounds.[59] The potential toxicity of oral retinoic acid limited the clinical applicability of these studies. It is well established that significant toxicity is associated with the use of oral retinoids but not with topical retinoid use because the systemic absorption of topically applied retinoids is minimal. In fact, one controlled study in which 0.025% tretinoin gel was applied daily to the face, neck, and upper part of the chest for 14 d showed fluctuations in plasma levels of endogenous retinoids to be lower than those due to diurnal and nutritional factors.[60]

Topical retinoids showed a similar wound healing profile. Several studies indicate that the application of tretinoin prior to procedures that remove the epidermis, such as dermabrasion,[61] chemical peels,[62] and laser surgery[63] and to full-thickness wounds[64] can significantly accelerate wound healing. One study examined the effects of tretinoin cream 0.05% applied to the face for 2 weeks before dermabrasion for the management of acne scarring. The group that received tretinoin experienced complete healing within 5 to 7 d, as evidenced by reepithelialization. The nontreated group healed in 7 to 11 days. In addition, pretreatment with tretinoin yielded fewer areas of crusting, erythema, and discomfort.[61] Tretinoin apparently primes the epithelium to heal more rapidly. Another study examined the effect of pretreatment with tretinoin on wound healing in wound sites on severely photoaged dorsal forearm skin.[64] Patients applied tretinoin cream 0.05% to one arm and a vehicle control to the other arm for 16 weeks. Full thickness punch biopsies (4 mm) were taken from both arms before the treatment, and full-thickness (2 mm) punch biopsies were taken after treatment. The biopsy site wounds were excised on day 11 of treatment. Histologic assessment and polarized light photography indicated that the wound areas in the tretinoin-treated arms were significantly smaller by 35 to 37% on days 1 and 4, and 47 to 50% smaller on days 6, 8, and 11. Tretinoin facilitated a more rapid reepithelialization and was shown to dramatically accelerate wound healing in photodamaged skin.[55] Similar results were seen in a double-blinded, placebo-controlled, prospective, randomized study which assessed the effects of tretinoin pretreatment on healing after 35% trichloroacetic acid (TCA) chemical peel. Patients were treated with 0.1% tretinoin on half of their faces 2 weeks before the chemical peel. The pretreated group showed a more even and earlier frosting. In addition, 75% of the pretreated group was healed within 7 d, compared with 31% of the nontreated group.[62]

Retinoids have also been used and shown to be helpful in chronic wound therapy. One recent study involved five patients with at least a 1-year-old chronic leg wound, which was treated with 10 min of topical 0.05% tretinoin solution to the wound bed daily for 4 weeks. The researchers found that as early as 1 week after treatment, an increased amount of granulation tissue was evident at the wound's edge. After 4 weeks of therapy with tretinoin, there was further stimulation of granulation tissue, new vascular tissue, and new collagen formation.[65] Another recent study compared the effects of tretinoin and adapalene on wound healing by measuring wound surface area after treatment. A decrease in wound surface area and histologic findings of improved wound healing were observed in both groups.[66]

Timing of application is another important factor when applying topical retinoids to wounds. In contrast to application of topical retinoids prior to dermatologic treatment or injury, studies have shown that topical application after a dermatologic procedure prolongs wound healing and actually in some cases inhibits the ability of the wound to heal. Using the Eaglstein and Mertz[67,68] porcine wound healing model, researchers studied the effects of topical tretinoin on epithelial wound healing. Tensile strength, quantity of granulation tissue formation, and the rate of healing of full-thickness wounds were evaluated. Pretreatment with 0.05% tretinoin cream once a day for 10 d was done prior to wounding, and treatment continued once daily on half of the group post injury. Treatment with topical tretinoin before wounding was shown to accelerate wound healing. Vascular dilatation, epithelial proliferation, and decreased transit time were observed. Continued daily treatment with 0.05% tretinoin had an adverse effect, however. Minimal epithelialization and epithelial defects were observed. Biopsy specimens of these wounds revealed progressive inflammation and a disorganized, noncohesive epithelium.[69] The increased inflammatory response may be associated with the destabilizing effect of retinoids on lysosomal membranes, which can cause the release of lysosomal enzymes.[70]

A single-blinded, randomized, placebo-controlled pilot study at the Mayo Clinic investigated high-tension excisional wounds and full-thickness skin grafts treated perioperatively with 0.1% tretinoin cream. The conclusion from the study was that perioperative treatment with tretinoin of high tension excisional wounds had no apparent benefit, but an adverse effect was observed on the full-thickness skin grafts.[71] A possible explanation may involve collagenase. Several studies have concluded that collagenase is necessary for tissue remodeling and reorganization.[72,73] Retinoids have been shown to decrease collagenase production, perhaps disrupting the wound healing remodeling process in those wounds treated with retinoids post injury.[58]

Many mechanisms must be present for retinoids to have such an impact on the wound healing process, some of which have been previously described. What is currently known is that retinoids exert their effects by binding to specific receptors in both the nucleus and cytoplasm. Research suggests that retinoids affect both epidermal and dermal aspects of wound healing.[74] It is thought that retinoids stimulate epidermal migration by decreasing epidermal tonofilaments and epidermal desmosomal attachments. Retinoids stimulate epidermal turnover, resulting in faster epithelialization of the epidermis.[55] In addition, the angiogenic properties of retinoids enhance wound healing by increasing oxygen delivery to the tissue. Papillary dermal vascularization after retinoid treatment to the skin has been documented by light microscopy and laser Doppler velocimetry.[69]

A recent study looked at the effects of retinoic acid on epidermal keratinocytes. This study demonstrated the upregulation of cell-associated plasminogen activation by retinoic acid. The activation of the proteolytic plasminogen activator system is essential for the reepithelialization of wounds as well as in regards to pericellular fibrinolysis required during wound healing.[75] Histologically, retinoids enable the stratum corneum to become thin and compact. The atypia of the stratum granulosum decreases, as does the disturbed polarity.[76] In the dermis, there is an increase in the quantity of dilated capillaries. Increases in the numbers of advential cells and fibroblasts in the dermis are seen as well.[55] Histologically, retinoid therapy causes normalization of the epidermis, neo-vascularization, and an increased presence of repair cells.[55]

17.4 NEW USES OF RETINOIDS

The natural history and clinical course of striae are similar to those of scar development. Striae may be a form of dermal scarring, as suggested by both light and electron microscopy.[77] These disfiguring marks are usually caused by excessive stretching of the skin. This occurs during pregnancy, growth spurts, and obesity.[77] These marks are usually benign but can have a psychological impact on the patient. They initially appear with erythema and no surface depression. Over time, the lesions develop a normal-to-lighter skin color, accompanied by surface depression and the development of fine wrinkles.[78]

Clinical investigations have demonstrated that retinoids can effectively treat striae. These studies indicate that topical tretinoin 0.1% halts and potentially reverses the progression of striae.[79] In a recent double-blinded, randomized, vehicle-controlled trial, 22 patients applied either 0.1% tretinoin or vehicle daily for 6 months to the affected area of striae. After 6 months of treatment, 80% of the treated group had marked improvement of their striae compared to the vehicle-treated group. In addition, decreases in the mean length and width of the striae were observed.[80] The authors further concluded that topical tretinoin improved the clinical appearance of early stretch marks during the active stage.[81] The cellular changes that caused the clinical improvement were undetermined. Further research is needed to determine if topical tretinoin would have the same beneficial effect on striae not in their early active stage.

17.5 SUMMARY

Over the last several decades, retinoids have become among the most important agents in the dermatologic armamentarium. The pharmacologic and clinical properties of retinoids have expanded their use to nondermatologic fields as well. Retinoids have secured their place in the treatment of acne, photoaging, hyperkeratotic disorders, and skin malignancies. Their evolving role in the areas of cutaneous wound healing and striae are seen in the literature as well. New advances and new discoveries into the benefits and mechanisms of action will lead to greater clinical specificity of retinoid therapy. Ongoing research will provide the development of new, more receptor specific, less toxic, and thus more effective retinoid agents.

REFERENCES

1. Karrer, P., Morf, R., and Schopp, K., Zur Kenntnis des vitamin A aus Fischtranin, *Helv. Chim. Acta,* 14, 1431, 1931.
2. Stuttgen G., Zur Lokalbehandlung von keratosen mit vitamin-A-Saure, *Dermatologica,* 124, 65, 1962.
3. Kligman, A., The growing importance of topical retinoids in clinical dermatology: a retrospective and prospective analysis, *J. Am. Acad. Dermatol.,* 39, S2, 1998.
4. Kligman, A.M., Fulton, J.E., and Plewig, G., Topical vitamin A acid in acne vulgaris, *Arch. Dermatol.,* 99, 469–476, 1969.
5. Chandraratna, R.A., Tazarotene — first of a new generation of receptor-selective retinoids, *Br. J. Dermatol.,* 135, 18, 1996.
6. Millikan, L.E., Adapalene: an update on newer comparative studies between the various retinoids, *Int. J. Dermatol.,* 39, 784, 2000.
7. Weiss, J.S., Current options for topical treatment of acne vulgaris, *Pediatr. Dermatol.,* 14, 480, 1997.
8. Chytil, F. and Ong. D., Cellular retinoid-binding proteins, in *The Retinoids,* vol. 2., Sporn, M.B., Roberts, A., and Goodman, D., Eds., Academic Press, Orlando, FL, 1984, p. 89.
9. Giguere, V., Ong, E.S., Segui, P. et al., Identification of a receptor for the morphogen retinoic acid, *Nature,* 330, 624, 1987.
10. Petkovich, M., Brand, N.J., Krust, A. et al., A human retinoic acid receptor which belongs to the family of nuclear receptors, *Nature,* 330, 444, 1987.
11. Kligman, L. and Kligman, A.M., Photoaging — retinoids, alpha hydroxy acids, and antioxidants, in *Dermatopharmacology of Topical Preparations,* Gabard, B., Elsner, P., Surber, C., and Treffel, P., Eds., Springer-Verlag, New York, 2000, p. 383.

12. Pfahl, M., The molecular mechanism of retinoid action — retinoids today and tomorrow, *Retinoids Dermatol.*, 44, 2, 1996.

13. Petkovich, M., Regulation of gene expression by vitamin A: the role of nuclear retinoic acid receptors, *Annu. Rev. Nutr.*, 12, 443, 1992.

14. Chambon, P., A decade of molecular biology of retinoic acid receptors, *FASEB J.*, 10, 940, 1996.

15. Nagpal, S. and Chandraratna, R.A., Recent developments in receptor-selective retinoids, *Curr. Pharm. Des.*, 6, 919, 2000.

16. Lippman, S. and Lotan, R., Advances in the development of retinoids as chemopreventive agents, *J. Nutr.*, 130, 479S, 2000.

17. Chandraratna, R.A., Future trends: a new generation of retinoids, *J. Am. Acad. Dermatol.*, 39, S149, 1998.

18. Mangelsdorf, D.J. et al., The retinoid receptors, in *The Retinoids: Biology, Chemistry, and Medicine*, 2nd ed., Sporn, M.B., Roberts, A.B., and Goodman, D.S., Eds., Raven Press, New York, 1994, p. 319.

19. Peck, G.L, DiGiovanna, J.J., The retinoids, in: *Fitzpatrick's Dermatology in General Medicine*, 5th ed., Freeberg, I.M., Eisen, A.Z., Fitzpatrick, T.B., et al., Eds., McGraw-Hill, 1999, pp. 2810–1819.

20. Stoll, S.W. and Elder, J.T., Retinoid regulation of heparin-binding EGF-like growth factor gene expression in human keratinocytes and skin, *Exp. Dermatol.*, 7, 391, 1998.

21. Mackenzie, I.C. and Gao, Z., KGF expression in human gingival fibroblasts and stimulation of gene expression by retinoic acid, *J. Periodontol.*, 72, 445, 2001.

22. Varani, J. et al., Vitamin A antagonizes decreased cell growth and elevated collagen-degrading MMPs and stimulates collagen accumulation in aged human skin, *J. Invest. Dermatol.*, 114, 480, 2000.

23. Leville, C. et al., All-*trans*-retinoic acid decreases vein graft intimal hyperplasia and MMP, *J. Surg. Res.*, 90, 183, 2000.

24. Cunliffe, W.J., *Acne,* Martin Dunitz, London, 1989.

25. Leyden, J.J. and Shalita, A.. Rational therapy for acne vulgaris, *J. Am. Acad. Dermatol.*, 15, 907, 1986.

26. Benard, B.A., Adapalene, a new chemical entity with retinoid activity, *Skin. Pharmacol.*, 5 (suppl), 51, 1993

27. Webster, G.F., Berson, D., Stein, L.F., Fivenson, D.P., Tanghetti, E.A., and Ling, M., Efficacy and tolerability of once-daily tazarotene 0.1% gel versus once-daily tretinoin 0.025% gel in the treatment of facial acne vulgaris: a randomized trial, *Cutis,* 67 (6 Suppl), 4, 2001.

28. Bershad, S., Kranjac Singer, G., Parente, J.E., Tan, M.H., Sherer, D.W., Persaud, A.N., and Lebwohl, M., Successful treatment of acne vulgaris using a new method: results of a randomized vehicle-controlled trial of short-contact therapy with 0.1% tazarotene gel, *Arch. Dermatol.*, 138, 481, 2002.

29. Webster, G.F., Guenther, L., Poulin, Y.P., Solomon, B.A., Loven, K., Webster, G.F., Guenther, L., Poulin, Y.P., Solomon, B.A., and Loven, K., A multicenter, double-blind, randomized comparison study of the efficacy and tolerability of once-daily tazarotene 0.1% gel and adapalene 0.1% gel for the treatment of facial acne vulgaris, *Cutis,* 69 (2 Suppl), 4, 2002.

30. Leyden, J.J., Tanghetti, E.A., Miller, B., Ung, M., Berson, D., and Lee, J.. Once-daily tazarotene 0.1 % gel versus once-daily tretinoin 0.1 % microsponge gel for the treatment of facial acne vulgaris: a double-blind randomized trial, *Cutis,* 6 (2 Suppl), 12, 2002.

31. Bergfeld, W.F., The evolving role of retinoids in the management of cutaneous conditions, *Clinician: The Cleveland Clinic Foundation Supplement* 16, 8–13, 1998.

32. Hood, A.F., Kwan, T.H., Mihm, M.C. Jr., et al., Neoplastic patterns of the epidermis, *Primer of Dermatopathology,* 2nd ed., Farmer, E.R. and Hood, A.F., Eds., Little Brown, Boston, 1993, p. 112–115.

33. Fisher, G.J. et al., Retinoic acid inhibits induction of c-Jun protein by ultraviolet radiation that occurs subsequent to activation of mitogen-activated protein kinase pathways in human skin *in vivo, J. Clin. Invest.,* 101, 1432, 1998.

34. Thorne, E.G., Long term clinical experience with a topical retinoid, *Br. J. Dermatol.,* 127, 31, 1992.

35. Kligman, A.L. and Thorne, E.G., Topical therapy of actinic keratoses with tretinoin, in *Retinoids in Cutaneous Malignancy,* Marks, R., Ed., Blackwell Scientific Publications, Oxford, 1991, p. 66.

36. Bodsworth, N.J., Bloch, M., Bower, M., Donnell, D., and Yocum, R., International Panretin Gel KS Study Group. Phase III vehicle-controlled, multi-centered study of topical alitretinoin gel 0.1% in cutaneous AIDS-related Kaposi's sarcoma, *Am. J. Clin. Dermatol.,* 2, 77–87, 2001.

37. Rudkin, G.H., Carlsen, B.T., Chung, C.Y., Huang, W., Ishida, K., Anvar, B., Yamaguchi, D.T., and Miller, T.A., Retinoids inhibit squamous cell carcinoma growth and intercellular communication, *J. Surg. Res.,* 103, 183, 2002.

38. Lippman, S.M. and Meyskens, F.L., Treatment of advanced squamous cell carcinoma of the skin with isotretinoin, *Ann. Intern. Med.,* 107, 499, 1987.

39. Niles, E.M., Recent advances in the use of vitamin A (retinoids) in the prevention and treatment of cancer, *Nutrition,* 16, 1084, 2000.

40. Niles, E.M., The use of retinoids in the prevention and treatment of skin cancer, *Expert Opin. Pharmacother.,* 3, 299, 2002.

41. McNamara, I.R., Muir, J., and Galbraith, A.J., Acitretin for prophylaxis of cutaneous malignancies after cardiac transplantation, *J. Heart Lung Transplant.,* 21, 1201, 2002.

42. Bergfeld, W.F., The evolving role of retinoids in the management of cutaneous conditions, *Clinician: The Cleveland Clinic Foundation Supplement,* 16, 16, 1998.

43. Fisher, G.J., Datta, S.C., Talwar, H.S. et al., Molecular basis of sun-induced premature skin ageing and retinoid antagonism, *Nature,* 379, 335, 1996.

44. Kligman, A.M., Grove, G.L., Hirose, R. et al., Topical tretinoin for photoaged skin, *J. Am. Acad. Dermatol.,* 15, 836, 1986.

45. Weiss, J.S., Ellis, C.N., Headington, J.T. et al., Topical tretinoin improves photoaged skin: a double-blind vehicle-controlled study, *JAMA,* 259, 527, 1988.

46. Griffiths, C.E., Kang, S., Ellis, C.N. et al., Two concentrations of topical tretinoin (retinoic acid) cause similar improvement of photoaging but different degrees of irritation. A double-blind, vehicle-controlled comparison of 0.1% and 0.025% tretinoin creams, *Arch. Dermatol.,* 131, 1037, 1995.

47. Fisher, G.J., Wang, Z.Q., Datta, S.C. et al., Pathophysiology of premature skin aging induced by ultraviolet light, *N. Engl. J. Med.,* 337, 1419, 1997.

48. Fisher, G., Datta, S., Wang, Z. et al., c-Jun-dependent inhibition of cutaneous procollagen transcription following ultraviolet irradiation is reversed by all-*trans* retinoic acid, *J. Clin. Invest.,* 106, 663, 2000.

49. Fisher, G.J., Talwar, H.S., Lin, J. et al., Molecular mechanisms of photoaging in human skin *in vivo* and their prevention by all-*trans* retinoic acid, *Photochem. Photobiol.,* 69, 154, 1999.

50. Woodley, D.T., Zelickson, A.S., Briggaman, R.A. et al., Treatment of photoaged skin with topical tretinoin increases epidermal-dermal anchoring fibrils. A preliminary report, *JAMA*, 263, 3057, 1990.

51. Ovington, L.G., Overview of MMP modulation and growth factor protection in wound healing, *Wounds*, 14, 3S, 2002.

52. Eaglstein, W.H., Wound healing and aging, *Dermatol. Clin.*, 4, 481, 1986.

53. Frazier, C.N. and Hu, C.K., Cutaneous lesions associated with deficiency of vitamin A in man, *Arch. Intern. Med.*, 48, 507, 1931.

54. Kennedy, M.C., Shin, L.M. et al., Modulation of rabbit keratinocyte production of collagen, glycosaminoglycans and fibronectin by retinoic acid, *Biochem. Biophys. Acta*, 889, 156, 1991.

55. Elson, M.L., The role of retinoids in wound healing, *J. Am. Acad. Dermatol.*, 39, S79, 1998.

56. Ehrlich, H.P. and Hunt, T.K., Effect of cortisone and vitamin A on wound healing, *Ann. Surg.*, 167, 324, 1968.

57. Kligman, L.H., Effects of all-*trans* retinoic acid on the dermis of hairless mice, *J. Am. Acad. Dermatol.*, 15, 779, 1986.

58. Lever, L., Kumar, P., and Marks, R., Topical retinoic acid in the treatment of elastotic degeneration, *Br. J. Dermatol.*, 122, 91, 1991.

59. Lee, K.H. and Tong, T.G., Mechanism of action of retinyl compounds on wound healing, *J. Pharm. Sci.*, 59, 1195, 1970.

60. Buchan, P., Eckhoff, C., Caron, D. et al., Repeated topical administration of all-*trans*-retinoic acid and plasma levels of retinoic acids in humans, *J. Am. Acad. Dermatol.*, 30, 428, 1994.

61. Mandy, S., Tretinoin in the preoperative and postoperative management of dermabrasion, *J. Am. Acad. Dermatol.*, 15, 848, 1986.

62. Hevia, O., Nemeth, A.J., and Taylor, J.R., Tretinoin accelerates healing after trichloracetic acid chemical peel, *Arch. Dermatol.*, 127, 678, 1991.

63. McDonald, W.S., Beasley, D., and Jones, C., Retinoic acid and CO_2 laser resurfacing, *Plast. Reconstr. Surg.*, 104, 2229, 1999.

64. Popp, C., Kligman, A.M., and Stoudemayer, T.J., Pretreatment of photoaged forearm skin with topical tretinoin accelerates healing of full-thickness wounds, *Br. J. Dermatol.*, 132, 46, 1995.

65. Paquette, D., Badiavas, E., and Falanga, V., Short contact topical tretinoin therapy to stimulate granulation tissue in chronic wounds, *J. Am. Acad. Dermatol.*, 45, 382, 2001.

66. Basak, P.Y. et al., Comparison of the effects of tretinoin, adapalene and collagenase in an experimental model of wound healing, *Eur. J. Dermatol.*, 12, 145, 2002.

67. Eaglstein, W.H. and Mertz, P.M, A new method for assessing epidermal wound healing. The effects of trimacinolone acetonide and polyethylene film occlusion, *J. Invest. Dermatol.*, 71, 381, 1978.

68. Mertz, P.M. and Eaglstein, W.H., A porcine model for evaluating epidermal wound healing, in *Swine in Biomedical Research*, Tumbleson, M., Ed., Plenum Press, New York, 1986, p. 291.

69. Hung, V.C., Lee, J.Y., Zitelli, J.A., and Hebda, P.A., Topical tretinoin and epithelial wound healing, *Arch. Dermatol.*, 12, 56, 1989.

70. Klein, P., Vitamin A acid in wound healing, *Acta Dermatol. Venereol.*, 7 (suppl), 171, 1975.

71. Otley, C.C. et al., Preoperative and postoperative topical tretinoin in high tension excisional wounds and full-thickness skin grafts in a porcine model, *Dermatol. Surg.*, 25, 716, 1999.

72. Grillo, H.C. and Gross, J., Collagenolytic activity during mammalian wound repair, *Devel. Biol.,* 15, 300, 1967.

73. Eisen, A.Z., Human skin collagenase: localization and distribution in normal human skin, *J. Invest. Dermatol.,* 52, 442, 1969.

74. Oikarinen, A., Oikarinen, H., and Uitto, J., Demonstration of cellular retinoic acid binding protein in cultured human skin fibroblasts, *Br. J. Dermatol.,* 113, 529, 1985.

75. Braungart, E. et al., Retinoic acid upregulates the plasminogen activator system in human epidermal keratinocytes, *J. Invest. Dermatol.,* 116, 778, 2001.

76. Elias, P.M. and Williams, M.L., Retinoid effects on epidermal differentiation, in *Retinoids: New Trends in Research and Therapy,* Saurat, J.H., Ed., S. Karger, Basel, Switzerland, 1985, p. 138.

77. Zheng, P., Larker, R.M., and Kligman, A.M., Anatomy of striae, *Br. J. Dermatol.,* 112, 185, 1985.

78. Bergfeld, W.F., The evolving role of retinoids in the management of cutaneous conditions, *Clinician: The Cleveland Clinic Foundation Supplement,* 16, 20, 1998.

79. Elson, M.L., Treatment of striae distensae with topical tretinoin, *J. Dermatol. Surg. Oncol.,* 16, 3, 1990.

80. Kang, S. et al., Topical tretinoin improves early stretch marks, *Arch. Dermatol.,* 132, 519, 1996.

18 Optimizing Epidermal Regeneration in Facial Skin Following Aesthetic Procedures

Greg Skover, James M. Spencer, and Mitchel P. Goldman

CONTENTS

18.1 INTRODUCTION

The aesthetic skincare market is one of the most dynamic and innovative areas in the personal skin care industry. Skin rejuvenation continues to be the growth leader at a pace of 13% per year and is projected to expand from $13 billion to $25 billion in 2005.* An aging population, a desire to preserve youthfulness, and changing social mores are making cosmetic procedures more acceptable. In 2001, over 14 million cosmetic procedures were performed, producing more than $8.5 billion in physician revenue, a growth of 48% over 2000.** Technological progress is keeping pace with the demand, leading to the introduction of new techniques that deliver on the desire to minimize the effects of intrinsic and extrinsic aging, photodamage, and scar repair. These procedures directly influence the epidermis, the dermis, or both simultaneously.

Clinical outcome requirements for these procedures are substantially different from the prevailing wound healing standards for chronic ulceration and acute traumatic wounds. These procedures use unique methods toward a common pursuit: inducing a controlled repair response in the epidermis and/or dermis that delivers a

---

* Moretti, M., The Skin Rejuvenation Technology Market, Version 3. Medical Insight, Inc.®
** American Society for Aesthetic Plastic Surgery 2001 Annual Survey.

0-8493-1561-1/04/$0.00+$1.50

superior cosmetic outcome. To complicate matters further, the wound is typically on the most visible body location, resulting in greatly increased patient expectations. New demands have changed the goal from simple wound closure to functionally regenerative repair.

18.2 SUPERFICIAL INTERVENTION

Aluminum oxide crystal microdermabrasion is a noninvasive, nonsurgical procedure used to revitalize and rejuvenate the skin. The instrumentation and technique were developed in Italy in 1985. This method is the least invasive of the mechanical skin rejuvenation systems that focus primarily on the exfoliation of the stratum corneum.[1] Microdermabrasion has become one of the leading cosmetic procedures for the superficial correction of fine rhytides, photoaging, mild surgical and acne scars, active acne, dyschromias, and melasma. The device gently pulls the skin into a hand piece via mild suction. Once the hand piece contacts the skin and the circuit is closed, the controlled flow of corundum particles begins. The subsequent impact of the particles on the skin's surface removes dirt, oil, surface debris, and dead skin cells. Setting the vacuum and particle flow rate controls the proximity of the skin's surface to the flowing particles and the quantity of particles passing over the skin. These factors combine with the speed of the hand piece over the surface of the skin and the number of passes to determine the degree of exfoliation (Table 18.1).

The treatments are typically performed in a series of 4 to 12 weekly visits taking 30 to 45 minutes each. After the procedure, there is a mild, transient erythema, increased surface temperature, and a sensation described as a slight sunburn or windburn (Color Figure 18.1).*

Repetitive abrasion of the skin with a cream preparation containing aluminum oxide granules has been shown to cause an increase in desquamation rate, cutaneous blood flow, epidermal thickness, and skin extensibility. However, no significant

TABLE 18.1
Aluminum Oxide Crystal Microdermabrasion and Factors Affecting the Degree of Exfoliation

Particle Flow	Vacuum Pressure	Number of Passes	Depth of Exfoliation
Low	Low Moderate	1 or 2	Stratum corneum to stratum lucidum (5 to 15 μm)
Moderate	Low Moderate High	3 or 4	Stratum corneum to stratum granulosum (5 to 25 μm)
High	Moderate High	4 to 6	Stratum granulosum to basal cell layer (25 to 75 μm)

* Color figures follow page 110.

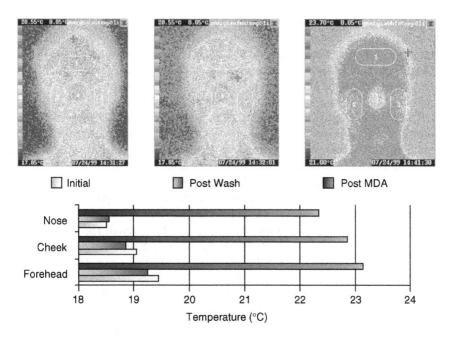

FIGURE 18.1 Skin surface thermography before and after microdermabrasion. The amount of physiological activity of the skin is measured by the amount of infrared radiation emanating from the surface using 600 lines of spatial resolution with 30° field of view at 30 frames/sec of real-time imaging. The instrument is internally referenced and self-calibrating to absolute zero with a resolution of 0.05°C at 35°C (TIP-200, Boston, MA). Scale is temperature, °C. (See color figure following page 110.)

inflammation or change in the degree of elastosis was detected histologically.[2] After a series of microdermabrasion treatments, the following have been reported: slight fibrotic changes in the upper dermis,[3] normalization of the stratum corneum, epidermal thickening, and increased collagen deposition in the papillary dermis.[2,3,9] In addition, it is postulated that new collagen and glycosaminoglycan deposition can occur.[9]

Lu et al. reported good to excellent improvements of post-acne, traumatic, and chicken pox scars in 41 patients treated with microdermabrasion.[4] Hernandez-Perez reported improvement after five treatments in women with mild to moderate photodamage. Posttreatment biopsy specimens showed mild improvement in elastosis, edema, and inflammation. The greatest change was observed in epidermal thickness, improving from 10 to 60 μm.[5] As reported by both physician and self evaluation, the majority of patients who were treated with a series of five to six weekly treatments of aluminum oxide crystal microdermabrasion with four passes at 30 mmHg experienced a mild but noticeable improvement in the appearance of facial skin.[6] An increase in skin roughness, a slight flattening of wrinkles, and a significant decrease in sebum content can occur after each treatment. However, these changes were transient and did not remain over the course of therapy or for the duration of the study.

Histological analysis showed some epidermal changes consistent with abrasion, but more dramatic changes were present in the reticular dermis and may include a vascular component. Perivascular mononuclear cell infiltrate, vascular ectasia, and dermal edema are all seen one week after the final treatment. This may produce the color change and improved appearance noted by patients and physicians.

Biomechanical assessment with the Dynamic Skin Analyzer (BTC 2000, Surgical Research Laboratory, Inc., Nashville, TN) recorded changes consistent with these histological observations. This instrument was designed to measure the elastic deformation of skin during dynamic stress. It applies a linear negative pressure at a predetermined rate until a maximum pressure is achieved for a specified number of cycles. An infrared targeting laser detects the vertical deformation of the skin, enabling the instrument to automatically calculate and display pressure and deformation in real time. Skin stiffness is defined as the slope of the stress/deformation curve. As the slope increases, so does the stiffness of the material. The more resistant a material is to stress, the greater its perceived hardness. Skin compliance or energy absorption is the integrated area under the stress/deformation curve. The compliance of a material describes its softness or firmness. As energy absorption increases, so does the softness of the material, which is inversely proportional to skin stiffness.

A significant decrease in skin stiffness with a reciprocal increase in skin compliance was also seen during the course of the study (Figure 18.2). This change persisted 1 week after the last treatment and is consistent with increased edema and hydration of the skin, similar to a stiff dry sponge becoming a soft, pliable sponge as it becomes hydrated. The depth of these changes is well below the level of direct abrasion. It is very likely that this technique may involve a mechanism other than abrasion. The aspiration system used to suck away the used aluminum oxide crystals may help promote tissue blood supply.[1] It may be possible that the negative pressure results in the vascular changes observed in our study and is responsible for the improved appearance noted by physicians and patients.[6]

18.3 NONABLATIVE LASER INTERVENTION

Microdermabrasion is a painless, bloodless, noninvasive procedure that removes portions of the epidermis. Depending upon the degree of exfoliation achieved, epidermal regeneration occurs rapidly with associated changes in the dermis, producing subtle changes in the appearance of the skin.[7] When the severity of damage warrants more invasive techniques, laser or laser-like photothermal rejuvenation induces structural changes in the skin. These methods have been popularized recently due to availability and an increase in the number of patients requesting improved outcomes without pain and with minimal recuperation time. Goldberg describes four basic approaches, those that:

1. Ablate the epidermis, cause dermal wounding, and provide a significant thermal effect
2. Ablate the epidermis, cause dermal wounding, and provide minimal thermal effects

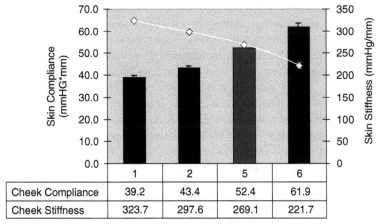

	1	2	5	6
Cheek Compliance	39.2	43.4	52.4	61.9
Cheek Stiffness	323.7	297.6	269.1	221.7

Treatment Week

FIGURE 18.2 Biomechanical properties of skin change following microdermabrasion. Skin stiffness and compliance were measured before and after the procedure (BTC 2000, Surgical Research Laboratory, Inc., Nashville, TN). The handpiece containing the suction chamber and targeting laser were positioned over the malar process on the right and left cheek. The instrument applies a linear negative pressure at a rate of 10 mmHg/sec over 1 cm of skin until 150 mmHg is achieved. An infrared targeting laser measures the vertical displacement of the skin during the cycle. Pressure and deformation are graphically displayed on the monitor, and embedded biomechanical algorithms determine the aforementioned parameters based on the average of three repetitive cycles (*P .001 stiffness [week 1] vs. stiffness [week 6]).

3. Ablate the epidermis, cause dermal wounding, and provide variable thermal effects
4. Do not ablate the epidermis, cause dermal wounding, and provide minimal thermal effects

Each of the four modalities has been shown to be effective in promoting facial rejuvenation.[10] Lasers perform this function by a process described as photothermolysis: selective absorption of light by pigmented targets, inducing a thermal-mediated injury in the desired tissue. Common targets include melanin, blood, ink, protein, and water. Cutaneous rejuvenation through laser vaporization of the skin has been demonstrated safe and effective since its introduction in 1994.

Nonablative laser and light source techniques have recently been introduced as treatments that selectively heat the upper dermis, inducing a wound healing response in the papillary and upper reticular dermis without epidermal ablation.[11–15] Histological studies have shown that new collagen synthesis and accumulation results from such procedures, and that removal of the epidermis and portions of the dermis are not required for neocollagenesis and collagen remodeling.[11,13]

Intense Pulsed Light (IPL™) is a filtered, broad spectrum light. The wavelengths are limited by various "cut-off" filters and treatment heads, which emit a broad spectrum of light from approximately 560 to 1200 nm. This range of noncoherent light is nonablative, using low energy to effect vascular and pigmentary changes associated with photodamage, lentigines, telangiectasia, and symptoms of rosacea.[16-18] Minimally invasive "rejuvenative" techniques, including IPL, were originally developed to treat telangiectasia; however, they were also found to be effective in treating dyspigmentation, dark hair, and perhaps shallow wrinkles and enlarged pores.[19,20] Today, higher wavelength sources are delivering energy deeper into the skin, producing selective dermal scarring that appears to be minimizing the appearance of photodamage and acne scarring by stimulating collagen remodeling while avoiding epidermal damage.[21-23] Histological studies have shown that new collagen production and deposition result from such procedures. This is similar to the results of ablative laser techniques that remove the epidermis and portions of the dermis by vaporization;[24] however, compelling visible evidence remains elusive.

We evaluated two different laser systems using three-dimensional *in situ* optical skin imaging to objectively quantify the effect of multiple treatment sessions and dynamic cooling on the appearance of periorbital wrinkles. One arm of the study used the Q-Switched Nd:YAG Laser (Medlite™ IV, Hoya ConBio, Fremont, CA) (λ = 1064 nm) for a pulse duration of 4 to 6 nsec and with a spot size of 6 mm at a fluence of 3 to 3.5 J/cm^2. This was compared to the 1320-nm Nd:YAG Laser (CoolTouch™, Roseville, CA), which used a 30-msec cryogen cooling spurt followed by a 20-msec pulse and a spot size of 10 mm at a fluence of 14 to 18 J/cm^2. Multiple passes with the laser were performed to the periorbital regions until a clinical end point of erythema was obtained (Color Figure 18.3). Treatments were performed in a series of four to five procedures at 2- to 3-week intervals. Data were acquired over 6 months with a noninvasive, three-dimensional optical profiling

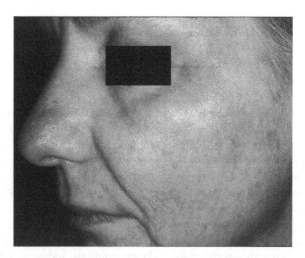

FIGURE 18.3 Immediately after 1064 nm Q-switched Nd:YAG laser treatment. The end point of erythema without blistering was achieved with the Q-Switched Nd:YAG Laser (Medlite IV, Hoya ConBio, Fremont, CA) (λ = 1064 nm), for a pulse duration of 4–6 nsec, with a spot size of 6 mm at a fluence of 3–3.5 J/cm^2. Skin was treated five times over a three-month period. (See color figure following page 110.)

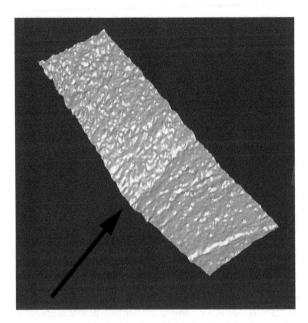

FIGURE 18.4 Pretreatment assessment of periorbital area. The image is a reconstructed, surface profile acquired with the PRIMOS 32 × 32 mm imaging system (PRIMOS Imaging System, GFM Teltow, Germany). Subjects were positioned in front of the light projector with the head position fixed using a head restraint. Periorbital skin was treated five times over a 3-month period. The dimensions of the wrinkle were determined with a trench evaluation software program prior to treatment. The depth of the furrow is 0.23 mm and the average volume/length is 0.142 mm. Arrow indicates measurement area.

system (PRIMOS, GFM, Teltow, Germany). The instrument projects phase shift patterns of light onto the skin surface via a digital micromirror device and records the entire surface image with a charge-coupled device (CCD) camera. One million pixels are captured in a 32 × 32 mm area and are used to recreate a three-dimensional surface profile with a resolution of 3 μm.[27] During the treatment period, it was observed that both systems actually induced an increase in skin roughness, and in some cases, the systems led to a deepening of the wrinkle by the end of the therapy (Figures 18.4 and 18.5).

Figure 18.5 clearly demonstrates an increase in wrinkle depth, even though the skin adjacent to the furrow appears to be remarkably smoother than at baseline. The healing response induced by the thermal insult is unpredictable, which possibly leads to skin contracture forming between native collagen and newly synthesized collagen in the furrow. However, close inspection of the image shows an increase in skin smoothness between the wrinkles. Furthermore, profilimetry data clearly indicates an increase in skin smoothness 6 months after the end of treatment (Figure 18.6). The 1320-nm laser, using higher energies and dynamic cooling, appears to induce a more profound improvement; however, it is not significantly different from the results obtained with the Q-switched 1064-nm laser (see Figure 18.7).[28] Although we did not measure for the presence of biomolecular signals, it can be hypothesized

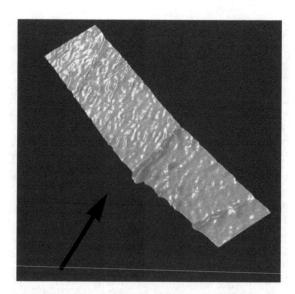

FIGURE 18.5 Increase in wrinkle depth follwing five treatments with the 1064 nm Q-switched Nd/YAG laser. Image is a reconstructed, surface profile acquired with the PRIMOS 32×32 mm imaging system. Subject was repositioned in head restraint in front of the light projector. Periorbital skin was treated five times over a 3-month period. The dimensions of the wrinkle were determined with a trench evaluation software program. The depth of the furrow is 0.37 mm and the average volume/length is 0.768 mm. Arrow indicates measurement area.

that the changing microenvironment produced a sequence of events that led to a decrease in inflammatory mediators and a concomitant decrease in matrix degrading enzymes, resulting in the net increase in matrix material.[29]

These findings suggest that minimally invasive lasers rejuvenate the skin to some extent. Nonablative devices that spare the epidermis and induce dermal remodeling, while provoking a limited thermal response, are currently in vogue not so much for what they do, but for what they do not do. This area of technology is still evolving, but it is clear from patients that they are willing to accept much less improvement if pain and inconvenience are minimized. However, a variety of ablative systems have been developed that deliver a precise amount of intense energy, causing vaporization of the target tissue with minimal heat absorbed by the surrounding tissue.[30-33] This event creates a partial-thickness burn wound that primarily removes photodamaged epidermal and dermal components while minimizing residual injury to the deeper connective tissue of the face. Furthermore, it heats the remaining collagen to the point of unwinding, which produces a tightening effect when the local tissue temperature returns to annealing temperatures.[32]

Different lasers accomplish this by different methods. Ultrapulse CO_2 lasers use a noncontinuous burst of energy, whereas scanning lasers move a continuous beam at a constant velocity over a predetermined area. Individual results are dependent on the energy-absorbing target: water. The first pass of the laser results in the vaporization of the superficial layers of the epidermis. Subsequent passes vaporize

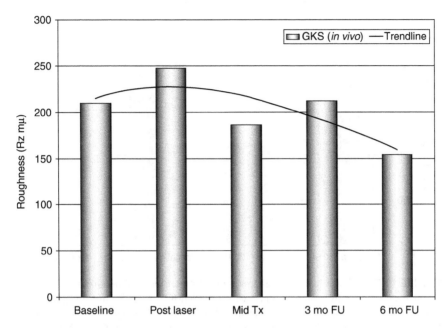

FIGURE 18.6 Decrease in skin roughness 6 months after the final treatment. Three-dimensional microtopography was performed with the PRIMOS 32×32 mm imaging system. Skin roughness (R_z mμ) was calculated from phase-shift algorithms embedded in the software. Roughness (R_z) is the mean peak-to-valley height and is the arithmetic average of the maximum peak-to-valley height of the roughness values Y1 to Y5 of five consecutive sampling sections over the filtered profile. Sixteen profile lines arranged in a radial display were used to compute the average surface roughness. Time points: Baseline, pretreatment; Post Laser, immediately after laser treatment; Mid Tx, measurement before the fourth laser treatment; 3 mo FU and 6 mo FU, 3 and 6 months after five laser treatments. Solid black line indicates a third order polynomial, best-fit line through the roughness points.

residual water located in the basal epidermis and papillary dermis. CO_2 lasers vaporize the epidermis, denature the dermis, and induce a significant thermal effect. As a result, they seem to be most useful for individuals with intrinsic and extrinsic skin damage.[32] Lasers of this type provide the greatest degree of dermal remodeling described as skin tightening; however, in some cases, it is residual thermal damage that leads to prolonged healing.[33] Alternatively, the short-pulsed Er:YAG lasers may enable healing because they promote minimal residual thermal damage. Unfortunately, the trade-offs are bleeding or a limited degree of perceptible improvement.

18.4 PHOTOTHERMAL LASER ABLATION

Combining modalities, CO_2/Er:YAG lasers, variable-pulsed Er:YAG lasers, and ablative radiofrequency devices lead to an effect somewhere in between that of pulsed CO_2 lasers and short-pulsed Er:YAG lasers.[30,34] Irrespective of the device, the resulting wound is highly reproducible and the extent of injury is dependent on the extent

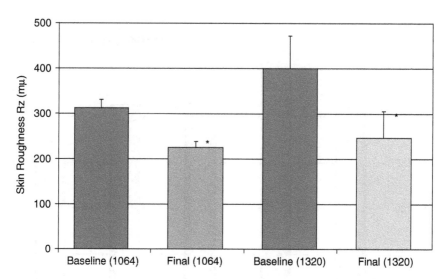

FIGURE 18.7 Decrease in skin roughness 6 months after the final treatment. Three-dimensional microtopography was performed with the PRIMOS 32 × 32 mm imaging system. Average skin roughness (R_z mμ) was calculated from phase-shift algorithms at baseline and 6 months after the final visit. Treatment groups: 1064, Q-switched 1064 nm Nd/YAG laser (n = 10); 1320, 1320 nm Nd/YAG laser with dynamic cooling (n = 8).* = P < 0.01: t-test comparing final to respective baseline.

of damage, number of passes, power density, and the skill of the surgeon. Controlling these variables produces a typical partial-thickness burn that is uniform in size, shape, and depth. Further passes can induce greater residual heat in the dermis, causing a more serious burn with nonaesthetic consequences. These wounds heal through a series of sequential, overlapping stages, which have been stratified for acute wounds as the inflammatory, proliferative, and maturation phases.[35] We can continue to use the same nomenclature; however, due to the combined nature of these wounds, the patient population, and the regenerative capacity of the facial epidermis, the standard curve shifts slightly to the left (Figure 18.8).

Unfortunately, no product or wound management regimen exists that delivers the specific requirements of regenerating skin at various times during the repair and maturation process. It is reasonable to suppose that the benefits of occlusive dressings apply to laser wounds, and a number of physicians have developed personal algorithms and regimens optimizing their use. However, comparative studies providing relevant data are scant.[36–40] The use of moisture-retentive dressings enhances wound healing by creating the cellular environment necessary for healing to proceed at an optimal rate. Principally, these dressings maintain temperature, humidity, and pH during the repair sequence.[41]

Furthermore, certain dressings localize the wound fluid supplying the regenerating skin with growth factors that stimulate cell proliferation, migration, and protein synthesis.[42,43] On the other hand, the local environment created by these dressings also provides an excellent culture medium for bacteria; however, results indicate that it does not consequently lead to infection and delayed healing.[44] Moreover,

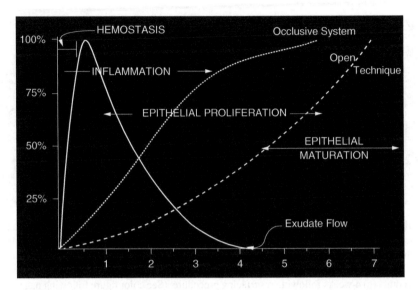

FIGURE 18.8 Schematic healing sequence following laser resurfacing. Wound healing progresses rapidly over the initial days (X axis) through the specific phases. Exudate flow is highest during the first few days and diminishes over time if no adverse events occur. Epidermal regeneration can be optimized (Y axis) with an appropriate wound healing system (dotted line), in comparison to using a semi-occlusive ointment (dashed line).

clinical trials have determined that these dressings actually minimize the possibility of infection.[45] Although the rationale has yet to be determined, the practical benefits of moisture-retentive dressings include pain reduction, excess fluid absorption and protection from exogenous contamination.[46] An optimal dressing is specific for the phases of wound healing, optimizing each stage. Specifically, the initial dressing would promote hemostasis and absorb exudate (inflammatory phase), followed by a dressing to promote epithelial migration (proliferative phase), and lastly one to support maturation and remodeling of the epidermis.[47]

We evaluated healing in a prospective, controlled, randomized, single-blinded outcome clinical trial in patients undergoing laser resurfacing for intrinsic and extrinsic skin damage. Prior to surgery, patients were randomized to either the treatment group (a multi-step dressing system), an occlusive dressing group (Silon-TSR® Dressing, Bio Med Sciences, Inc., Allentown, PA) or an ointment group (Aquaphor® ointment/Purpose® Dual Action Moisturizer regimen, Beiersdorf, Charlotte, N.C.). All patients were treated with either the UltraPulse CO_2 laser (Lumens, Ltd., Palo Alto, CA) alone or with the UltraPulse CO_2 followed by an erbium:YAG laser (Derma-20 ESC Sharplan, Inc., Needham, MA) and/or a blended CO_2/Er:YAG laser (Derma-K laser, ESC Sharplan, Inc., Needham, MA) or a variable pulse erbium:YAG laser (Contour, Sciton Laser Corp, Palo Alto, CA). The computer utilizes a pattern generator set at a density of five or six and an energy setting of 300 mJ. The number of passes varied from one to four depending on the patient's facial skin damage (Color Figure 18.9).

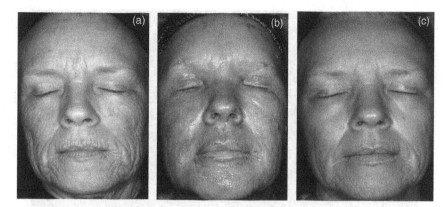

FIGURE 18.9 Epithelialization of facial skin following CO_2 laser resurfacing. Representative patient (#107) in the treatment group, treated with three passes of the UltraPulse CO_2 laser (Coherent Technologies, Palo Alto, CA) utilizing a computer pattern generator set at a density of 6 and an energy setting of 300 mJ. (a) Pretreatment image, (b) 2 d following resurfacing procedure, (c) 4 weeks following resurfacing procedure. (See color figure following page 110.)

Patients enrolled in the treatment group were managed with two primary dressings used in sequence. The first was Fibracol® collagen–alginate wound dressing (Johnson & Johnson Medical, Inc., Arlington, TX), which was applied immediately after surgery (Color Figure 18.10a). Fibracol wound dressing is a combination of alginate with bovine collagen in the form of a flexible, lyophilized sponge that intimately conforms to facial contours and transforms into a gel on contact with fluid. Fibracol protects the wounded skin, absorbs exudate, facilitates epidermal regeneration, and creates a provisional dermal matrix.[48,49] After 48 h the healing skin is less exudative, enabling a change to the second treatment, a crosslinked hydrogel dressing. This dressing is 96% water, providing an environment that optimizes epidermal proliferation and migration, which enables epidermal regeneration to proceed at an optimal rate. Both dressings were covered with an absorbent cover and held in place with securement goggles. The absorbent cover provides a fluid capacity for over 10 g of experimental fluid, and the securement goggles hold the dressing in place as well as protect the skin around the eyes from desiccation.

Removal of occlusive dressing therapy on Day 3 (Color Figure 18.10b) and beginning open therapy with the protective ointment created an air–water interface necessary for epidermal maturation.[50,51] The ointment is composed of petrolatum and as few additional ingredients as possible to minimize irritation potential. Depending on the individual's rate of epidermal turnover, the ointment was switched to an emulsion with glycerin between Days 5 and 8 to enhance barrier formation while permitting adequate vapor transmission (Color Figure 18.10c). Patients in the occlusive therapy group were managed with Silon-TSR for the initial 6 d and were followed with Aquaphor ointment when an occlusive dressing was no longer necessary. Patients enrolled in the ointment group were dressed with a film coating of Aquaphor ointment over the entire face for 36 to 48 h. The subjects were instructed

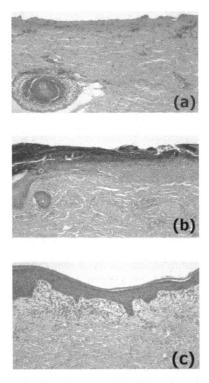

FIGURE 18.10 Histology of skin following CO_2 laser procedure. Representative section of skin treated with three passes of the UltraPulse CO_2 laser (Coherent Technologies, Palo Alto, CA) utilizing a computer pattern generator set at a density of 6 and an energy setting of 300 mJ. (a) Immediately after procedure, (b) 3 d post procedure, (c) 5 d post procedure. (H&E stain at $100 \times$ magnification). (See color figure following page 110.)

to soak their faces for 15 min every 2 h while they were awake and reapply the ointment as necessary.

Pain is a major outcome following this procedure and was assessed on a 5-point scale: a score of 5 indicates no pain, whereas, a score of 1 indicates severe pain. Subjects in the treatment group and the occlusive dressing group experienced significantly less pain than subjects in the ointment group on both Day 2 ($P \le .03$) and Day 3 ($P \le .04$). Eighty percent of the subjects in the treatment and occlusive dressing groups experienced "minimal" to "no pain," whereas 40% of subjects in the ointment group experienced "severe pain" on Day 2.

Skin surface microbial flora was assessed after dressing removal and before cleanup of any residue or remnant material on the skin surface. The skin of subjects in the treatment group had numerically higher bacterial colonization throughout the study; however, the difference was not statistically significant. These data suggest that microbial colonization of the skin occurs in a similar manner regardless of the whether the wound is covered with an occlusive dressing or managed with an "open" dressing regimen. Colonization reached an inflection point earlier in the healing process in the treatment group, suggesting either that the skin was regaining its

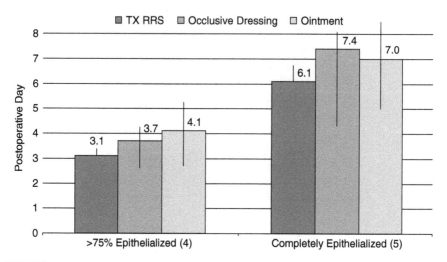

FIGURE 18.11 Epithelialization of facial skin following laser resurfacing. Epithelialization was evaluated on Day 2, Day 3, and Day 6 or Day 7 through 10 using a subjective, six-point scale: 5 = Skin completely epithelialized, 4 = Skin >75% epithelialized and does not require a dressing, 3 = Skin > 75% epithelialized but requires a dressing, 2 = Skin >50% epithelialized, 1 = Wound is greater than 25% epithelialized, appearance of epithelial islands, 0 = No presence of epithelial islands. Scoring was based on the overall presence of epidermal regeneration. The critical time points were the day dressings were no longer required (Epithelialization score = 4) and the day the skin was judged to be completely epithelialized (Epithelialization score = 5). Black bars indicate patients enrolled in the treatment group (n = 31); dark gray bars indicate patients enrolled in the occlusive dressing group (n = 21); light gray bars indicate patients enrolled in the ointment dressing group (n = 10).

barrier properties more quickly or that nutrients required to sustain microbial growth were diminishing. This is consistent with clinical evidence that demonstrates a decrease in wound infections while using occlusive dressings.[45]

The high level of colonization observed early in the healing process was composed mostly of an overgrowth of skin flora. *Staphylococcus* was the most frequently isolated microorganism, followed by *Streptococcus* and Gram-negative bacilli. These microorganisms continue to be the most prevalent species isolated from contaminated and infected wounds.[52] No bacterial skin infections were confirmed in either group; however, all subjects were managed with prophylactic antibiotics, suggesting that appropriate antibiotic therapy is effective in minimizing the risk of infection during a period of high microbial colonization. Epithelialization was evaluated on Day 2, Day 3, and Day 6 or 7 using a subjective, 5-point scale by a clinical observer unaware of the wound management therapy (Figure 18.11). Scoring was based on the overall presence of epidermal regeneration. The critical time points were the day when dressings were no longer required (Epithelialization score = 4) and the day the skin was judged to be completely epithelialized (Epithelialization score = 5).

The average day that the skin was greater than 75% epithelialized and did not require a dressing was 3.1 d in the treatment group, 3.7 d in the occlusive dressing group and 4.1 d in the ointment group. This produced a 95% confidence interval of

0.25 d in the treatment group and 0.68 d in the ointment group. Statistical analysis indicates that subjects in the treatment group achieved this level of healing significantly faster than subjects in the ointment group did ($P < .05$). This difference remained statistically significant for the day when the subjects' skin was judged as completely epithelialized (Epithelialization score = 5). Subjects in the treatment group were completely epithelialized in an average of 6.1 d, whereas subjects in the ointment group were completely epithelialized in 7.0 d ($P < .04$). Complete epithelialization occurred in 7.4 d in the occlusive therapy group ($P < .02$). This produced a 95% confidence interval of 0.42 d in the treatment group, 0.70 d in the occlusive dressing group, and 0.81 d in the ointment group. These results indicate that subjects in the treatment group healed more quickly and with less variability than subjects in the control group.

Unfortunately, wound repair is a unique event subject to uncontrolled complications. Not all wound sites are created equal, dressing fixation is sometimes a problem, and the development of a rich tissue culture environment will benefit microorganisms as well as host cells. Creating a second-degree burn on the face further complicates these dependent events.[53] In addition, tissue ischemia is also an obstacle to epidermal healing and was thought to deter the combination of laser resurfacing with rhytidectomy.[55] We challenged this precept by adding a rhytidectomy procedure prior to the resurfacing procedure in a subset of patients. The division of patients into two groups, a surgical group and a resurfacing group, demonstrated epithelialization as comparable, irrespective of the dressing system (7.2 d vs. 6.6 d, p < .3, Figure 18.12). Furthermore, the multi-dressing approach

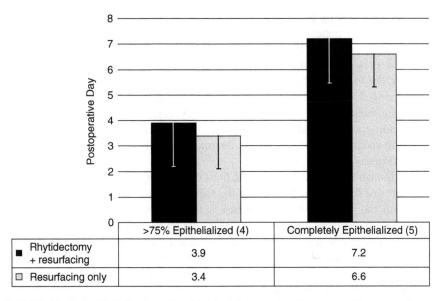

FIGURE 18.12 Epithelialization of facial skin following rhytidectomy and laser resurfacing. Epithelialization was evaluated as described (Figure 18.11). Black bars indicate patients receiving rhytidectomy and resurfacing (n = 11); gray bars indicate patients receiving resurfacing only (n = 31).

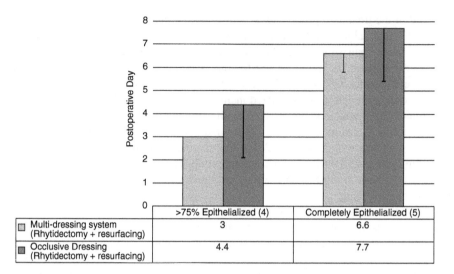

FIGURE 18.13 Epithelialization of facial skin following rhytidectomy and laser resurfacing. Epithelialization was evaluated as described (Figure 18.11). Light gray bars indicate patients enrolled in the treatment group after rhytidectomy and resurfacing (n = 5); dark gray bars indicate patients enrolled in the occlusive dressing group after rhytidectomy and resurfacing (n = 6).

appeared to neutralize the interruption in blood supply. Patients with both rhytidectomy and resurfacing were completely epithelialized in 6.6 d, whereas subjects who only had a resurfacing procedure healed in 6.3 d (Figure 18.13).

Although the patients who were managed with an occlusive dressing healed about a day slower than those in the multi-system group, the rate was similar to those with presurgery rhytidectomy and laser resurfacing followed by Silon-TSR.[56] However, the variability between those managed with an occlusive dressing versus those managed with a multi-dressing system provided a substantial difference. The confidence interval was 1.2 d vs.7 d, respectively, corroborating the finding that by implementing a multiple-dressing regimen, both the healing duration and the variability are reduced irrespective of the treatment site, laser used, or procedure performed (Figure 18.13).[57]

The human face presents one of the most challenging dressing assignments, due to contours of the face and because of the requirements to retain vision, and permit respiration and food ingestion. Nevertheless, these wounds heal in a very short time with few complications due to the numerous epidermal appendages. Wound repair following aesthetic resurfacing procedures is a finely orchestrated sequence of events resulting in functionally regenerated skin. Ongoing research in the functional dynamics of repair has enhanced our understanding of these processes and of the cellular and molecular mechanisms that govern the outcome.[54]

As we have shown, superficial irregularities can be modified by microdermabrasion. If the damage is more severe, alternative laser and nonlaser solutions to achieve specific outcome goals exist. Understanding the type and severity of damage as well as the most appropriate intervention enables the physician to maximize the body's healing mechanisms to regenerate skin that is not only functionally enhanced but also aesthetically appealing.

REFERENCES

1. Hopping, S., The power peel: its emergence and future in cosmetic surgery, *Int. J. Cosmet. Surg.,* 6, 98–100, 1999.
2. Marks, R., Hill, S., and Barton, S.P., The effects of an abrasive agent on normal skin and on photoaged skin in comparison with topical tretinoin, *Br. J. Dermatol.,* 123, 457–466, 1990.
3. Tsai, R.Y., Wang, C.N., and Chan, H.L., Aluminium oxide crystal microdermabrasion, a new technique for treating facial scarring, *Dermatol. Surg.,* 21, 539–542, 1995.
4. Lu, C.F., Chan, H.L., Yu, H.S., The physical effect and repair process of skin after AOCM, 19th Annual Meeting of the Chinese Dermatological Society, Taipei, November 13–14, 1993.
5. Hernandez-Perez, E. and Ibiett, E.V., Gross and microscopic findings in patients undergoing microdermabrasion for facial rejuvenation, *Dermatol. Surg.,* 27, 637–640, 2001.
6. Tan, M.H., Spencer, J.M., Pires, L.M., and Skover, G.R., The evaluation of aluminum oxide crystal microdermabrasion for photodamage, *Dermatol. Surg.,* 27, 943–949, 2001.
7. Freedman, M.S., Microdermabrasion. *Fac. Plast. Surg. Clin. North. Am.,* 9, 257–266, 2001.
8. Warmuth, I.P., Bader, R., Scarborough, D.A., and Bisaccia, E., Herpes simplex infection after microdermabrasion, *Cosmet, Dermatol.,* 12, 13, 1999.
9. Rubin. M.G. and Greenbaum, S.S., Histologic effects of aluminum oxide microabrasion on facial skin, *J. Aesthet. Dermatol. Cosmet. Surg.,* 1, 237–239, 2000.
10. Goldberg, D., Lasers for facial rejuvenation, *Am. J. Clin. Dermatol.,* 4, 225–234, 2003.
11. Kelly, K.M., Nelson, J.S., Lask, G., Geronemus, R.G., and Bernstein, L.J., Cryogen spray cooling in combination with nonablative laser treatment of facial rhytids, *Arch. Dermatol.,* 135, 691–694, 1999.
12. Zelickson, B.D., Kilmer, S.L., Bernstein, E., Chotzen, V.A., Dock, J., Mehregan, D., and Coles, C., Pulsed dye laser therapy for sun damaged skin, *Lasers Surg. Med.,* 25, 229–236, 1999.
13. Menaker, G.M., Wrone, D.A., Williams, R.M., and Moy, R.L., Treatment of facial rhytids with a nonablative laser: a clinical and histologic study, *Dermatol. Surg.,* 25, 440–444, 1999.
14. Goldberg, D.J. and Metzler, C., Skin resurfacing utilizing a low fluence Nd:YAG laser, *J. Cutan. Laser Ther.,* 1, 23–27, 1999.
15. Goldberg, D.J. and Whitworth, J., Laser skin resurfacing with the Q-Switched Nd:YAG laser, *Dermatol. Surg.,* 23, 903–907, 1997.
16. Weiss, R.A., Goldman, M.P., and Weiss, M.A., Treatment of poikiloderma of Civatte with an intense pulsed light source, *Dermatol. Surg.,* 26, 823–827, 2000.
17. Bitter, P.H., Noninvasive rejuvenation of photodamaged skin using serial, full-face intense pulsed light treatments, *Dermatol. Surg.,* 26, 835–842, 2000.
18. Hernandez-Perez, E. and Ibiett, E.V., Gross and microscopic findings in patients submitted to nonablative full face resurfacing using intense pulsed light, *Dermatol. Surg.,* 28, 651–655, 2002.

19. Prieto, V.G., Sadick, N.S., Lloreta, J., et al., Effects of intense pulsed light on sun-damaged human skin, routine, and ultrastructural analysis, *Lasers Med. Surg.,* 30, 82–85, 2002.

20. Negishi, K., Wakamatsu, S., Kushikata, N. et al., Full-face photorejuvenation of photodamaged skin by intense pulsed light with integrated contact cooling, *Lasers Surg. Med.,* 30, 298–305, 2002.

21. Trelles, M.A., Allones, I., and Luna, R., Facial rejuvenation with 1320 nm Nd:YAG laser, *Dermatol. Surg.,* 27, 111, 2001.

22. Goldberg, D.J. and Silapunt, S., Q-switched Nd:YAG laser non-ablative dermal remodeling, *J. Cutan. Laser Ther.,* 2, 157, 2000.

23. Bjerring, P. et al., Non-ablative laser rejuvenation, *J. Cutan. Laser Ther.,* 2, 9, 2000.

24. Ravinder, D., Lam, S.M., and Williams, E.F., III., A systematic histologic analysis of nonablative laser therapy in a porcine model using pulsed dye laser, *Arch. Facial Plast. Surg.,* 5, 218–223, 2003.

25. Friedman, P.M., Skover, G.R., Payonk, G.S., and Geronemus, R.G., Quantitative evaluation of nonablative laser technology, *Sem. Cutan. Med. Surg.,* 21, 266–273, 2001.

26. Bowes, L.E., Goldman, M.P., Payonk, G.S., and Skover, G.R., Quantitative assessment of rejuvenated skin using biomechanical characterization and three-dimensional microtopography, *Lasers Surg. Med.,* Suppl 13, 33, 2001.

27. Jaspers, S., Hopermann, H., Sauermann, G., Hoppe, U., Lunderstädt, R., and Ennnen, J., Rapid *in vivo* measurement of the topography of human skin by active image triangulation using a digital micromirror device, *Skin Res. Technol.,* 5, 195–207, 1999.

28. Skover, G.R., Bowes, L.E., Friedman, P.M., Payonk, G.S., Goldman, M.P., and Geronemus, R.G., *In-vivo* 3D imaging is more predictive of outcome than replica profilometry in photodamaged skin following non-ablative laser treatment, *Lasers Surg. Med.,* Suppl 14, 28, 2002.

29. Rhie, G., Shin, M.H., Seo, J.Y. et al., Aging- and photoaging-dependent changes of enzymic and nonenzymic antioxidants in the epidermis and dermis of human skin *in vivo, J. Invest. Dermatol.,* 117, 1212–1217, 2001.

30. Grekin, R., Tope, W., et al., Electrosurgical facial resurfacing, *Arch. Dermatol.,* 136, 1309–1316, 2000.

31. Fitzpatrick, R.E., Goldman, M.P., Satur, N.M., and Tope, W.D., Ultrapulse CO_2 laser resurfacing of photoaged skin, *Arch. Dermatol.,* 132, 395–402, 1996.

32. Goldman, M.P. and Fitzpatrick, R.E., Eds., *Cutaneous Laser Resurfacing: The Art and Science of Selective Photothermolysis,* 2nd Ed., Mosby, St. Louis, 1999.

33. Fitzpatrick, R.E. and Goldman, M.P., *Cosmetic Laser Surgery,* Mosby, St. Louis, 2000.

34. Goldman, M.P. and Manuskiatti, W., Combined laser resurfacing with the $UPCO_2$ & Er:YAG lasers, *Dermatol. Surg.,* 25, 160–163, 1999.

35. Singer, A.J. and Clark, R.A.F., Cutaneous wound healing, *N. Engl. J. Med.,* 341, 738–746, 1999.

36. Ruiz-Esparza, J., Barba Gomez, J.M., and Gomez de la Torre, O.L., Wound care after laser skin resurfacing. A combination of open and closed methods using a new polyethylene mask, *Dermatol. Surg.,* 24, 79–81, 1998.

37. Suarez, M. and Fulton, J.E., A novel occlusive dressing for skin resurfacing, *Dermatol. Surg.,* 24, 567–570, 1998.

38. VanderKam, V.M., Achauer, B.M., and Finnie, G., Use of a semipermeable dressing (Biobrane) following laser resurfacing of the face, *Plast. Surg. Nurs.,* 17, 177–179, 1997.

39. Newman, J.P., Koch, R.J., and Goode, R.L., Closed dressings after laser skin resurfacing, *Arch. Otolaryngol. Head Neck Surg.*, 124, 751–757, 1998.

40. Concannon, M.J., Malaney, K.B., Wiemer, M.S., and Puckett, C.L., Omiderm: an inexpensive dressing after CO_2 laser resurfacing, *Plast. Reconstr. Surg.*, 101, 1981–1983, 1998.

41. Alvarez, O.M., Pharmacological and environmental modulation of wound healing, in *Connective Tissue Disease. Molecular Pathology of the Extracelllular Matrix,* Uitto, J. and Perejda, A.J., Eds., Marcel Dekker, New York, 1987, pp. 367–384.

42. Katz, M., Alvarez, A., Kirsner, R., Eaglstein, W.H., and Falanga, V., Human wound fluid from acute wounds stimulates fibroblast and endothelial cell growth, *J. Am. Acad. Dermatol.*, 25, 1054, 1991.

43. Jalkanen, M., Haapanen, T., Lyytikainen, A.M., and Larjava, H., Wound fluids mediate granulation tissue growth phases, *Cell Biol. Int. Rep.*, 7, 745–753, 1983.

44. Mertz, P.M. and Eaglstein, W.H., The effect of a semiocclusive dressing on the microbial population in superficial wounds, *Arch. Surg.*, 119, 287–289, 1984.

45. Hutchinson, J.J. and McGuckin, M., Occlusive dressings: a microbiological and clinical review, *Am. J. Infect. Control*, 18, 257–268, 1990.

46. Eaglstein, W.H., Occlusive dressings, *J. Dermatol. Surg. Oncol.*, 19, 716–721, 1993.

47. Goldman, M.P. and Skover, G.R., Optimizing wound healing in the post-laser abrasion face, *Cosmet. Dermatol.*, 12, 123–156, 2000.

48. Van Gils, C.C., Roeder, B., Chesler, S.M., and Mason, S., Improved healing with a collagen-alginate dressing in the chemical matricectomy, *J. Am. Podiatr. Med. Assoc.*, 88, 452–456, 1998.

49. Donaghue, V.M., Chrzan, J.S., Rosenblum, B.I., Giurini, J.M., Habershaw, G.M., and Veves, A., Evaluation of a collagen-alginate wound dressing in the management of diabetic foot ulcers, *Adv. Wound Care*, 11, 114–119, 1998.

50. Rheinwald, J.G. and Green, H., Epidermal growth factor and the multiplication of cultured human epidermal keratinocytes, *Nature*, 265, 421–424, 1977.

51. Sun, T.T. and Green, H., Differentiation of the epidermal keratinocyte in cell culture: formation of the cornified envelope, *Cell*, 9, 511–521, 1976.

52. Holzapfel, L., Jacquet-Francillon, T., Rahmani, J., Achard, P., Marcellin, E., Joffre, T., Lallement, P.Y., Bousquet, A., Devaux, S., and Coupry, A., Microbiological evaluation of infected wounds of the extremities in 214 adults, *J. Accid. Emerg. Med.*, 16, 32–34, 1999.

53. Zawacki, B.E., The natural history of reversible burn injury, *Surg. Gynecol. Obstet.*, 139, 867–872, 1974.

54. Martin, P., Wound healing — aiming for perfect skin regeneration, *Science*, 276, 75–81, 1997.

55. Guyuron, B., Michelow, B., Schmelzer, R., Thomas, T., and Ellison, M.A., Delayed healing of rhytidectomy flap resurfaced with CO_2 laser [see comments], *Plast. Reconstr. Surg.*, 101, 816–819, 1998.

56. Graf, R.M., Bernardes, A., Auerswald, A., and Noronha, L., Full-face laser resurfacing and rhytidectomy, *Aesthet. Plast. Surg.*, 23, 101–106, 1999.

57. Goldman, M.P., Roberts, T.L. III, Skover, G.R., Letteri, J.T., and Fitzpatrick, R.E., Optimising wound healing in the face after laser abrasion, *J. Am. Acad. Dermatol.*, 46, 399–407, 2002.

19 Active Treatments for Acute and Chronic Wounds*

Carlos A. Charles and William H. Eaglstein

CONTENTS

* Partially supported by the Dermatology Foundation of South Florida, Miami.

19.1 INTRODUCTION

During the last decade, scientists, clinical investigators and device and drug companies have worked hard to translate scientific discoveries into products for improving wound healing. This chapter outlines the current status of those attempts, especially those consequent upon new understanding of the chemical signals known collectively as growth factors and cellular and matrix materials, whose manipulation and application toward therapy have come to be known as tissue engineering. As will be seen, the translational effort has been successful with the introduction of matrix, cellular, and growth factor products. However, there have been a disquietingly large number of failed attempts, which emphasize our still-too-sketchy understanding of how to properly utilize much of the laboratory-based information underlying both failed and successful attempts.

In selecting material for this chapter, which deals with new and potential wound healing products, we have emphasized the products that are either available to clinicians today or that may be available in the foreseeable future. Numerous ongoing efforts are currently underway, which hopefully will bring about new products in the near future.

Generally speaking, we can take comfort in the safety profile of all recorded attempts thus far. Many of the theoretic adverse outcomes that have been speculated upon have not been realized. For example, a decade ago there was great concern that growth factors might, in fact, stimulate the development of cancers or promote their early, unrecognized growth, a theoretical phenomenon that has not been recognized. The potential transmission by tissue-engineered products of recognized or unrecognized disease-causing agents such as viruses or prions has not occurred, and most clearly, acute rejection reactions have not been demonstrated, although current evidence suggests that tissue-engineered products are quickly replaced by host tissue. It is to be hoped that in the future the work of the past decade or so and the less-than-ideal products developed so far will be seen as the first stages in a revolution in our ability to stimulate and control healing and repair.

19.2 TISSUE-ENGINEERED SKIN PRODUCTS

19.2.1 BACKGROUND

Over the last 25 years, the science collectively known as tissue engineering and the use of tissue-engineered skin for tissue therapy has progressed at an extremely rapid rate. Many years ago, the idea of cultivating tissues to replace or to stimulate the regeneration of human skin was merely theoretical. When tissue therapy with skin regeneration was clinically indicated for chronic and acute wounds of diverse etiologies, the only alternatives were split- or full-thickness skin grafts, free tissue transfers, or tissue flaps.[1] Today, a wide range of tissue-engineered products have been approved for use by the U.S. Food and Drug Administration (FDA) and a number of others are currently undergoing testing through well-structured clinical trials. There are many advantages to tissue-engineered products as opposed to autologous skin grafting, including the option of giving tissue therapy without requiring a donor site and the potential for faster healing with improved cosmetic results.[2]

The concept of tissue engineering was first defined in 1987 by the National Science Foundation bioengineering panel meeting in Washington, D.C., as "the application of the principles and methods of engineering and the life sciences toward the development of biological substitutes to restore, maintain, or improve function." The exact mechanism by which tissue-engineered skin products aid in healing acute and chronic wounds is not completely understood; however, they may function by providing the needed matrix materials, cells, or cell products such as growth factors to stimulate the healing process.[3] Clinical studies focusing on genetic modifications of transplanted cells and novel systemic gene product delivery mechanisms are broadening the field of tissue engineering.[4]

In this chapter, the term tissue-engineered skin refers to skin products produced from cells, extracellular matrix materials, or a combination, and sometimes includes nonbiologic materials.

19.2.2 Products with Living Cells

19.2.2.1 Combined Epidermal and Dermal Layers

19.2.2.1.1 Apligraf® (Graftskin) — Living Allogeneic Bilayered Skin Construct

Apligraf® is a living human skin equivalent derived by combining a gel type I bovine collagen with living neonatal allogeneic fibroblasts along with an overlying cornified epidermal layer of neonatal allogeneic keratinocytes. This technique was first described by Bell et al.[5] over 20 years ago. Apligraf closely resembles human skin histologically and is currently the most sophisticated commercially available tissue-engineered product. *In vivo,* Apligraf makes matrix proteins and growth factors; additionally, if wounded, Apligraf has the capacity to heal itself.[6] Apligraf is thought to stimulate healing from the wound margins or appendage structures within the wound. However the exact mechanism for Apilgraf's efficacy is not completely understood. In a study using polymerase chain reaction analysis to determine the longevity of the allogeneic fibroblasts and keratinocytes of Apligraf in venous leg ulcers, investigators found that allogeneic deoxyribonucleic acid (DNA) was present in two of eight specimens at 1 month after initial grafting, while neither of the two patients showed persistence of the allogeneic DNA at 2 months after initial grafting.[7] Even in an acute neonatal epidermolysis bullosa wound, evidence of allogeneic DNA survival could not be detected beyond 4 months.[14] These results suggest that allogeneic cells from Apligraf do not survive permanently after grafting, although they may play a role in stimulating healing. Other mechanisms of action that may be important for the efficacy of Apligraf include cytokine release and matrix-induced cell migration and activation. Apligraf has gained FDA approval for the treatment of venous and diabetic ulcers, and it is commercially available in a ready-to-use form with a shelf life of 5 days.

A prospective, controlled, randomized, multicenter study showed that significantly more patients achieved complete wound closure of venous ulcers when treated with Apligraf plus compression therapy compared to compression therapy alone (ulcer healing rate of 63 vs. 49%). Additionally, patients treated with Apligraf healed more rapidly (61 vs. 185 days).[8] These findings were further confirmed in a prospective randomized study by Sabolinski et al.[9] evaluating the efficacy of Apligraf in healing venous ulcers. The tissue-engineered product was three times more effective than compression therapy alone in achieving complete wound closure at 8 weeks.[10]

Apligraf has been studied as treatment for acute wounds. A prospective, multi-center, open study of 107 patients with acute partial- or full-thickness excisional wounds made mostly by excision of skin cancer suggested that Apligraf is safe, useful, and well tolerated.[11] The study found no evidence of clinical or laboratory rejection. In a study by Muhart et al., 20 patients each with three donor site wounds treated with three different devices were investigated to compare the healing time, pain relief, and cosmetic outcomes between Apligraf, autografts, and polyurethane film. The study demonstrated that Apligraf appeared to clinically take and that it was as effective and as well tolerated as autograft in acute donor sites.[12] Additionally, both Apligraf and autograft were superior to polyurethane film. Apligraf has also been used successfully in the treatment of acute and chronic wounds of epidermolysis bullosa.[13,14] Apligraf has many advantages in that it is easy to use, does not require a surgical procedure for use, and can be applied in the outpatient setting. The major disadvantages of Apligraf include its cost and short shelf life (5 days).

19.2.2.1.2   OrCel® — Composite Cultured Skin

Composite cultured skin is a living skin equivalent consisting of allogeneic fibroblasts and keratinocytes grown *in vitro* and attached to opposing sides of a bilayered matrix of bovine collagen.[15] The bovine collagen matrix is composed of a cross-linked collagen sponge that is completely covered by a superimposed layer of pepsinized insoluble collagen. The composite is constructed by seeding keratinocytes over one side of a nonporous collagen gel and fibroblasts on the opposing aspect of the porous collagen sponge. After seeding, it is cultured for 10 to 15 days. The final "product" has a thin, two- or three-cell-layer thick "epidermis" overlying a fibroblast-infiltrated collagen sponge. At present, composite cultured skin is FDA approved for use over donor sites in the surgical repair of syndactyly and flexion contractures of the digits of children with recessive dystrophic epidermolysis bullosa,[16] and has been used as a partial substitution for autografts. In epidermolysis bullosa repairs, morphologic and functional results were judged to be good to excellent with the application of composite cultured skin. Furthermore, the average time to recurrence of hand malformations was increased approximately twofold, and smaller autografts needed to be used. Treated donor sites proved superior for further skin graft harvesting.

Composite cultured skin has many theoretical advantages such as immediate availability and ease of use. However, the efficacy of composite cultured skin in chronic wounds has not yet been proven or described, and few clinical data are available to support its use. Multicenter clinical trials are currently in progress to investigate its effectiveness and tolerability in chronic wounds such as refractory venous leg ulcers.

19.2.2.2 Epidermal Layer

19.2.2.2.1   Epicel® — Cultured Autologous Keratinocyte Construct

The clonal *in vitro* growth of human keratinocytes was first described more than 20 years ago.[17] This technique permits the development of confluent sheets of epidermal keratinocytes *in vitro*, which can be applied to wounds of various etiologies. The application of cultured autologous human keratinocytes to wound healing has been described in chronic leg ulcers,[18] burns,[19] epidermolysis bullosa,[20] wounds resulting from the excision of giant pigmented nevi,[21] vitiligo,[22] chronic mastoiditis,[23] congenital hypospadias,[24] pressure ulcers,[25] corneal replacement,[26] and neonatal scalp necrosis.[27] Optimal wound bed preparation is important for the treatment of wounds with cultured epidermal autografts. Techniques such as pregrafting the wound with an allograft[28] and the application of a dermal bed of allogeneic[29] or autologous dermis[30] have all demonstrated enhanced take.

Although they may stimulate and speed healing, cultured autologous epidermal keratinocyte sheets result in an unstable epithelium, giving rise to spontaneous blister formation many months after grafting. This can often lead to scarring and contraction.[31]

The use of autologous cultured epidermal keratinocytes has many advantages including fast pain relief, the provision of permanent wound coverage, rapid coverage of the wound, and a decreased requirement for donor sites. However, cultured epidermal keratinocytes are expensive and require a high level of skilled labor for their production and application. Furthermore, the requirement for one to multiple skin biopsies, up to a 3-week delay for graft cultivation, and the lack of a dermal component are disadvantages of this technique.

19.2.2.3 Dermal Layer

19.2.2.3.1   Dermagraft® Living Allogeneic Dermal Construct

Dermagraft is a living cryopreserved dermal skin equivalent derived from neonatal foreskin fibroblasts cultured on a bioabsorbable polymer scaffold (polyglactin-910 or polyglycolic acid, Vicryl™ or Dexon™, respectively). The dermal fibroblasts are seeded on the bioabsorbable mesh in a sterile bag with circulating nutrients. This technique, developed by Cooper et al.,[32] allows the neonatal fibroblasts to become confluent within the polymer mesh and secrete growth factors as well as dermal matrix proteins, thereby creating a human living dermal structure.[33] *In vitro* studies have demonstrated that the fibroblasts of Dermagraft produce vascular endothelial growth factor (VEGF) and hepatocyte growth factor/scatter factor (HGF/SF), which are thought to aid in the wound healing process.[34] VEGF stimulates the proliferation of endothelial cells[35] and, with HGF/SF, is an effective inducer of angiogenesis *in vivo* and acts as a mitogen *in vitro*. HGF/SF has been shown to stimulate the repair of wounds in endothelial cell monolayers, promote neovascularization, and stimulate the scattering of endothelial cells grown in three-dimensional collagen gels.[36] The exact action of these and the many other growth factors and cytokines produced by the fibroblasts within Dermagraft *in vivo* is not completely understood and is currently under investigation. Nonetheless, it is believed that Dermagraft stimulates the ingrowth of fibrovascular tissue from the wound bed while promoting reepithelialization from the wound edges. Additionally, studies examining the expression of molecules associated with activation of the immune system in acute rejection found little induction of these molecules in scaffold-based three-dimensional *in vitro* cultures, suggesting that the interaction of the fibroblasts within Dermagraft and the fibroblast-derived extracellular matrix is critical to mitigating the acute immune response.[37]

Dermagraft is FDA approved for the treatment of chronic foot ulcers in patients with diabetes.[38,39] The recent findings from one center of a prospective, multicenter, randomized, controlled 12-week study evaluating the effectiveness of a Dermagraft for treating diabetic foot ulcers demonstrated that patients treated with Dermagraft showed a statistically significant higher percent of wound closure by week 12 than control patients who were treated with saline-moistened gauze dressing.[40] The percent of patients who experienced an infection of the study wound was less in the Dermagraft treatment group than in the control group. In the surgical arena, Dermagraft has been used beneath meshed split-thickness skin grafts for full-thickness wounds[41] and as an alternative to skin grafting to achieve complete closure in fasciotomy wounds.[42] Advantages over other bioengineered skin equivalents include relatively long shelf life in its cryopreserved state, ease of use, and lack of clinical rejection.[43,44]

19.2.3 PRODUCTS WITH NONLIVING MATRIX MATERIALS

19.2.3.1 AlloDerm® — Allogeneic Acellular Dermal Matrix

AlloDerm® is a human cadaveric skin product that is processed with high salt to remove the epidermis, treated with a solution to remove the dermal cellular material, and then cryopreserved, resulting in a nonimmunogenic acellular dermal matrix complex with an intact basement membrane. AlloDerm is used as a dermal graft and has been approved by the FDA since 1992 for the treatment of burn wounds. In a multicenter study of 67 burn patients with full-thickness or deep partial-thickness burns, wounds were excised and treated with AlloDerm plus a thin split-skin graft versus a thick split-skin graft alone.[45] This study demonstrated that outcomes associated with the use of thin split-thickness autografts plus AlloDerm were equivalent to those obtained with the use of thicker split-thickness autografts alone. Case reports have also described the successful use of AlloDerm in conjunction with ultra-thin meshed split-skin grafts over the dorsum of three hands and one ankle with deep wound from thermal burns.[46] These reports describe good to excellent cosmetic and functional results with an early recovery and no residual functional deficit after the use of AlloDerm grafts with thin autografts. Additionally, the use of AlloDerm has been reported in the otolaryngologic literature as a viable alternative to split-thickness skin grafting for various flap surgical repairs.[47,48] AlloDerm has also been used successfully for the treatment of soft tissue defects, such as facial scarring, as well as for cosmetic purposes.[49,50] As an acellular and immunologically inert product AlloDerm is well tolerated and can effectively act as a template for epidermal regeneration. The main disadvantage to this allogeneic dermal product is the small yet present risk of transmitting infectious diseases.

19.2.3.2 Integra®— Extracellular Matrix of Collagen and Chondroitin-6-Sulfate

Integra® is an *in vitro* dermal replacement and is currently the most broadly accepted skin substitute for use in burn wounds. Developed by Burke and Yannas,[51,52] it is composed of an artificial dermal matrix of crosslinked bovine collagen and chondroitin-6-sulfate, along with a disposable silicone (silastic) membrane that provides some "epidermal" function. Following application to the wound bed, the collagen matrix layer becomes biointegrated with the wound, forming a vascularized "neodermis." This process can take anywhere from 3 to 6 weeks, and once the neodermis has formed, the disposable silastic layer is removed and replaced with a thin split-thickness skin graft. Integra received approval by the FDA in 1996 for use in burn wounds.

Initial clinical studies to evaluate the efficacy of Integra found problems with hematoma and seroma formation as well as premature separation of the temporary silastic layer.[53] However, in a subsequent controlled, randomized, multicenter clinical study in 106 burn patients, the median "take" for Integra was 85%, compared with take rates of 95% in control patients treated with split-thickness skin grafts.[54] These results were comparable to those for all nonautograft control materials. Furthermore, donor sites created in this study were thinner and generally healed 4 d sooner with better cosmetic results compared to control sites.

Since Integra requires a two-stage procedure for successful application, including a minimum of 3 weeks while the neodermis forms, the procedure can increase the time required to achieve complete wound healing. Boyce et al.[55] demonstrated an alternative therapy in which cultured epithelial autografts were successfully applied onto a pregrafted Integra in three burn patients.

Disadvantages to the use of Integra include relatively expensive cost as compared to cadaveric allograft skin, and high failure rates are often initially encountered when learning how to successfully use this skin product. The use of Integra is also associated with many advantages. First, it provides improved cosmetic outcome and elasticity compared to thin split-thickness grafts, as well as reduced donor site morbidity. Additionally, the risk of infectious disease transmission associated with allografts is eliminated.

19.2.3.3 Transcyte™ Extracellular Matrix of Allogeneic Human Dermal Fibroblasts

Transcyte™ is a temporary skin replacement composed of a collagen-coated nylon mesh, which is seeded with neonatal fibroblasts. The nylon mesh is not biodegradable and therefore cannot act as a permanent dermal substitute. The neonatal fibroblasts with Transcyte are cultured for 17 d, allowing them to produce fibronectin, type I collagen, proteoglycan, and growth factors. The entire complex is then frozen to –70°C, rendering the fibroblasts nonviable, and then stored at –20°C until the product is ready for use. In a multicenter, randomized, controlled study with 66 patients with 132 excised burn wounds, it was demonstrated that Transcyte was easier to remove, resulted in less bleeding, and was just as effective as an allograft.[56] Transcyte has also been studied in pediatric burn patients with involvement of greater than 7% total body surface. Transcyte-treated wounds required a lower percentage of split-thickness skin autografts than did wounds treated with standard therapy of anti-microbial ointments and hydrodebridement.[57] Transcyte is currently approved by the FDA for the treatment of burn wounds.

19.3 GROWTH FACTORS

19.3.1 BACKGROUND

For the past three decades, there has been a great amount of interest in evaluating the efficacy of growth factors in the active treatment of acute and chronic wounds. Growth factors, or cytokines, are biologically active polypeptides that function by both para-crine and autocrine mechanisms to modify the growth, differentiation, migration, and metabolism of target cells.[98] They exert their influence by binding to specific cell surface receptors leading to the induction of a complex cascade of signal transduction pathways. Growth factors are pleiotrophic, that is they influence a wide range of cellular behavior, and the majority affect several target cell populations.

The results of clinical trials investigating the topical application of growth factors to acute and chronic wounds have not been as dramatic as initially expected. This finding is probably best explained as a consequence of the complexity of the wound healing process and the pleiotrophic nature of each growth factor. To date, only platelet-derived growth factor has been approved by the FDA for use in the treatment of chronic human wounds. Many clinical trials are underway to identify their poten-tial role and to demonstrate the safety and efficacy of other topical growth factors in accelerating wound healing. Novel growth factor delivery systems are being investigated with promising results in *in vitro* and animal models.

19.3.2 APPROVED BY THE FDA FOR HUMAN USE

19.3.2.1 Platelet-Derived Growth Factor

Platelet-derived growth factor (PDGF) was first described in 1974 as a platelet-derived mitogen for smooth muscle cells and fibroblasts.[58] It is made up of two peptide chains, A and B, which are held together by disulfide bonds, and occurs naturally in heterodimeric and homodimeric forms: PDGF-AA, PDGF-AB, and PDGF-BB. These three isoforms bind two types of cell receptors (α and β),[59] with the α receptor having the capability to bind all three isoforms while the β receptor binds the BB homodimer with highest affinity, binds the AB heterodimer with lower affinity, and does not bind the AA homodimer.[60,61] The AB heterodimer is the most common isoform in human platelets.

PDGF is produced by platelets, monocytes, macrophages, vascular endothelium, and keratinocytes,[62,63] all of which are components of early wound healing. Platelets are the earliest and largest source of PDGF. It is released from their α granules during the clotting cascade. Although endothelial cells produce PDGF, they do not respond to the growth factor; instead, PDGF works in a paracrine manner to stimulate adjacent vascular smooth muscle cells. PDGF is both a potent chemoattractant and mitogen for keratinocytes, smooth muscle cells and fibroblasts; it acts synergistically with other growth factors such as transforming growth factor β (TGF-β) and epidermal growth factor and also stimulates the synthesis of fibronectin and hyaluronic acid.

Although not indicated by the FDA for pressure ulcers, the topical application of PDGF for pressure ulcers has been studied in clinical trials. A 20-patient, randomized, phase I/II, double-blind, placebo-controlled study of topically applied recombinant human BB homodimeric PDGF in chronic pressure ulcers demonstrated a reduction in wound volume of 94% vs. 78% with 28 days of treatment.[64] A second study demonstrated complete healing in 23% of 124 pressure ulcers treated with 100 μg/ml of PDGF at 16 weeks compared with none treated with placebo. Additionally, in the ulcers treated with PDGF, ulcer volume was reduced by 93% versus 73% in the control group.[65] A follow-up study was performed for this latter trial in which 12 ulcers treated with PDGF that did not heal were surgically closed.[66] The ulcers remained healed after 1 year in 11 of these 12 patients, while none of three patients who received placebo followed by surgical closure remained healed, suggesting that PDGF may influence the surgical outcome.

A retrospective analysis by Harrison-Balestra et al. investigated the application of recombinant human PDGF (rhPDGF) gel in the treatment of refractory chronic ulcers of various etiologies.[67] The study included ulcers of venous insufficiency, surgical and radiation induced wounds, and scleroderma-associated ulcers, as well as ulcers secondary to Werner's syndrome and Kaposi's sarcoma. Twelve patients with 14 ulcers were treated daily with rhPDGF gel 0.01%; nine of the 14 ulcers healed (64%), with a mean time to healing of 26 weeks. Two of the nine healed ulcers (22%) reopened during a 15-month follow-up period. No adverse effects of rhPDGF gel were observed. The authors concluded that the recombinant human PDGF gel is effective and well tolerated for the treatment of refractory ulcers of various etiologies. A double-blind controlled study of PDGF for the treatment of acute full-thickness punch biopsy wounds showed significantly faster healing rates for PDGF-treated wounds compared to antibiotic-treated control wounds.[68] In this study of seven healthy volunteers, two full-thickness wounds were made on each arm of each volunteer using a 4-mm skin punch biopsy instrument. Fourteen wounds were treated with PDGF gel and were compared with 14 wounds treated with antibiotic ointment. Healing was evaluated by visual determination of the global percentage healed and the wound depth. The investigators found that wounds treated with PDGF gel showed a significantly faster rate of healing on each of the initial six follow-up visits. The greatest difference was noted on day 10 of the study when PDGF-treated wounds were 71% healed compared with 28% for antibiotic-treated wounds ($P = .0005$). At days 22 and 24, 92.9 and 100% of the PDGF gel-treated wounds were healed, compared with 50 and 57%, respectively ($P = .0313$ and $P = .0313$), in the antibiotic ointment group. Additionally, PDGF decreased the wound depth compared with wounds treated with antibiotic ointment at days 8 and 10 with P values <.0313 and <.0020, respectively.

PDGF gel is FDA approved only for the treatment of neurotrophic diabetic foot ulcers. Numerous studies have examined the application of PDGF in the treatment of diabetic foot ulcers. In a prospective, multicenter, double-blinded, randomized study of 118 patients who received either topical PDGF 30 μg/g or placebo, complete ulcer healing was demonstrated in 48% of those treated with PDGF compared with 25% of the placebo group after 20 weeks ($P = .01$).[69] However, another randomized placebo-controlled trial of 379 patients found that the daily application of PDGF 30 μg/g had no effect on ulcer healing, but that 100 μg/g daily resulted in 50% of ulcers healed compared to placebo gel ($P = .007$) after 20 weeks of treatment.[70] Combined analysis of these and other studies suggests that the daily application of PDGF (beclapermin) 100-μg/g gel combined with surgical debridement is effective in improving diabetic foot ulcer healing.[71] Topical PDGF gel is commercially available as Regranex® (Ortho-McNeil, Princeton, N.J.) and is thus far the only growth factor application available for the treatment of wounds. Since PDGF is a protein and is therefore subject to heat denaturing, it is to be kept refrigerated and when applied it is to be kept moist which is thought to prolong its activity. These features plus its expense and the need for surgical debridement make its use more difficult than would be desired. Nevertheless, it is the first FDA-approved growth factor for wound healing and is an important advance in wound care.

19.3.3 PROVEN EFFICACY IN HUMAN TRIALS

19.3.3.1 Fibroblast Growth Factor

Fibroblast growth factor (FGF) encompasses a family of as many as ten heparin-bound growth factors. Most research studies have focused on FGF-1 (acidic FGF [aFGF]), FGF-2 (bFGF), and FGF-7 or keratinocyte growth factor (KGF). FGFs are mainly produced by fibroblasts, smooth muscle cells, endothelial cells, chondrocytes, and mast cells.[72] FGF-2 has been associated with the proliferation, differentiation, and migration of regenerated keratinocytes.[73] Furthermore, FGF-2 aids in angiogenesis in granulation tissue by stimulating the proliferation and migration of capillary endothelial cells,[74] and it also stimulates keratinocytes to produce collagenase, a protease involved in angiogenesis.[75] While FGFs play a critical role in the early cellular events of wound healing by stimulating the initiation of granulation tissue formation,[76] they are also involved in the later stages of wound healing associated with tissue remodeling.

In animal models, topical bFGF has been shown to improve the strength of ischemic wounds[77] and accelerate their rate of closure.[78] In diabetic rodents, bFGF restores the reduction of angiogenesis to levels found in nondiabetic rodents.[79] Additionally, it reverses the impairment in the strength of healing wounds seen in diabetic rats.[78] Other studies have demonstrated that aFGF may help to stimulate peripheral nerve regeneration.[80] The application of bFGF to small split-thickness skin graft donor sites in children failed to show a significant improvement in wound healing.[81] A clinical trial of topical bFGF in the treatment of 50 human subjects with pressure ulcers demonstrated a nonsignificant reduction in wound volume of 69% in the treatment group compared with 59% in those treated with placebo after a 30-day treatment period.[82] Additionally, a clinical trial studying the effects of bFGF on 17 patients with diabetic foot ulcers showed a healing rate of 33% in those treated with daily bFGF compared with 63% in those treated with placebo at 12 weeks.[83] In sum, these trials suggest that topical bFGF has no advantage over placebo; however, larger sample sizes must be studied to make definitive conclusions.

FGF-7 or keratinocyte growth factor (KGF) was discovered in 1989. Although KGF is found and produced only by fibroblasts, it stimulates keratinocytes, not fibroblasts. The expression of KGF is increased during reepithelialization of normal skin; additionally, it induces the proliferation and migration of keratinocytes. In a randomized, double-blind, parallel-group, placebo-controlled, multicenter study to evaluate the safety and efficacy of topical KGF treatment, for 12 weeks, in the healing of chronic venous ulcers in 94 patients, KGF was shown to accelerate wound healing, with significantly more patients achieving 75% wound closure with KGF than with placebo. Additionally, treatment with topical KGF was well tolerated. Subsequent trials of longer duration are currently underway to assess the potential of KGF to influence complete wound closure.

19.3.3.2   Granulocyte–Macrophage Colony-Stimulating Factor

Granulocyte–macrophage colony stimulating factor (GM-CSF) was discovered in 1971 in the study of granulocytopenia.[84] It primarily stimulates the proliferation and differentiation of hematopoietic progenitor cells in the myeloid and erythroid lineages into neutrophils, eosinophils, and macrophages. It also induces the release of neutrophils from the bone marrow to the peripheral blood and stimulates their proper functioning. The beneficial effects of GM-CSF in the treatment of patients with myelodepressive states associated with chemotherapy, radiation therapy, and bone marrow suppression are well described.

The role of GM-CSF in wound healing has recently been studied. Cell mediators released during the acute inflammatory phase of wound healing are integral in coordinating the early connective tissue repair process. GM-CSF regulates several biologic functions of the inflammatory cells, macrophages and neutrophils, associated with this critical phase of wound healing. In addition to modulating elements of the inflammatory processes, GM-CSF has been shown to act as a chemoattractant and mitogen for fibroblasts and endothelial cells *in vitro*.[85] Furthermore, these cells are also stimulated indirectly or synergistically by GM-CSF and other cytokines, such as interleukins 1, 6, and 8, as well as tumor necrosis factor-α.[85-87]

A number of studies have demonstrated promising clinical results with rapid healing of chronic wounds subsequent to perilesional or subcutaneous injections with recombinant human GM-CSF (rhGM-CSF). In a double-blind, placebo-controlled study of 25 patients with chronic venous leg ulcers,[88] patients were treated with a single 400-μg dose of rhGM-CSF or a saline placebo as subcutaneous perilesional injections. Three of 16 (19%) of the patients treated with rhGM-CSF had their ulcers healed by week 1, and eight of 16 (50%) were healed by week 8. In the placebo-treated group, only one of the nine patients (11%) had an ulcer heal during the study by week 8. Furthermore, reduction in ulcer size was significantly greater in the rhGM-CSF group ($P < 0.005$) compared to the placebo group, and no significant side effects or changes in laboratory parameters were observed with the rhGM-CSF treatment.

Subsequently, a double-blind, randomized, placebo-controlled trial was performed aimed at defining the dose-response relationship of rhGM-CSF and ascertaining the rate of healing.[89] Sixty patients with chronic venous leg ulcers were enrolled. They were treated with placebo or with 200 or 400µg of granulocyte-macrophage colony stimulating factor by perilesional injections for four weekly treatment episodes. The numbers of healed wounds in the placebo and the treated arms were significantly different ($P = 0.05$), with four of 21 (19%) in the placebo group having healed at week 13, as compared to 12 of 21 (57%) and 11 of 18 (61%), in the 200 and 400 µg groups, respectively. Additionally, there were only minor side effects attributable to the treatment, and follow-up at 6 months showed that none of the treated ulcers recurred during that period. These findings suggest that perilesionally injected GM-CSF may be a useful drug for the treatment of chronic venous leg ulcers.

19.3.3.3 Epidermal Growth Factor

Epidermal growth factor (EGF), the first growth factor to be discovered, led to the 1986 Nobel Prize in Physiology or Medicine for Stanley Cohen. It was first identified in mouse salivary glands in 1962 and gave rise to the idea that animals licking their wounds were treating them with EGF.[90] EGF is produced by platelets, monocytes, and macrophages, as well as by lacrimal, salivary, and duodenal glands and the kidney. It operates via the EGF receptor on epidermal cells and fibroblasts.[91] The primary role of EGF is to stimulate epithelial cells to grow across the wound; however, it also has effects on smooth muscle cells and fibroblasts. The family of growth factors to which EGF belongs also includes TGF-α, heparin-binding EGF, and amphiregulin.

Animal studies have demonstrated the efficacy of EGF in promoting wound healing. EGF significantly accelerated epidermal regeneration of partial- and full-thickness skin wounds in pigs;[92] additionally, continuous or prolonged EGF exposure increased tensile strength in rat skin wounds.[93] Human studies have also shown enhancement of wound healing by EGF. A prospective, randomized, double-blind clinical trial was performed using skin-graft-donor sites to determine whether epidermal growth factor would accelerate the rate of epidermal regeneration in humans.[94] The authors found that the donor sites treated with silver sulfadiazine containing EGF had an accelerated rate of epidermal regeneration in all patients as compared with paired donor sites treated with silver sulfadiazine alone. Furthermore, treatment with EGF and silver sulfadiazine significantly decreased the average length of time to 25 and 50 % healed by approximately 1 day, and to 75 and 100 % healed by approximately 1.5 days ($P < .02$), suggesting that EGF accelerates the rate of healing of partial-thickness skin wounds. Additionally, a small study of the treatment of venous ulcers with EGF demonstrated complete healing in 35% of those treated with EGF compared with 11% receiving placebo ($P = .1$), with reduction in ulcer size of 73 vs. 33% ($P = 0.32$) by 10 weeks.[95] The authors concluded that the topical application of EGF to venous ulcers in these studies was safe and that the greater reduction in ulcer size and the larger numbers of healed ulcers with the use of EGF were encouraging but not significant due to the small sample sizes.

19.3.4 PROVEN EFFICACY IN ANIMAL STUDIES

19.3.4.1 Transforming Growth Factor β

In 1983 TGF-β was first described for its ability to stimulate the growth of mouse embryo and normal rat kidney fibroblasts.[96] Since its original discovery, TGF-β has been described as a large family of related growth factors that play an important role in wound healing. In humans and all mammals, three isoforms have been described: TGF-β1, 2, and 3. The TGF-βs are produced by fibroblasts, keratinocytes, lymphocytes, platelets, and activated macrophages. Various cell types have receptors for the TGF-βs, and their actions may be inhibitory or stimulatory, depending on the presence of other growth factors or interaction with the extracellular matrix. At low concentrations, the TGF-βs stimulate fibroblast proliferation, while they induce differentiation at higher concentrations.[97]

TGF-β1 predominates in humans. It is released by the α granules of platelets, monocytes, and macrophages.[98] The release of TGF-β1 results in increased fibroblast migration and proliferation and the secretion of extracellular matrix components, such as fibronectin and collagen.[98] Studies in frozen sections of rat wound tissue have demonstrated that TGF-β1 is released early in the wound healing process, with a second peak in concentration at 5 to 7 d.[99] Additionally, the absence of TGF-β1 delays wound healing, as demonstrated by immunodeficient TGF-β1 knockout mice. Other animal studies have shown the involvement of the TGF-βs in wound healing and scarring; additionally, topical applications of TGF-β1 and 2 have improved healing.[100–102] The majority of the animal studies have characterized incisional acute wounds, which have demonstrated an initial increase in the levels of TGF-β1 and TGF-β2, with a delayed increase in TGF-β3 and a simultaneous reduction in TGF-β1.

Limited human data exist on the role of expression of the TGF-βs and their effect on wound healing. One study characterized the biosynthetic activity and response to TGF-β1 of dermal fibroblast cultures isolated from biopsies of venous ulcers and from normal thigh skin of seven patients.[103] This study detected no difference between ulcer and control fibroblasts in the synthesis of total TGF-β1, and the messenger RNA (mRNA) levels for alpha 1(I) procollagen and TGF-β1 were comparable in both groups. However, TGF-β1 enhanced collagen protein synthesis by more than 60% and in a dose-dependent manner in control fibroblast cultures, while failing to stimulate collagen production by venous ulcer fibroblasts. This unresponsiveness to TGF-β1 was associated with up to a fourfold decrease in TGF-β Type II receptors. The authors concluded that fibroblasts from the edge of non-healing venous ulcers are unresponsive to the action of TGF-β1, and that this blunted response may cause faulty deposition of the extracellular matrix needed for reepithelialization and wound healing. Studies characterizing the expression of the TGF-βs in acute and chronic pressure wounds have demonstrated a lack of expression of

TGF-β1 and 2 in the chronic wounds, while both of these factors were consistently identified in normal and acutely wounded skin.[104] Higley et al. found a similar lack of TGF-β1 within the early matrix of venous ulcers.[105] A recent study characterized the distribution of TGF-β1, 2, and 3 and TGF-β receptors in diabetic foot ulcers, diabetic skin, and normal skin. Additionally, the expression of the TGF-βs was compared with that seen in chronic venous ulcers. The authors found a lack of TGF-β1 up-regulation in both diabetic foot ulcers and venous ulcers, which may explain the impaired healing in these chronic wounds.

TGF-β1 appears to play a critical role in the healing process of both acute and chronic wounds. It acts as a potent chemoattractant for monocytes, lymphocytes, neutrophils, and fibroblasts, and it stimulates the release of cytokines from these cells.[106] Furthermore, TGF-β1 stimulates angiogenesis and is an important regulator of the extracellular matrix (ECM) by inhibiting ECM-degrading proteases and upregulating the synthesis of protease inhibitors.[107] Lastly, a study by Kane et al. demonstrated an increase in the expression of TGF-β1 by migrating keratinocytes at the margins of human cutaneous wounds.[108] This increase in TGF-β1 expression may be essential for the keratinocyte migration required for optimal wound healing. In sum, while future studies are warranted, the lack of TGF-β1 in chronic wounds, as well as pressure ulcers, may in part explain their poor healing compared to acute wounds.

19.3.4.2 Vascular Endothelial Growth Factor

Vascular endothelial growth factor (VEGF) was first described as a mediator of vascular permeability in the late 1970s. Five isoforms with different molecular mass have been identified in human tissue.[109] The expression of VEGF is potentiated in response to hypoxia, by activated oncogenes, and by a variety of cytokines, such as PDGF, FGF-2, and TGF-β1.[110] VEGF induces endothelial cell proliferation, promotes cell migration, and inhibits apoptosis. *In vivo* VEGF induces angiogenesis and increases the permeability of blood vessels, thereby playing a central role in the regulation of vasculogenesis.[111] VEGF is released by neutrophils and platelets,[112,113] and it acts through two tyrosine kinase receptors located predominantly on endothelial cells, but also on monocytes.[114] VEGF is similar in structure to PDGF. In wound healing, VEGF stimulates the formation of new blood vessels.[114] It stimulates monocyte migration; however, it does not affect fibroblasts or vascular smooth muscle cells. VEGF has been demonstrated to act synergistically with FGF-2. A study of the effects of topically applied VEGF in ischemic rabbit wounds[115] demonstrated improvement in granulation tissue formation. At present, no trials have been reported studying the effects of VEGF in human wound healing.

19.3.5 Novel Approaches for the Delivery of Growth Factors

The promising results of *in vitro* growth factor studies as well as the positive effects of growth factors in animal models of impaired healing have not always translated into positive human clinical trials. Of note, other than the clinical trials involving the subcutaneous injection of GM-CSF, all trials described thus far have utilized the topical application of growth factors. Concern about the probable rapid degradation of topically applied growth factors by enzymes or other elements in the wound bed environment has lead to the investigation of novel topical and nontopical mechanisms for growth factor delivery.

Gene therapy has been investigated as a way to provide a more persistent source of growth factor in various acute and chronic wound healing models. A recent study examined the ability of a subdermally injected adenovirus containing the platelet-derived growth factor-B transgene to improve the rate of wound healing around an excisional wound in ischemic rabbit skin through the induction of platelet-derived growth factor-B overexpression.[116] This procedure resulted in quicker wound healing than even nonischemic wounds ($P < 0.05$), thereby suggesting that the adenoviral-mediated gene transfer of platelet-derived growth factor-B overcame the ischemic defect in wound healing and could potentially play a role in the treatment of ischemic or other nonhealing wounds. Another recent study investigated the survival of ischemic experimental skin flaps after treatment with the gene encoding for vascular endothelial growth factor (VEGF).[117] Thirty Sprague-Dawley rats were studied in which anterior abdominal skin flaps supplied by the epigastric artery and vein were created. Ten animals were treated with a mixture of liposomes and the cDNA encoding the 121-amino acid isoform of VEGF. Another ten animals were treated with control plasmid DNA and liposome transfection medium; a third group of ten animals was given physiologic saline. Each solution was injected directly into the femoral artery distal to the origin of the epigastric pedicle supplying the flap. Four days after injection, the pedicle was ligated. Seven days later, the amount of viable tissue within the flap was measured by planimetry. The flaps receiving VEGF cDNA had significantly greater tissue viability at the end of 7 d compared with the control groups: 93.9 vs. 28.1% for the control plasmid DNA group and 31.9% for the saline group ($P < 0.05$). Additionally, immunohistochemical staining documented increased deposition of VEGF protein in flaps that were infused with the VEGF cDNA versus saline alone ($P < 0.05$). These results suggest that the survival of ischemic tissues can be enhanced by administration of a cDNA encoding VEGF. This delivery system may have future applications in promoting angiogenesis and granulation tissue formation in chronic wounds.

The encapsulation of recombinant basic fibroblast growth factor (bFGF) into a red blood cell delivery vehicle referred to as a "red blood cell ghost" applied topically to rat incisional wounds has been studied. This delivery system allows for delayed bFGF release at the site of application.[118] Wounds treated with bFGF in such vehicles were 50 % stronger measured by wound breaking load than paired control wounds receiving vehicle alone (388 ± 27 vs. 256 ± 28 g/cm^2, $P < 0.002$) 7 d after injury. Additionally, treated wounds were significantly more cellular at 4 d than paired control wounds. This study found that the topical application of bFGF at the time of injury exerts a positive effect on incisional wound strength only when a vector that delays release is used. It remains to be proven that the "red blood cell ghost" vehicle will allow more activity by the growth factor delivered.

While VEGF has been demonstrated to have strong stimulating effects on vascularization, it has a short half-life when administered by uncontrolled and nonspecific methods; on the other hand, delivered systemically in large doses it can cause harmful side effects. A study to determine the *in vitro* release behavior of VEGF from calcium alginate microspheres and the potency of this controlled release system in promoting localized neovascularization at the epigastric groin fascia of VEGF microsphere-implanted rats resulted in a high level of angiogenesis in surrounding tissue compared with no angiogenesis in a control group receiving empty control microspheres ($P < 0.03$).[119] Hopefully, the half-life of VEGF will be extended by this delivery mechanism.

Lastly, modified methods of treating with growth factors consisting of combined applications of tissue-engineered products and growth factors have also been investigated. One such study investigated cultured skin substitutes consisting of collagen–glycosaminoglycan substrates inoculated with human fibroblasts and either human keratinocytes genetically modified to overexpress VEGF or normal control keratinocytes.[120] Northern blot analysis demonstrated enhanced expression of VEGF mRNA in cultured skin substitutes prepared with the genetically modified cells. Additionally, the VEGF-modified cultured skin substitutes secreted greatly elevated levels of VEGF protein throughout the entire culture period. VEGF-modified and control cultured skin substitutes were grafted to full-thickness wounds on athymic mice, and elevated VEGF mRNA expression was detected in the modified grafts for at least 2 weeks after surgery. VEGF-modified grafts exhibited increased numbers of dermal blood vessels and decreased time to vascularization compared with controls. These results suggest that genetic modification of keratinocytes in cultured skin substitutes can potentially lead to increased VEGF expression, which could improve vascularization of cultured skin substitutes for wound healing applications. Another novel therapeutic investigation studying the combination of growth factors and tissue-engineered skin evaluated the incorporation of basic fibroblast growth factor (bFGF)-impregnated gelatin microspheres into an artificial dermis on the regeneration of dermis-like tissues.[121] The incorporation of bFGF into the artificial dermis accelerated fibroblast proliferation and capillary formation when implanted into full-thickness skin defects on the back of guinea pigs in a dose-dependent manner. While these results show promise for the treatment of chronic wounds with growth factors, at present, none of these systems has been tested in human clinical trials.

19.4 CONCLUSION

As evidenced by the material in this chapter, the active treatment of acute and chronic wounds has been the subject of considerable effort over the past few decades. With continued research to better understand the complex physiologic interactions and characteristics of acute and chronic wounds, new pharmacologic agents and tissue-engineered skin products will undoubtedly be generated. It is hoped that over time, as both researchers and clinicians broaden their knowledge base and become more proficient in the science of growth factor manipulation and delivery as well as tissue-engineering, these techniques will be more effective and less costly for the treatment of complex wounds.

REFERENCES

1. Pomahac, B., Svensjo, T., Yao, F. et al., Tissue engineering skin, *Crit. Rev. Oral Biol. Med.,* 9, 333–344, 1998.
2. Eaglstein, W.H., Iriondo, M., and Laszlo, K., A composite skin substitute (graftskin) for surgical wounds. A clinical experience, *Dermatol. Surg.,* 21, 839–843, 1995.
3. Falanga, V.J., Tissue engineering in wound repair, *Adv. Skin Wound Care,* 13 (2 Suppl), 15–19, 2000.
4. Supp, D.M., Bell, S.M., Morgan, J.R., and Boyce, S.T., Genetic modification of cultured skin substitutes by transduction of human keratinocytes and fibroblasts with platelet-derived growth factor-A, *Wound Repair Regen.,* 8, 26–35, 2000.
5. Bell, E., Ehrlich, H.P., Buttle, D.J., and Nakatsuji, T., Living tissue formed *in vitro* and accepted as skin-equivalent tissue of full thickness, *Science,* 211, 1052–1054, 1981.
6. Falanga, V., How to use Apligraf to treat venous ulcers, *Skin Aging,* 7, 30–36, 1999.
7. Phillips, T.J., Manzoor, J., Rojas, A., Isaacs, C., Carson, P., Sabolinski, M., Young, J., and Falanga, V., The longevity of a bilayered skin substitute after application to venous ulcers, *Arch. Dermatol.,* 138, 1079–1081, 2002.
8. Falanga, V., Margolis, D., Alvarez, O. et al., Rapid healing of venous ulcers and lack of clinical rejection with an allogeneic cultured human skin equivalent. Human Skin Equivalent Investigators Group, *Arch. Deramtol.,* 134, 293–300, 1998.
9. Sabolinski, M.L., Alvarez, O., Auletta, M., Mulder, G., and Parenteau, N.L., Cultured skin as a "smart material" for healing wounds: experience in venous ulcers, *Biomaterials,* 17, 311–320, 1996.
10. Falanga, V., Tissue engineering in wound repair, *Adv. Skin Wound Care,* 13 (2 Suppl.), 15–19, 2000.
11. Eaglstein, W.H., Alvarez, O.M., Auletta, M., Leffel, D., Rogers, G.S., Zitelli, J.A., Norris, J.E., Thomas, I., Irondo, M., Fewkes, J., Hardin-Young, J., Duff, R.G., and Sabolinski, M.L., Acute excisional wounds treated with a tissue-engineered skin (Apligraf), *Dermatol. Surg.,* 25, 195–201, 1999.
12. Muhart, M., McFalls, S., Kirsner, R.S., Elgart, G.W., Kerdel, F., Sabolinski, M.L., Hardin-Young, J., and Eaglstein, W.H., Behavior of tissue-engineered skin: a comparison of a living skin equivalent, autograft, and occlusive dressing in human donor sites, *Arch. Dermatol.,* 135, 913–918, 1999.
13. Falabella, A.F., Valencia, I.C., Eaglstein, W.H., and Schachner, L.A., Tissue-engineered skin (Apligraf) in the healing of patients with epidermolysis bullosa wounds, *Arch. Dermatol.,* 136, 1225–1230, 2000.
14. Falabella, A.F., Schachner, L.A., Valencia, I.C., and Eaglstein, W.H., The use of tissue-engineered skin (Apligraf) to treat a newborn with epidermolysis bullosa, *Arch. Dermatol.,* 135, 1219–1222, 1999.
15. Morgan, J. and Yarmush, M., Bioengineered skin substitutes, *Sci. Med.,* Jul/Aug 1997, pp. 6–15.
16. Eisenberg, M. and Llewelyn, D., Surgical management of hands in children with recessive dystrophic epidermolysis bullosa: use of allogeneic composite cultured skin grafts, *Br. J. Plast. Surg.,* 51, 608–613, 1998.
17. Rheinwald, J.G. and Green, H., Serial cultivation of strains of human epidermal keratinocytes: the formation of keratinizing colonies from single cells, *Cell,* 6, 331–343, 1975.

18. Leigh, I.M., Purkis, P.E., Navsaria, H.A., and Phillips, T.J., Treatment of chronic venous ulcers with sheets of cultured allogenic keratinocytes, *Br. J. Dermatol.,* 117, 591–597, 1987.
19. Carsin, H., Ainaud, P., Le Bever, H., Rives, J., Lakhel, A., Stephanazzi, J., Lambert, F., and Perrot, J., Cultured epithelial autografts in extensive burn coverage of severely traumatized patients: a five year single-center experience with 30 patients, *Burns,* 26, 379–387, 2000.
20. Carter, D.M., Lin, A.N., Varghese, M.C., Caldwell, D., Pratt, L.A., and Eisinger, M., Treatment of junctional epidermolysis bullosa with epidermal autografts, *J. Am. Acad. Dermatol.,* 7 (2 Pt 1), 246–250, 1987.
21. Gallico, G.G., 3rd, O'Connor, N.E., Compton, C.C., Remensnyder, J.P., Kehinde, O., and Green, H., Cultured epithelial autografts for giant congenital nevi, *Plast. Reconstr. Surg.,* 84, 1–9, 1989.
22. Plott, R.T., Brysk, M.M., Newton, R.C., Raimer, S.S., and Rajaraman, S., A surgical treatment for vitiligo: autologous cultured-epithelial grafts, *J. Dermatol. Surg. Oncol.,* 15, 1161–1166, 1989.
23. Premachandra, D.J., Woodward, B.M., Milton, C.M., Sergeant, R.J., and Fabre, J.W., Treatment of postoperative otorrhoea by grafting of mastoid cavities with cultured autologous epidermal cells, *Lancet,* 335, 365–367, 1990.
24. Romagnoli, G., De Luca, M., Faranda, F., Bandelloni, R., Franzi, A.T., Cataliotti, F., and Cancedda, R., Treatment of posterior hypospadias by the autologous graft of cultured urethral epithelium, *N. Engl. J. Med.,* 323, 527–530, 1990.
25. Phillips, T.J. and Pachas, W., Clinical trial of cultured autologous keratinocyte grafts in the treatment of longstanding pressure ulcers, *WOUNDS,* 6, 133–139, 1994.
26. Pellegrini, G., Traverso, C.E., Franzi, A.T., Zingirian, M., Cancedda, R., and De Luca, M., Long-term restoration of damaged corneal surfaces with autologous cultivated corneal epithelium, *Lancet,* 349, 990–993, 1997.
27. Morykwas, M.J., Beason, E.S., and Argenta, L.C., Scalp necrosis in a neonate treated with cultured autologous keratinocytes, *Plast. Reconstr. Surg.,* 87, 549–552, 1991.
28. Compton, C.C., Hickerson, W., Nadire, K., and Press, W., Acceleration of skin regeneration from cultured epithelial autografts by transplantation to homograft dermis, *J. Burn Care Rehabil.,* 14, 653–662, 1993.
29. Navsaria, H.A., Kangesu, T., Manek, S., Green, C.J., and Leigh, I.M., An animal model to study the significance of dermis for grafting cultured keratinocytes on full thickness wounds, *Burns,* 20 Suppl 1, S57–S60, 1994.
30. Nave, M., Wound bed preparation: approaches to replacement of dermis, *J. Burn Care Rehabil.,* 13, 147–153, 1992.
31. Hafemann, B., Ensslen, S., Erdmann, C., Niedballa, R., Zuhlke, A., Ghofrani, K., and Kirkpatrick, C.J., Use of a collagen/elastin-membrane for the tissue engineering of dermis, *Burns,* 25, 373–384, 1999.
32. Cooper, M., Hansbrough J., Spielvogel, R. et al., *In vivo* optimization of a living dermal substitute employing cultured human fibroblasts on a biodegradable polyglycolic acid or polyglactin mesh, *Biomaterials,* 12, 243–248, 1991.
33. Hansbough, J.F., Morgan, J., Greenleaf, G., and Underwood, J., Development of a temporary living skin replacement composed of human neonatal fibroblasts cultured in Biobrane, a synthetic dressing material, *Surgery,* 115, 633–644, 1994.
34. Jiang, W.G. and Harding, K.G., Enhancement of wound tissue expansion and angiogenesis by matrix-embedded fibroblast (Dermagraft), a role for hepatocyte growth factor/scatter factor, *Int. J .Mol. Med.,* 2, 203–210, 1998.

35. Folkmann, J., The role of angiogenesis in tumor growth, *Semin. Cancer Biol.,* 3, 65–71, 1992.
36. Bussolino, F., Di Renzo, M.F., Ziche, M., Bocchietto, E., Olivero, M., Naldini, L., Gaudino, G., Tamagnone, L., Coffer, A., and Comoglio, P.M., Hepatocyte growth factor is a potent angiogenic factor which stimulates endothelial cell motility and growth, *J. Cell Biol.,* 119, 629–641, 1992.
37. Kern, A., Liu, K., and Mansbridge, J., Modification of fibroblast gamma-interferon responses by extracellular matrix, *J. Invest. Dermatol.,* 117, 112–118, 2001.
38. Eaglstein, W.H., Dermagraft treatment of diabetic ulcers, *J. Dermatol.,* 25, 803–804, 1998.
39. Gentzkow, G.D., Iwasaki, S.D., Hershon, K.S., Mengel, M., Prendergast, J.J., Ricotta, J.J., Steed, D.P., and Lipkin, S., Use of dermagraft, a cultured human dermis, to treat diabetic foot ulcers, *Diabetes Care,* 19, 350–354, 1996.
40. Hanft, J.R. and Surprenant, M.S., Healing of chronic foot ulcers in diabetic patients treated with a human fibroblast-derived dermis, *J. Foot Ankle Surg.,* 4, 291–299, 2002.
41. Hansbrough, J.F., Dore, C., and Hansbrough, W.B., Clinical trials of a living dermal tissue replacement placed beneath meshed, split-thickness skin grafts on excised burn wounds, *J. Burn Care Rehabil.,* 13, 519–529, 1992.
42. Omar, A.A., Mavor, A.I., and Homer-Vanniasinkam, S., Evaluation of dermagraft as an alternative to grafting for open fasciotomy wounds, *J. Wound Care,* 11, 96–97, 2002.
43. Pollack, R.A., Edington, H., and Jensen, J., A human dermal replacement for the treatment of diabetic foot ulcers, *Wounds,* 9. 175. 1997.
44. Hansbrough, J.F., Status of cultured skin replacements, *Wounds,* 7, 30–36, 1995.
45. Wainwright, D., Madden, M., Luterman, A., Hunt, J., Monafo, W., Heimbach, D., Kagan, R., Sittig, K., Dimick, A., and Herndon, D., Clinical evaluation of an acellular allograft dermal matrix in full-thickness burns, *J. Burn Care Rehabil.,* 17, 124–136, 1996.
46. Lattari, V., Jones, L.M., Varcelotti, J.R., Latenser, B.A., Sherman, H.F., and Barrette, R.R., The use of a permanent dermal allograft in full-thickness burns of the hand and foot: a report of three cases, *J. Burn Care Rehabil.,* 18, 147–155, 1997.
47. Wax, M.K., Winslow, C.P., and Andersen, P.E., Use of allogenic dermis for radial forearm free flap donor site coverage, *J. Otolaryngol.,* 31(6), 341–345, 2002.
48. Ayshford, C.A., Shykhon, M., Uppal, H.S., and Wake, M., Endoscopic repair of nasal septal perforation with acellular human dermal allograft and an inferior turbinate flap, *Clin. Otolaryngol.,* 28, 29–33, 2003.
49. Achauer, B.M., VanderKam, V.M., Celikoz, B., and Jacobson, D.G., Augmentation of facial soft-tissue defects with Alloderm dermal graft, *Ann. Plast. Surg.,* 41, 503–507, 1998.
50. Rohrich, R.J., Reagan, B.J., Adams ,W.P. Jr., Kenkel, J.M., and Beran, S.J., Early results of vermilion lip augmentation using acellular allogeneic dermis: an adjunct in facial rejuvenation, *Plast. Reconstr. Surg.,* 105, 409–416, discussion 417–418, 2000.
51. Yannas, I.V. and Burke, J.F., Design of an artificial skin. I. Basic design principles, *J. Biomed. Mater. Res.,* 14, 65–81, 1980.
52. Yannas, I.V., Burke, J.F., Gordon, P.L., Huang, C., and Rubenstein, R.H., Design of an artificial skin. II. Control of chemical composition, *J. Biomed. Mater. Res.,* 14, 107–132, 1980.

53. Burke, J.F., Yannas, I.V., Quinby, W.C., Jr., Bondoc, C.C., and Jung, W.K., Successful use of a physiologically acceptable artificial skin in the treatment of extensive burn injury, *Ann. Surg.*, 194, 413–428, 1981.

54. Heimbach, D., Luterman, A., Burke, J., Cram, A., Herndon, D., Hunt, J., Jordan, M., McManus, W., Solem, L., Warden, G. et al., Artificial dermis for major burns. A multi-center randomized clinical trial, *Ann. Surg.*, 208, 313–320, 1988.

55. Boyce, S.T., Kagan, R.J., Meyer, N.A., Yakuboff, K.P., and Warden, G.D., The 1999 clinical research award. Cultured skin substitutes combined with Integra Artificial Skin to replace native skin autograft and allograft for the closure of excised full-thickness burns, *J. Burn Care Rehabil.*, 20, 453–461, 1999.

56. Purdue, G.F., Hunt, J.L., Still, J.M., Jr. et al., A multicenter clinical trial of a biosynthetic skin replacement, Dermagraft-TC, compared with cryopreserved human cadaver skin for temporary coverage of excised burn wounds, *J. Burn Care Rehabil.*, 18 (1 Pt 1), 52–57, 1997.

57. Lukish, J.R., Eichelberger, M.R., Newman, K.D. et al., The use of a bioactive skin substitute decreases length of stay for pediatric burn patients, *J. Pediatr. Surg.*, 36, 1118–1121, 2001.

58. Ross, R., Glomset, J., Kariya, B., and Harker, L., A platelet-dependent serum factor that stimulates the proliferation of arterial smooth muscle cells *in vitro. Proc. Natl. Acad. Sci. U.S.A.*, 71, 1207–1210, 1974.

59. Pierce, G.F., Mustoe, T.A., Altrock, B.W., Deuel, T.F., and Thomason, A., Role of platelet-derived growth factor in wound healing, *J. Cell Biochem.*, 45, 319–326, 1991.

60. Dvonch, V.M., Murphey, R.J., Matsuoka, J., and Grotendorst, G.R., Changes in growth factor levels in human wound fluid, *Surgery*, 112, 18–23, 1992.

61. Greenhalgh, D.G., The role of growth factors in wound healing, *J. Trauma*, 41, 159–167, 1996.

62. Lynch, S.E., Nixon, J.C., Colvin, R.B., Antoniades, H.N., Role of platelet-derived growth factor in wound healing: synergistic effects with other growth factors, *Proc. Natl. Acad. Sci. U.S.A.*, 84, 7696–7700, 1987.

63. Ansel, J.C., Tiesman, J.P., Olerud, J.E., Krueger, J.G., Krane, J.F., Tara, D.C., Shipley, G.D., Gilbertson, D., Usui, M.L., and Hart, C.E., Human keratinocytes are a major source of cutaneous platelet-derived growth factor, *J. Clin. Invest.*, 92, 671–678, 1993.

64. Robson, M.C., Phillips, L.G., Thomason, A., Robson, L.E., and Pierce, G.F., Platelet-derived growth factor-BB for the treatment of chronic pressure ulcers, *Lancet*, 33, 23–25, 1992.

65. Rees, R.S., Robson, M.C., Smiell, J.M., and Perry, B.H., Becaplermin gel in the treatment of pressure ulcers: a phase II randomized, double-blind, placebo-controlled study, *Wound Repair Regen.*, 7, 141–147, 1999.

66. Kallianinen, L.K., Hirshberg, J., Marchant, B., Rees, R.S., Role of platelet-derived growth factor as an adjunct to surgery in the management of pressure ulcers, *Plast. Reconstr. Surg.*, 106, 1243–1248, 2000.

67. Harrison-Balestra, C., Eaglstein, W.H., Falabela, A.F., and Kirsner, R.S., Recombinant human platelet-derived growth factor for refractory nondiabetic ulcers: a retrospective series, *Dermatol. Surg.*, 28, 755–759, 2002.

68. Cohen, M.A. and Eaglstein, W.H., Recombinant human platelet-derived growth factor gel speeds healing of acute full-thickness punch biopsy wounds, *J. Am. Acad. Dermatol.*, 45, 857–862, 2001.

69. Steed, D.L., Clinical evaluation of recombinant human platelet-derived growth factor for the treatment of lower extremity diabetic ulcers. Diabetic Ulcer Study Group, *J. Vasc. Surg.*, 21, 71–78, 1995.

70. Weiman, T.J., Smiell, J.M., and Su, Y., Efficacy and safety of a topical gel formulation of recombinant human platelet-derived growth factor-BB (Beclapermin) in patients with chronic neuropathic ulcers. A phase III randomised placebo-controlled double-bind study, *Diabetes Care,* 21, 822–837, 1998.
71. Smiell, J.M., Wieman, T.J., Steed, D.L., Perry, B.H., Sampson, A.R., and Schwab, B.H., Efficacy and safety of becaplermin (recombinant human platelet-derived growth factor-BB) in patients with nonhealing, lower extremity diabetic ulcers: a combined analysis of four randomized studies, *Wound Repair Regen.,* 7, 335–346, 1999.
72. Reed, J.A., Albino, A.P., and McNutt, N.S., Human cutaneous mast cells express basic fibroblast growth factor, *Lab. Invest.,* 72, 215–222, 1995.
73. Kibe, Y., Takenaka, H., and Kishimoto, S., Spatial and temporal expression of basic fibroblast growth factor protein during wound healing of rat skin, *Br. J. Dermatol.,* 143, 720–727, 2000.
74. Steed, D.L., Modifying the wound healing response with exogenous growth factors, *Clin. Plast. Surg.,* 25, 397–405, 1998.
75. Sasaki, T., The effects of basic fibroblast growth factor and doxorubicin on cultured human skin fibroblasts: relevance to wound healing, *J. Dermatol.,* 19, 664–666, 1992.
76. Gibran, N.S., Isik, F.F., Heimbach, D.M., and Gordon, D., Basic fibroblast growth factor in the early human burn wound, *J. Surg. Res.,* 56, 226–234, 1994.
77. Quirinia, A. and Viidik, A., The effect of recombinant basic fibroblast growth factor (bFGF) in fibrin adhesive vehicle on the healing of ischaemic and normal incisional skin wounds, *Scand. J. Plast. Reconstr. Surg. Hand Surg.,* 32, 9–18, 1998.
78. Uhl, E., Barker, J.H., Bondar, I., Galla, T.J., Leiderer, R., Lehr, H.A., and Messmer, K., Basic fibroblast growth factor accelerates wound healing in chronically ischaemic tissue, *Br. J. Surg.,* 80, 977–980, 1993.
79. Okumura, M., Okuda, T., Nakamura, T., and Yajima, M., Acceleration of wound healing in diabetic mice by basic fibroblast growth factor, *Biol. Pharm. Bull.,* 19, 530–535, 1996.
80. Lee, Y.S., Hsiao, I., and Lin, V.W., Peripheral nerve grafts and aFGF restore partial hindlimb function in adult paraplegic rats, *J. Neurotrauma,* 19, 1203–1216, 2002.
81. Greenhalgh, D.G., The role of growth factors in wound healing, *J. Trauma,* 41, 159–167, 1996.
82. Robson, M.C., Phillips, L.G., Lawrence, W.T., Bishop, J.B., Youngerman, J.S., Hayward, P.G., Broemeling, L.D., and Heggers, J.P., The safety and effect of topically applied recombinant basic fibroblast growth factor on the healing of chronic pressure sores, *Ann. Surg.,* 216, 401–406, 1992.
83. Richard, J.L., Parer-Richard, C., Daures, J.P., Clouet, S., Vannereau, D., Bringer, J., Rodier, M., Jacob, C., and Comte-Bardonnet, M., Effect of topical basic fibroblast growth factor on the healing of chronic diabetic neuropathic ulcer of the foot. A pilot, randomized, double-blind, placebo-controlled study, *Diabetes Care,* 18, 64–69, 1995.
84. Shadduck, R.K. and Nagabhushanam, N.G., Granulocyte colony stimulating factor. I. Response to acute granulocytopenia, *Blood,* 38, 559–568, 1971.
85. Bussolino, F., Wang, J.M., Defilippi, P., Turrini, F., Sanavio, F., Edgell, C.J., Aglietta, M., Arese, P., and Mantovani, A., Granulocyte- and granulocyte-macrophage-colony stimulating factors induce human endothelial cells to migrate and proliferate, *Nature,* 337, 471–473, 1989.
86. Jones, T.C., The effects of rhGM-CSF on macrophage function, *Eur. J. Cancer,* 29A Suppl 3, S10–S13, 1993.
87. Hancock, G.E., Kaplan, G., and Cohn, Z.A., Keratinocyte growth regulation by the products of immune cells, *J .Exp. Med.,* 168, 1395–1402, 1988.

88. Da Costa, R.M., Jesus, F.M., Ancieto, C., and Mendes, M.A., Double-blind randomized placebo-controlled trial of the use of granulocyte-macrophage colony-stimulating factor in chronic leg ulcers, *Am. J. Surg.,* 173, 165–168, 1997.

89. Da Costa, R.M., Ribeiro Jesus, F.M., Aniceto, C., and Mendes, M., Randomized, double-blind, placebo-controlled, dose-ranging study of granulocyte-macrophage colony stimulating factor in patients with chronic venous leg ulcers, *Wound Repair Regen.,* 7, 17–25, 1999.

90. Cohen, S., Isolation of a mouse submaxillary gland protein accelerating incisor eruption and eyelid opening in the newborn animal, *J. Biol. Chem.,* 237, 1555–1562, 1962.

91. Nanney, L.B., Epidermal and dermal effects of epidermal growth factor during wound repair, *J. Invest. Dermatol.,* 94, 624–629, 1990.

92. Brown, G.L., Curtsinger, L., 3rd, Brightwell, J.R., Ackerman, D.M., Tobin, G.R., Polk, H.C. Jr,, George-Nascimento, C., Valenzuela, P., and Schultz, G.S., Enhancement of epidermal regeneration by biosynthetic epidermal growth factor, *J. Exp. Med.,* 163, 1319–1324, 1986.

93. Brown, G.L., Curtsinger, L.J., White, M., Mitchell, R.O., Pietsch, J., Nordquist, R., von Fraunhofer, A., and Schultz, G.S., Acceleration of tensile strength of incisions treated with EGF and TGF-beta, *Ann. Surg.,* 208, 788–794, 1988.

94. Brown, G.L., Nanney, L.B., Griffen, J., Cramer, A.B., Yancey, J.M., Curtsinger, L.J., 3rd, Holtzin, L., Schultz, G.S., Jurkiewicz, M.J., and Lynch, J.B., Enhancement of wound healing by topical treatment with epidermal growth factor, *N. Engl. J. Med.,* 321, 76–79, 1989.

95. Falanga, V., Eaglstein, W.H., Bucalo, B., Katz, M.H., Harris, B., and Carson, P., Topical use of human recombinant epidermal growth factor (h-EGF) in venous ulcers, *J. Dermatol. Surg. Oncol.,* 18, 604–606, 1992.

96. Frolik, C.A., Dart, L.L., Meyers, C.A., Smith, D.M., and Sporn, M.B., Purification and initial characterization of a type beta transforming growth factor from human placenta, *Proc. Natl. Acad. Sci. U.S.A.,* 80, 3676–3680, 1983.

97. Massague, J., The transforming growth factor-beta family, *Annu. Rev. Cell Biol.,* 6, 597–641, 1990.

98. Steed, D.L., The role of growth factors in wound healing, *Surg. Clin. North Am.,* 77, 575–586, 1997.

99. Yang, L., Qiu, C.X., Ludlow, A., Ferguson, M.W., and Brunner, G., Active transforming growth factor-beta in wound repair: determination using a new assay, *Am. J. Pathol.,* 154, 105–111, 1999.

100. Broadley, K.N., Aquino, A.M., Hicks, B., Ditesheim, J.A., McGee, G.S., Demetriou, A.A., Woodward, S.C., and Davidson, J.M., The diabetic rat as an impaired wound healing model: stimulatory effects of transforming growth factor-beta and basic fibroblast growth factor, *Biotechnol. Ther.,* 1, 55–68, 1989–1990.

101. Shah, M., Foreman, D.M., and Ferguson, M.W., Control of scarring in adult wounds by neutralising antibody to transforming growth factor beta, *Lancet,* 339, 213–214, 1992.

102. Roberts, A.B., Transforming growth factor: activity and efficacy in animal models of wound healing, *Wound Repair Regen.,* 3, 408–418, 1996.

103. Hasan, A., Murata, H., Falabella, A., Ochoa, S., Zhou, L., Badiavas, E., and Falanga, V., Dermal fibroblasts from venous ulcers are unresponsive to the action of transforming growth factor-beta 1, *J. Dermatol. Sci.,* 16, 59–66, 1997.

104. Schmid, P., Cox, D., Bilbe, G., McMaster, G., Morrison, C., Stahelin, H., Luscher, N., and Seiler, W., TGF-beta s and TGF-beta type II receptor in human epidermis: differential expression in acute and chronic skin wounds, *J. Pathol.,* 171, 191–197, 1993.

105. Higley, H., Persichitte, K., Chu, S., Waegell, W., Vancheeswaran, R., and Black, C., Immunocytochemical localization and serologic detection of transforming growth factor beta 1. Association with type I procollagen and inflammatory cell markers in diffuse and limited systemic sclerosis, morphea, and Raynaud's phenomenon, *Arthritis Rheum.*, 37, 278–288, 1994.

106. Roberts, A.B. and Sporn, M.B., The transforming growth factors βs, in *Handbook of Experimental Pharmacology: Peptide Growth Factors and Their Receptors,* Vol. 95, Sporn, M.B. and Roberts, A.B., Eds., Springer-Verlag, New York, 1990, 419–472.

107. O'Kane, S. and Ferguson, M.W., Transforming growth factor beta s and wound healing. *Int. J. Biochem. Cell Biol.,* 29, 63–78, 1997.

108. Kane, C.J., Hebda, P.A., Mansbridge, J.N., and Hanawalt, P.C., Direct evidence for spatial and temporal regulation of transforming growth factor beta 1 expression during cutaneous wound healing, *J. Cell Physiol.,* 148, 157–173, 1991.

109. Neufeld, G., Cohen, T., Gengrinovitch, S., and Poltorak, Z., Vascular endothelial growth factor (VEGF) and its receptors, *FASEB J.,* 13, 9–22, 1999.

110. Howdieshell, T.R., Riegner, C., Gupta, V., Callaway, D., Grembowicz, K., Sathyanarayana, and McNeil, P.L., Normoxic wound fluid contains high levels of vascular endothelial growth factor, *Ann. Surg.,* 228, 707–715, 1998.

111. Li, J., Zhang, Y.P., and Kirsner, R.S., Angiogenesis in wound repair: angiogenic growth factors and the extracellular matrix, *Microsc. Res. Tech.,* 60, 107–114, 2003.

112. McCourt, M., Wang, J.H., Sookhai, S., and Redmond, H.P., Proinflammatory mediators stimulate neutrophil-directed angiogenesis, *Arch. Surg.,* 134, 1325–1332, 1999.

113. Weltermann, A., Wolzt, M., Petersmann, K., Czerni, C., Graselli, U., Lechner, K., and Kyrle, P.A., Large amounts of vascular endothelial growth factor at the site of hemostatic plug formation *in vivo, Arterioscler. Thromb. Vasc. Biol.,* 19, 1757–1760, 1999.

114. Dvorak, H.F., VPF/VEGF and the angiogenic response, *Semin. Perinatol.,* 24, 75–78, 2000.

115. Nissen, N.N., Polverini, P.J., Koch, A.E., Volin, M.V., Gamelli, R.L., and DiPietro, L.A., Vascular endothelial growth factor mediates angiogenic activity during the proliferative phase of wound healing, *Am. J. Pathol.,* 152, 1445–1452, 1998.

116. Liechty, K.W., Nesbit, M., Herlyn, M., Radu, A., Adzick, N.S., and Crombleholme, T.M., Adenoviral-mediated overexpression of platelet-derived growth factor-B corrects ischemic impaired wound healing, *J. Invest. Dermatol.,* 113, 375–383, 1999.

117. Taub, P.J., Marmur, J.D., Zhang, W.X., Senderoff, D., Nhat, P.D., Phelps, R., Urken, M.L., Silver, L., and Weinberg, H., Locally administered vascular endothelial growth factor cDNA increases survival of ischemic experimental skin flaps, *Plast. Reconstr. Surg.,* 102, 2033–2039, 1998.

118. Slavin, J., Hunt, J.A., Nash, J.R., Williams, D.F., and Kingsnorth, A.N., Recombinant basic fibroblast growth factor in red blood cell ghosts accelerates incisional wound healing, *Br. J. Surg.,* 79, 918–921, 1992.

119. Elcin, Y.M., Dixit, V., and Gitnick, G., Extensive *in vivo* angiogenesis following controlled release of human vascular endothelial cell growth factor: implications for tissue engineering and wound healing, *Artif. Organs,* 25, 558–565, 2001.

120. Supp, D.M., Supp, A.P., Bell, S.M., and Boyce, S.T., Enhanced vascularization of cultured skin substitutes genetically modified to overexpress vascular endothelial growth factor, *J. Invest. Dermatol.,* 114, 5–13, 2000.

121. Kawai, K., Suzuki, S., Tabata, Y., Ikada, Y., and Nishimura, Y., Accelerated tissue regeneration through incorporation of basic fibroblast growth factor-impregnated gelatin microspheres into artificial dermis, *Biomaterials,* 21, 489–499, 2000.

Index

A

Acne, 314, 317–319
Acticoat® dressing, 171
Actinic keratosis, 319–320
Actisorb® Plus, 229, 231
Activator protein-1 (AP-1), 34, 65
Acute biopsies, 96
Acute burns, 97, 166
Acute wounds vs. chronic wounds, 26–29, 156, 168, 255–256
Acylated homoserine lactone (actyl-HSL), 157
Adapalene, 317–319
Adenoviral therapy, 248, 273–274
Adherens junctions (AJ), 37
Adhesion, keratinocyte, 36–37
Aesthetic procedures
    nonablative laser intervention, 334–339
    photothermal laser ablation, 339–347
    superficial intervention, 332–334
Aesthetic skin care market, 331–332
Albumin, 202
Alcohols, 162
Alginate dressings, 220–221
Alginic acid, 219–221
Allergic contact dermatitis, 144–145
AlloDerm®, 356–357
Aluminum oxide crystal microdermabrasion, 332–334
Aminoglycosides, 162–163
Ammonium hydroxide (AH), 145
Anabolic agents, 208–209
Anabolic steroid, 208–209
Anaerobes, 160
Angiogenesis, 74, 190, 205–206, 259
Anilides, 162
Animals, 141–143, 147–149, 300, 363–364
Antimicrobials, 118–120
Antiseptics, 162–163, 258
Apligraf™, 251, 353–354
Aquaphor® ointment, 341, 342
Arginine, 204
Ascorbic acid, 205
Avage™, 321
Avance™, 229–230
Ayurvedic medicine, 90

B

Bacteria, 118–120, 156–157
    antiseptic effect on, 162–163
    control within chronic wounds, 257–259
    importance within wounds, 157–158
    iodine compounds effect on, 163–165, 171, 229, 258
    management, 161–174, 228–230
    sampling techniques, 159–161
    silver compounds effect on, 171, 172–173, 229–230, 258
Bacteroides sp., 230
Basal keratinocytes, 36, 246
Baynton, Thomas, 91
Bed preparation, wound
    acute vs. chronic, 255–256
    advanced therapies, 256
    background, 255–256
    bacterial burden control, 257–259
    biological microenvironment management and, 261–262
    control of exudate in, 259–261
    debridement of necrotic tissue in, 259
    introduction, 256–257
    matrix metalloproteinases (MMPs) and, 256–257
    systemic approaches to, 263
Beta-galactosidase, 29
Biguanides, 162
Biochemical signaling
    epidermal migration and, 61–63
    maturation, 64
    mitosis, 63–64
    onset of, 60–66
    signal transduction and transcription factors in, 64–66
Biofilms, 118–120, 156–157
Biological microenvironment management, 261–262
Biopsies
    acute, 96
    determining microbial load during, 159
Bisphenols, 162
Blisters, 145–146
Blood perfusion, 183–184, 192–193, 196
Breasted, James, 90

Milton Keynes UK
Ingram Content Group UK Ltd.
UKHW021827071024
449327UK00021B/1456